Molecular Diagnostics in Cytopathology

Sinchita Roy-Chowdhuri
Paul A. VanderLaan
John M. Stewart
Gilda da Cunha Santos
Editors

Molecular Diagnostics in Cytopathology

A Practical Handbook for the Practicing Pathologist

Springer

Editors
Sinchita Roy-Chowdhuri
MD Anderson Cancer Center
The University of Texas
Houston, TX
USA

Paul A. VanderLaan
Beth Israel Deaconess Medical Center
Harvard Medical School
Boston, MA
USA

John M. Stewart
MD Anderson Cancer Center
The University of Texas
Houston, TX
USA

Gilda da Cunha Santos
Department of Laboratory Medicine
University of Toronto
Toronto, ON
Canada

ISBN 978-3-319-97396-8 ISBN 978-3-319-97397-5 (eBook)
https://doi.org/10.1007/978-3-319-97397-5

Library of Congress Control Number: 2018957088

This Springer imprint is published by the registered company Springer Nature Switzerland AG
The registered company address is: Gewerbestrasse 11, 6330 Cham, Switzerland

Preface

This book is a compilation of high-yield molecular pathology topics relevant to the field of cytopathology in a user-friendly format that can be used as a reference handbook by training and practicing pathologists and laboratory personnel dealing with, and interested in, this evolving field.

Molecular diagnostics are increasingly used to help guide targeted therapy in solid organ tumors and hematologic malignancies. A large proportion of molecular testing is performed on limited-volume samples obtained via minimally invasive techniques, such as fine needle aspiration. Increasingly, cytopathologists play an essential role in this process, both in the triage of specimens during rapid on-site evaluation and in the evaluation of archival samples to determine suitability for ancillary testing. Therefore, it is imperative that practicing cytopathologists stay abreast of up-to-date diagnostic, prognostic, and predictive ancillary tests that can be used on limited cytologic material. This is a challenge since the landscape of known genomic alterations is constantly evolving and the subsequent set of testing options is ever expanding. In addition, many practicing cytopathologists have not had substantial molecular pathology training during residency or fellowship; therefore, the basic core principles of molecular testing may remain elusive.

The main focus of this book is to provide an overview of the principles of molecular diagnostics in context of cytopathology specimens together with a basic understanding and working knowledge of the available technology, platforms, and clinical applications. The initial sections of the book summarize the pre-analytic aspects of molecular testing, including cytology specimen preparation and handling, specimen selection and evaluation, and workflow algorithms as well as the analytic considerations for a variety of nucleic acid and protein-based testing. The remaining section focuses on disease-specific molecular testing for various organ-based applications.

Molecular cytopathology is an expanding and evolving field. With the increasing demand for molecular testing on small specimens, cytopathologists need to understand how to efficiently select and triage the best tissue for testing as well as interpret the molecular test results in context of the morphology to cement the role of cytopathology as an independent and essential component of diagnostic and precision medicine.

We hope this book will serve as a practical handbook of clinical molecular diagnostics in context of the cytopathology specimen.

Houston, TX, USA Sinchita Roy-Chowdhuri
Boston, MA, USA Paul A. VanderLaan
Houston, TX, USA John M. Stewart
Toronto, ON, Canada Gilda da Cunha Santos

Acknowledgment

We would like to sincerely thank all coauthors for contributing their time and expertise to this project, without whom this book would not have happened. We are also indebted to all the pathologists, cytotechnologists, and trainees, who inspire us every day, and to our families, friends, and loved ones for standing by us and dealing with the long hours spent away from them. We also want to thank our publishing team at Springer, especially Stephanie Frost, our editorial coordinator, for her efforts and assistance with this book.

Contents

Contributors

Zubair W. Baloch, MD, PhD Department of Pathology and Laboratory Medicine, Hospital of the University of Pennsylvania, Philadelphia, PA, USA

Güliz A. Barkan, MD Department of Pathology and Laboratory Medicine, Loyola University Medical Center, Maywood, IL, USA

Julia A. Bridge, MD, FACMG Departments of Pathology/Microbiology, Pediatrics and Orthopedic Surgery, University of Nebraska Medical Center/Nebraska Medicine, Omaha, NE, USA

Miriam Cieri, MD Department of Public Health, University of Naples "Federico II", Naples, Italy

Gilda da Cunha Santos, MD, PhD, FIAC Department of Laboratory Medicine, University of Toronto, Toronto, ON, Canada

Maren Y. Fuller, MD Department of Pathology, Children's Hospital of Pittsburgh of University of Pittsburgh Medical Center (UPMC), Pittsburgh, PA, USA

Ming Guo, MD Department of Pathology, The University of Texas MD Anderson Cancer Center, Houston, TX, USA

Vickie Y. Jo, MD Harvard Medical School, Department of Pathology, Brigham and Women's Hospital, Boston, MA, USA

Rashmi Kanagal-Shamanna, MD Department of Hematopathology and Molecular Diagnostics, The University of Texas MD Anderson Cancer Center, Houston, TX, USA

Jeffrey F. Krane, MD, PhD Department of Pathology, Harvard Medical School, Brigham and Women's Hospital, Boston, MA, USA

Umberto Malapelle, PhD Department of Public Health, University of Naples "Federico II", Naples, Italy

Ross A. Miller, MD, FCAP, FASCP Memorial Pathology Consultants, P.A., Kingwood, TX, USA

Sara E. Monaco, MD Department of Pathology, University of Pittsburgh Medical Center, Children's Hospital of Pittsburgh of UPMC, Pittsburgh, PA, USA

Michiya Nishino, MD, PhD Department of Pathology, Beth Israel Deaconess Medical Center, Harvard Medical School, Boston, MA, USA

Stefan E. Pambuccian, MD Department of Pathology and Laboratory Medicine, Loyola University Medical Center, Maywood, IL, USA

Francesco Pepe, PhD Department of Public Health, University of Naples "Federico II", Naples, Italy

Pasquale Pisapia, MD Department of Public Health, University of Naples "Federico II", Naples, Italy

Martha Bishop Pitman, MD Department of Pathology, Harvard Medical School, Massachusetts General Hospital, Boston, MA, USA

Xiaohua Qian, MD, PhD Harvard Medical School, Department of Pathology, Brigham and Women's Hospital, Boston, MA, USA

Liza M. Quintana, MD Department of Pathology, Beth Israel Deaconess Medical Center, Boston, MA, USA

Michael H. Roh, MD, PhD Department of Laboratory Medicine and Pathology, Anatomic Pathology, Mayo Clinic, Rochester, MN, USA

Esther Diana Rossi, MD, PhD, MIAC Division of Anatomic Pathology and Histology, Fondazione Policlinico Unviersitario "A. Gemelli", Catholic University of Sacred Heart, Rome, Italy

Sinchita Roy-Chowdhuri, MD, PhD MD Anderson Cancer Center, The University of Texas, Houston, TX, USA

Eleanor Russell-Goldman, MD, PhD Department of Pathology, Harvard Medical School, Brigham and Women's Hospital, Boston, MA, USA

Mauro Ajaj Saieg, MD, PHD, MIAC Head, Cytopathology, AC Camargo Cancer Center, São Paulo, SP, Brazil

John M. Stewart, MD, PhD MD Anderson Cancer Center, The University of Texas, Houston, TX, USA

Ashwyna Sunassee, MD Department of Pathology and Genomic Medicine, Houston Methodist Hospital, Houston, TX, USA

Laura J. Tafe, MD Laboratory for Clinical Genomics and Advanced Technologies, Department of Pathology and Laboratory Medicine, Dartmouth-Hitchcock Medical Center, Lebanon, NH, USA

Giancarlo Troncone, MD, PhD Department of Public Health, University of Naples "Federico II", Naples, Italy

Karen D. Tsuchiya, MD Department of Laboratories, Seattle Children's Hospital, Seattle, WA, USA

Paul A. VanderLaan, MD, PhD Beth Israel Deaconess Medical Center, Harvard Medical School, Boston, MA, USA

Mingjuan Lisa Zhang, MD Department of Pathology, Massachusetts General Hospital, Boston, MA, USA

Part I
Overview of Molecular Cytopathology

Chapter 1
Introduction: Overview of Current Molecular Diagnostic Testing on Cytology Samples

Michael H. Roh and Rashmi Kanagal-Shamanna

Abbreviations

ALK	Anaplastic lymphoma kinase or ALK receptor tyrosine kinase
BRAF	v-raf murine sarcoma viral oncogene homolog B
CEP	Centromeric probe
DDIT3	DNA damage-inducible transcript 3
EGFR	Epidermal growth factor receptor
EWSR1	Ewing sarcoma breakpoint region 1
FISH	Fluorescence *in situ* hybridization
FNA	Fine-needle aspiration
FOXO1	Forkhead box O1
FUS	Fused in sarcoma

M. H. Roh (✉)
Department of Laboratory Medicine and Pathology, Anatomic Pathology, Mayo Clinic, Rochester, MN, USA
e-mail: roh.michael@mayo.edu

R. Kanagal-Shamanna
Department of Hematopathology and Molecular Diagnostics, The University of Texas MD Anderson Cancer Center, Houston, TX, USA
e-mail: rkanagal@mdanderson.org

S. Roy-Chowdhuri et al. (eds.), *Molecular Diagnostics in Cytopathology*, https://doi.org/10.1007/978-3-319-97397-5_1

GNA11	Guanine nucleotide-binding protein subunit alpha-11
GNAQ	Guanine nucleotide-binding protein G(q) subunit alpha
HER2	Human epidermal growth factor receptor 2 (*ERBB2*)
HPV	Human papillomavirus
KIT	KIT proto-oncogene receptor tyrosine kinase
KRAS	Kirsten rat sarcoma viral oncogene homolog
MDM2	Mouse double minute 2 homolog or E3 ubiquitin protein ligase homolog (mouse)
MEK1	Mitogen-activated protein kinase kinase 1
MYCN	v-myc myelocytomatosis viral oncogene homolog, neuroblastoma derived
NRAS	Neuroblastoma RAS viral oncogene
PDGFB	Platelet-derived growth factor β
PDGFRA	Platelet-derived growth factor receptor A
Pter	Terminal of chromosome short arm
Qter	Terminal of chromosome long arm
RNA	Ribonucleic acid
ROS1	ROS proto-oncogene 1, receptor tyrosine kinase
SS18	Synovial sarcoma translocation chromosome 18
TFE3	Transcription factor binding to immunoglobulin heavy constant

Key Points

- Molecular testing plays a critical role in the work-up of both solid tumors and hematological malignancies for the purposes of diagnosis and biomarker identification for assessment of prognosis and therapeutic targets
- Pathologists have a central role in integrating appropriate molecular ancillary testing into routine cytopathology workflow to enable personalized medicine

During this continuously evolving era of precision medicine, there have been tremendous advances in our understanding of the molecular genetic aberrations (e.g., mutations, gene amplifications, and gene rearrangements) that underlie and drive the growth and spread of various cancers. This has been complemented by advances in molecular diagnostic technologies available to pathologists and laboratory personnel to interrogate and detect these genetic abnormalities. Concurrent advances in minimally invasive interventional procedures have resulted in an increasing reliance on small biopsies along with exfoliative and fine-needle aspiration (FNA) cytology specimens not only for diagnostic purposes but also for ancillary molecular testing to guide the increasingly "personalized" management of patients with cancer [1–4]. In addition, the rapid development of new high-throughput and multiplex molecular testing modalities holds the promise to address the issue of simultaneously testing for a multitude of different genomic abnormalities utilizing cytology samples and small biopsies [5–8]. Furthermore, the recognition of tumor heterogeneity at the molecular level places an increasing demand for these procedures, as will the need to analyze multiple samples from the same patient over time in order to monitor the pattern of evolution of molecular abnormalities [9]. This would serve to reevaluate patients with cancers which have stopped responding to targeted therapy in order to identify new alterations which may be amenable to a switch in a targeted therapeutic regimen. Consequently, the importance of effectively integrating molecular ancillary testing with anatomic pathology workflow, particularly with regard to cytologic and small biopsy specimens, has never been greater.

Section II of this book will broadly address the practical considerations of cytology specimen processing in the molecular laboratory. Namely, chapters will be dedicated to the types of preparatory protocols and platforms utilized for molecular ancillary testing (Chap. 2), sample acquisition and test requisition (Chap. 3), specimen assessment/selection along with triaging workflows for this purpose (Chap. 4), technical aspects of the various molecular diagnostic techniques and the practical implications for each (Chaps. 5, 6, and 7), and the interpretation of molecular diagnostic results along with how they correlate with cytopathologic diagnoses (Chap. 8).

Section III of this book will discuss the clinical settings in which molecular testing dovetails with the evaluation of cytology and small biopsy specimens, with respect to specific organ systems. In one aspect, molecular ancillary tests can be seen as adjuncts to aid in the diagnosis of small biopsies and cytology specimens [10–19]. Some key examples, not intended to be exhaustive, are listed in Table 1.1. The classic example is human papillomavirus (HPV) testing applied to gynecologic cytology specimens, which can be particularly useful to help guide the management of patients with indeterminate Pap test results [20]. HPV testing is also being increasingly applied in the diagnostic work-up of head and neck squamous cell carcinomas [21–24]. Detailed discussion of these applications will be addressed in Chaps. 9 and 10. Next, a variety of molecular diagnostic approaches have emerged to aid in the diagnosis of indeterminate thyroid FNAs [10, 15–17, 25–29]. These include high-throughput analysis of gene mutations and gene rearrangements, gene expression classifier analysis, and microRNA expression profiling (Chap. 12). Fluorescence *in situ* hybridization (FISH) analysis has also emerged as a useful diagnostic adjunct in the evaluation of pancreatobiliary brushings (Chap. 15) and urinary tract cytology specimens (Chap. 16) [11, 12, 18]. FISH testing also serves an instrumental role in the diagnosis and subclassification of salivary gland neoplasms (Chap. 14) and sarcomas (Chap. 18) in FNA and small biopsy samples [14, 30, 31].

Alternatively, molecular diagnostic adjuncts can be utilized to interrogate biomarkers that provide information pertinent to prognosis and/or targeted therapeutic strategies [1, 32–43]. Salient examples are listed in Table 1.2 and include molecular testing of non-small cell lung carcinomas for *EGFR* and *BRAF* gene mutations along with *ALK* and *ROS1* gene rearrangements (Chap. 11); testing of metastatic

TABLE 1.1 Examples of molecular testing as diagnostic adjuncts applied to cytology and small biopsy specimens

Context	**Molecular diagnostic adjuncts**
Liquid-based cervical cytology	HPV testing
Head and neck squamous cell carcinoma	HPV testing
Thyroid FNA cytology	Gene mutation and rearrangement analysis Gene expression classifier testing microRNA analysis
Urine cytology	FISH probe set (CEP3, CEP7, CEP17, 9q21)
Pancreatobiliary brushing cytology	FISH probe set (CEP3, CEP7, CEP17, 9q21) FISH probe set (1q21, 7p12, 8q24, 9p21)
Renal cell carcinoma (examples below)	FISH probes
• Clear cell renal cell carcinoma	3pter/3qter
• Papillary renal cell carcinoma	CEP1, CEP7, CEP17
• Chromophobe renal cell carcinoma	CEP1, CEP7, CEP17
• Translocation-associated renal cell carcinoma	*TFE3*
Soft tissue tumors (examples below)	FISH probes and RT-PCR assays
• Alveolar rhabdomyosarcoma	*FOXO1*
• Alveolar soft part sarcoma	*TFE3*

(continued)

Table 1.1 (continued)

Context	**Molecular diagnostic adjuncts**
• Clear cell sarcoma	*EWSR1*
• Dermatofibrosarcoma protuberans	*PDGFB*
• Desmoplastic small round cell tumor	*EWSR1*
• Ewing sarcoma	*EWSR1*
• Myxoid/round cell liposarcoma	*DDIT3/FUS*, *DDIT3/EWSR1*
• Synovial sarcoma	*SS18*
• Well-differentiated liposarcoma	*MDM2*
Small B-cell lymphomas	
• Lymphoplasmacytic lymphoma	*MYD88*, *CXCR4* mutation analysis
• Follicular lymphoma	t(14;18)(q32;q21) *IGH/BCL2*
• Mantle cell lymphoma	t(11;14)(q13;q32) *CCND1/IGH*
• Hairy cell leukemia	*BRAF* mutation analysis
• Extranodal marginal zone lymphoma	t(11;18)(q21;q21) *BIRC3/MALT1*; t(14;18)(q32;q21) *IGH/MALT1*; t(3;14)(p14.1;q32) *FOXP1/IGH*; t(1;14)(p22;q32) *BCL10/IGH*
Burkitt lymphoma	t(8;14)(q24;q32) *MYC/IGH*
Extranodal NK/T-cell lymphoma, nasal type	EBV testing
ALK-positive T-cell lymphoma	*ALK* rearrangement

TABLE 1.2 Examples of molecular testing as prognostic/theranostic adjuncts applied to cytology and small biopsy specimens

Context	Molecular diagnostic adjuncts
Non-small cell lung carcinoma	*EGFR* and *BRAF* mutation testing *ALK* and *ROS1* rearrangement testing PD-L1 testing
Melanoma	*BRAF*, *KIT*, *GNAQ*, *GNA11*, *NRAS*, *MEK1* mutation testing
Colon adenocarcinoma	*KRAS*, *BRAF* mutation testing
Breast carcinoma	*ERBB2* amplification
Gastroesophageal adenocarcinoma	*ERBB2* amplification
Gastrointestinal stromal tumor	*KIT* and *PDGFRA* mutation testing
Neuroblastoma	*MYCN* amplification
Inflammatory myofibroblastic tumor	*ALK* rearrangement
Papillary thyroid carcinoma	*BRAF* mutation testing
Lymphoplasmacytic lymphoma	*MYD88*, *CXCR4* mutation testing
Diffuse large B-cell lymphoma	*MYC* rearrangement FISH testing Gene expression classifier testing Gene mutation analysis for *CARD11*, *CD79A*, *CD79B*, *EZH2*, *MYC*, *MYD88*, *TP53*, etc.
High-grade B-cell lymphoma	*MYC*, *BCL2*, *BCL6* rearrangement

(continued)

Table 1.2 (continued)

Context	Molecular diagnostic adjuncts
Chronic lymphocytic leukemia/small lymphocytic lymphoma	Deletions of *ATM*, D13S319, and *TP53*; trisomy 12 Gene mutation analysis for *ATM*, *BIRC3*, *TP53*, *NOTCH1*, *SF3B1*, etc. Drug resistance mutation testing for *BTK*, *PLCG2* genes
Myeloid sarcomas	FISH testing for multiple rearrangements Gene mutation analysis including *ASXL1*, *CALR*, *DNMT3A*, *FLT3*, *IDH1/2*, *JAK2*, *KIT*, *MPL*, *NPM1*, *RUNX1*, *SF3B1*, *SRSF2*, *TET2*, *TP53*, etc.

melanomas for various mutations including *BRAF*, *NRAS*, and *KIT* gene mutations; *ERBB2* gene amplification testing for breast (Chap. 13) and gastroesophageal carcinomas; and a multitude of molecular testing for pediatric tumors (Chap. 19) for which *MYCN* gene amplification testing in neuroblastomas represents a classic example.

Similar to solid tumors, molecular testing is a critical adjunct for diagnosis and personalized therapy in hematological malignancies [44]. This is reflected in the recently revised 2017 WHO classification system for lymphoid and myeloid disorders where genetic results form a basis for diagnosis and classification in multiple disease groups [45, 46]. Cytology FNA is routinely used for work-up of tissue-based hematological malignancies including lymphomas and leukemias and provides ample opportunity for molecular testing [5, 47]. Typical scenarios are summarized below, while Chap. 17 will address these in greater detail.

Differentiation of low-grade lymphomas and reactive lymphoid proliferations is, by far, the most challenging task for pathologists. Molecular tools can be extremely helpful to identify clonal markers that can facilitate this distinction. These include detection of monoclonal VDJ rearrangements in immunoglobulin heavy chain (*IgH*), T-cell receptor (*TCR*) beta or gamma receptor genes, as well as specific gene rearrangements and gene mutations in B-cell and T-cell lymphomas [47–56]. In the right clinical and morphologic context, FISH or PCR studies for characteristic gene rearrangements are helpful in sub-typing of small B-cell lymphomas [such as t(11;14)(q13;q32) *IGH/CCND1* in mantle cell lymphoma, t(14;18)(q32;q21) *IGH@-BCL2* in follicular lymphoma, etc.], certain large B-cell lymphomas such as Burkitt lymphoma [t(8;14)(q24;q32) *MYC-IGH@*], and *ALK*-positive T-cell lymphomas [t(2;5)(p23;q35)] [47, 51, 57, 58]. Assessment of translocations by PCR enables evaluation of measurable (minimal) residual disease [59]. Molecular testing is essential to identify biomarkers to assess prognosis and determine the choice of therapy. Some examples, which are in no way comprehensive, include molecular testing of lymphoplasmacytic lymphoma for mutations in *MYD88* and *CXCR4* [60]; testing of large B-cell lymphomas for *MYC* gene rearrangement as well as gene expression profile for distinguishing between germinal center and activated B-cell phenotype [61, 62]; testing of high-grade B-cell lymphomas for rearrangements and copy number changes in *MYC*, *BCL2*, and *BCL6* genes [63, 64]; testing of T-cell lymphomas for *ALK* gene rearrangement (58); and testing of myeloid sarcomas for recurrent genetic translocations such as t(15;17) and t(9;22) *BCR/ABL* and various gene mutations such as *FLT3* and *IDH1/2* [46, 65, 66]. Further, in the context of newly developed targeted therapies, testing for gene mutations that confer resistance to drugs such as *BTK* mutations in chronic lymphocytic leukemia/small lymphocytic lymphomas is emerging as a standard modality [67]. In most cases, mutation testing for multiple genes is best done using a multi-gene sequencing assay such as next-generation sequencing. Molecular testing for malignancy associated viruses, specifically Epstein-Barr virus, plays an important role in diagnosis and monitoring of a variety of hematological conditions including Hodgkin and non-Hodgkin lymphoma, immunodeficiency-associated lymphoproliferative disorders including post-stem cell transplant [68, 69]. These applications will be further elaborated in Chap. 17.

Although some molecular tests serve more as diagnostic aids (Table 1.1) and others serve more to provide prognostic/theranostic information (Table 1.2), as mentioned above, these two roles of molecular diagnostic tests applied to cytology specimens and small biopsies should not be seen as necessarily mutually exclusive. As the repertoire of targeted therapeutic regimens expands, based on our evolving scientific knowledge surrounding molecular biomarkers and targets, these two roles will become increasingly intertwined.

The objective of this book is several-fold. First, the advantages and limitations of cytology specimens will be discussed to assist in the understanding, on the part of pathologists and laboratory personnel, of how best to leverage these patient samples for diagnosis and molecular testing. Second, practical knowledge surrounding the acquisition and laboratory processing of these specimens, along with triage and workflow algorithms, will be shared. This information will be cemented by providing details surrounding the actual testing methodologies utilized for molecular diagnostic evaluation of these samples (Section II). Finally, clinically relevant contexts in which molecular diagnostics and cytopathology are becoming increasingly intertwined will be discussed (Section III).

It is the hope of the editors of this book and the individual chapter authors that the reader can utilize this book as a practical guide to develop best practice algorithms by which molecular testing is applied to the diagnosis and work-up of cytology and small biopsy specimens. Understanding the pre-analytic and analytic aspects of molecular testing for cytology samples will enable pathologists and laboratory personnel to best determine how samples are managed and triaged to successfully obtain the optimum amount of diagnostic, prognostic, and theranostic information for each patient sample.

References

1. Aisner DL, Sams SB. The role of cytology specimens in molecular testing of solid tumors: techniques, limitations, and opportunities. Diagn Cytopathol. 2012;40(6):511–24.
2. Clark DP. Seize the opportunity: underutilization of fine-needle aspiration biopsy to inform targeted cancer therapy decisions. Cancer. 2009;117(5):289–97.
3. Knoepp SM, Roh MH. Ancillary techniques on direct-smear aspirate slides: a significant evolution for cytopathology techniques. Cancer Cytopathol. 2013;121(3):120–8.
4. Krishnamurthy S. Applications of molecular techniques to fine-needle aspiration biopsy. Cancer. 2007;111(2):106–22.
5. Kanagal-Shamanna R, Portier BP, Singh RR, Routbort MJ, Aldape KD, Handal BA, et al. Next-generation sequencing-based multi-gene mutation profiling of solid tumors using fine needle aspiration samples: promises and challenges for routine clinical diagnostics. Mod Pathol. 2014;27(2):314–27.
6. Killian JK, Walker RL, Suuriniemi M, Jones L, Scurci S, Singh P, et al. Archival fine-needle aspiration cytopathology (FNAC) samples: untapped resource for clinical molecular profiling. J Mol Diagn. 2010;12(6):739–45.
7. Rekhtman N, Roy-Chowdhuri S. Cytology specimens: a goldmine for molecular testing. Arch Pathol Lab Med. 2016;140(11):1189–90.
8. Roy-Chowdhuri S, Chow CW, Kane MK, Yao H, Wistuba II, Krishnamurthy S, et al. Optimizing the DNA yield for molecular analysis from cytologic preparations. Cancer Cytopathol. 2016;124(4):254–60.
9. Beca F, Schmitt F. Growing indication for FNA to study and analyze tumor heterogeneity at metastatic sites. Cancer Cytopathol. 2014;122(7):504–11.
10. Alexander EK, Kennedy GC, Baloch ZW, Cibas ES, Chudova D, Diggans J, et al. Preoperative diagnosis of benign thyroid nodules with indeterminate cytology. N Engl J Med. 2012;367(8):705–15.
11. Barr Fritcher EG, Kipp BR, Halling KC, Clayton AC. FISHing for pancreatobiliary tract malignancy in endoscopic brushings

enhances the sensitivity of routine cytology. Cytopathology. 2014;25(5):288–301.
12. Barr Fritcher EG, Voss JS, Brankley SM, Campion MB, Jenkins SM, Keeney ME, et al. An optimized set of fluorescence in situ hybridization probes for detection of pancreatobiliary tract cancer in cytology brush samples. Gastroenterology. 2015;149(7):1813–24. e1.
13. Barroca H, Bom-Sucesso M. Fine needle biopsy with cytology in paediatrics: the importance of a multidisciplinary approach and the role of ancillary techniques. Cytopathology. 2014;25(1):6–20.
14. Dal Cin P, Qian X, Cibas ES. The marriage of cytology and cytogenetics. Cancer Cytopathol. 2013;121(6):279–90.
15. Nikiforov YE, Carty SE, Chiosea SI, Coyne C, Duvvuri U, Ferris RL, et al. Highly accurate diagnosis of cancer in thyroid nodules with follicular neoplasm/suspicious for a follicular neoplasm cytology by ThyroSeq v2 next-generation sequencing assay. Cancer. 2014;120(23):3627–34.
16. Nikiforov YE, Carty SE, Chiosea SI, Coyne C, Duvvuri U, Ferris RL, et al. Impact of the multi-gene ThyroSeq next-generation sequencing assay on cancer diagnosis in thyroid nodules with atypia of undetermined significance/follicular lesion of undetermined significance cytology. Thyroid. 2015;25(11):1217–23.
17. Nikiforov YE, Ohori NP, Hodak SP, Carty SE, LeBeau SO, Ferris RL, et al. Impact of mutational testing on the diagnosis and management of patients with cytologically indeterminate thyroid nodules: a prospective analysis of 1056 FNA samples. J Clin Endocrinol Metab. 2011;96(11):3390–7.
18. Reynolds JP, Voss JS, Kipp BR, Karnes RJ, Nassar A, Clayton AC, et al. Comparison of urine cytology and fluorescence in situ hybridization in upper urothelial tract samples. Cancer Cytopathol. 2014;122(6):459–67.
19. Savic S, Franco N, Grilli B, Barascud Ade V, Herzog M, Bode B, et al. Fluorescence in situ hybridization in the definitive diagnosis of malignant mesothelioma in effusion cytology. Chest. 2010;138(1):137–44.
20. Massad LS, Einstein MH, Huh WK, Katki HA, Kinney WK, Schiffman M, et al. 2012 updated consensus guidelines for the management of abnormal cervical cancer screening tests and cancer precursors. J Low Genit Tract Dis. 2013;17(5 Suppl 1):S1–S27.
21. Guo M, Khanna A, Dhillon J, Patel SJ, Feng J, Williams MD, et al. Cervista HPV assays for fine-needle aspiration

specimens are a valid option for human papillomavirus testing in patients with oropharyngeal carcinoma. Cancer Cytopathol. 2014;122(2):96–103.
22. Guo M, Khanna A, Feng J, Patel S, Zhang W, Gong Y, et al. Analytical performance of cervista HPV 16/18 in SurePath pap specimens. Diagn Cytopathol. 2015;43(4):301–6.
23. Kerr DA, Pitman MB, Sweeney B, Arpin RN 3rd, Wilbur DC, Faquin WC. Performance of the Roche cobas 4800 high-risk human papillomavirus test in cytologic preparations of squamous cell carcinoma of the head and neck. Cancer Cytopathol. 2014;122(3):167–74.
24. Kerr DA, Sweeney B, Arpin RN 3rd, Ring M, Pitman MB, Wilbur DC, et al. Automated extraction of formalin-fixed, paraffin-embedded tissue for high-risk human papillomavirus testing of head and neck squamous cell carcinomas using the roche cobas 4800 system. Arch Pathol Lab Med. 2016;140(8):844–8.
25. Agretti P, Ferrarini E, Rago T, Candelieri A, De Marco G, Dimida A, et al. MicroRNA expression profile helps to distinguish benign nodules from papillary thyroid carcinomas starting from cells of fine-needle aspiration. Eur J Endocrinol. 2012;167(3):393–400.
26. Dettmer M, Vogetseder A, Durso MB, Moch H, Komminoth P, Perren A, et al. MicroRNA expression array identifies novel diagnostic markers for conventional and oncocytic follicular thyroid carcinomas. J Clin Endocrinol Metab. 2013;98(1):E1–7.
27. Keutgen XM, Filicori F, Crowley MJ, Wang Y, Scognamiglio T, Hoda R, et al. A panel of four miRNAs accurately differentiates malignant from benign indeterminate thyroid lesions on fine needle aspiration. Clin Cancer Res. 2012;18(7):2032–8.
28. Nikiforova MN, Tseng GC, Steward D, Diorio D, Nikiforov YE. MicroRNA expression profiling of thyroid tumors: biological significance and diagnostic utility. J Clin Endocrinol Metab. 2008;93(5):1600–8.
29. Shen R, Liyanarachchi S, Li W, Wakely PE Jr, Saji M, Huang J, et al. MicroRNA signature in thyroid fine needle aspiration cytology applied to "atypia of undetermined significance" cases. Thyroid. 2012;22(1):9–16.
30. Bajaj J, Gimenez C, Slim F, Aziz M, Das K. Fine-needle aspiration cytology of mammary analog secretory carcinoma masquerading as low-grade mucoepidermoid carcinoma: case report with a review of the literature. Acta Cytol. 2014;58(5):501–10.

31. Hudson JB, Collins BT. MYB gene abnormalities t(6;9) in adenoid cystic carcinoma fine-needle aspiration biopsy using fluorescence in situ hybridization. Arch Pathol Lab Med. 2014;138(3):403–9.
32. Aisner DL, Marshall CB. Molecular pathology of non-small cell lung cancer: a practical guide. Am J Clin Pathol. 2012;138(3):332–46.
33. Beltran H. The N-myc oncogene: maximizing its targets, regulation, and therapeutic potential. Mol Cancer Res. 2014;12(6):815–22.
34. Bergethon K, Shaw AT, Ou SH, Katayama R, Lovly CM, McDonald NT, et al. ROS1 rearrangements define a unique molecular class of lung cancers. J Clin Oncol. 2012;30(8):863–70.
35. Bernacki KD, Betz BL, Weigelin HC, Lao CD, Redman BG, Knoepp SM, et al. Molecular diagnostics of melanoma fine-needle aspirates: a cytology-histology correlation study. Am J Clin Pathol. 2012;138(5):670–7.
36. da Cunha Santos G, Saieg MA, Geddie W, Leighl N. EGFR gene status in cytological samples of nonsmall cell lung carcinoma: controversies and opportunities. Cancer Cytopathol. 2011;119(2):80–91.
37. Griewank KG, Scolyer RA, Thompson JF, Flaherty KT, Schadendorf D, Murali R. Genetic alterations and personalized medicine in melanoma: progress and future prospects. J Natl Cancer Inst. 2014;106(2):djt435.
38. Howell GM, Nikiforova MN, Carty SE, Armstrong MJ, Hodak SP, Stang MT, et al. BRAF V600E mutation independently predicts central compartment lymph node metastasis in patients with papillary thyroid cancer. Ann Surg Oncol. 2013;20(1):47–52.
39. Joensuu H, Hohenberger P, Corless CL. Gastrointestinal stromal tumour. Lancet. 2013;382(9896):973–83.
40. Pang NK, Nga ME, Chin SY, Ismail TM, Lim GL, Soong R, et al. KRAS and BRAF mutation analysis can be reliably performed on aspirated cytological specimens of metastatic colorectal carcinoma. Cytopathology. 2011;22(6):358–64.
41. Sipos JA, Shah MH. Thyroid cancer: emerging role for targeted therapies. Ther Adv Med Oncol. 2010;2(1):3–16.
42. Tothova Z, Wagner AJ. Anaplastic lymphoma kinase-directed therapy in inflammatory myofibroblastic tumors. Curr Opin Oncol. 2012;24(4):409–13.
43. Yoon HH, Sukov WR, Shi Q, Sattler CA, Wiktor AE, Diasio RB, et al. HER-2/neu gene amplification in relation to expression of

HER2 and HER3 proteins in patients with esophageal adenocarcinoma. Cancer. 2014;120(3):415–24.
44. Kanagal-Shamanna R, Singh RR, Routbort MJ, Patel KP, Medeiros LJ, Luthra R. Principles of analytical validation of next-generation sequencing based mutational analysis for hematologic neoplasms in a CLIA-certified laboratory. Expert Rev. Mol Diagn. 2016;16(4):461–72.
45. Swerdlow SH, Campo E, Pileri SA, Harris NL, Stein H, Siebert R, et al. The 2016 revision of the World Health Organization classification of lymphoid neoplasms. Blood. 2016;127(20):2375–90.
46. Arber DA, Orazi A, Hasserjian R, Thiele J, Borowitz MJ, Le Beau MM, et al. The 2016 revision to the World Health Organization (WHO) classification of myeloid neoplasms and acute leukemia. Blood. 2016;127:2391–405; blood-2016-03-643544.
47. Ochs RC, Bagg A. Molecular genetic characterization of lymphoma: application to cytology diagnosis. Diagn Cytopathol. 2012;40(6):542–55.
48. Bagg A. Immunoglobulin and T-cell receptor gene rearrangements: minding your B's and T's in assessing lineage and clonality in neoplastic lymphoproliferative disorders. J Mol Diagn. 2006;8(4):426–9; quiz 526–7.
49. Zhang S, Abreo F, Lowery-Nordberg M, Veillon DM, Cotelingam JD. The role of fluorescence in situ hybridization and polymerase chain reaction in the diagnosis and classification of lymphoproliferative disorders on fine-needle aspiration. Cancer Cytopathol. 2010;118(2):105–12.
50. Maroto A, Martinez M, Martinez MA, de Agustin P, Rodriguez-Peralto JL. Comparative analysis of immunoglobulin polymerase chain reaction and flow cytometry in fine needle aspiration biopsy differential diagnosis of non-Hodgkin B-cell lymphoid malignancies. Diagn Cytopathol. 2009;37(9):647–53.
51. Venkatraman L, Catherwood MA, Patterson A, Lioe TF, McCluggage WG, Anderson NH. Role of polymerase chain reaction and immunocytochemistry in the cytological assessment of lymphoid proliferations. J Clin Pathol. 2006;59(11):1160–5.
52. Peluso AL, Ieni A, Mignogna C, Zeppa P. Lymph node fine-needle cytology: beyond flow cytometry. Acta Cytol. 2016;60(4):372–84.
53. Grosso LE, Collins BT. DNA polymerase chain reaction using fine needle aspiration biopsy smears to evaluate non-Hodgkin's lymphoma. Acta Cytol. 1999;43(5):837–41.
54. Langerak AW, Groenen PJ, Brüggemann M, Beldjord K, Bellan C, Bonello L, et al. EuroClonality/BIOMED-2 guidelines for

interpretation and reporting of Ig/TCR clonality testing in suspected lymphoproliferations. Leukemia. 2012;26(10):2159.
55. Evans P, Pott C, Groenen P, Salles G, Davi F, Berger F, et al. Significantly improved PCR-based clonality testing in B-cell malignancies by use of multiple immunoglobulin gene targets. Report of the BIOMED-2 Concerted Action BHM4-CT98–3936. Leukemia. 2007;21(2):207.
56. Patel KP, Pan Q, Wang Y, Maitta RW, Du J, Xue X, et al. Comparison of BIOMED-2 versus laboratory-developed polymerase chain reaction assays for detecting T-cell receptor-γ gene rearrangements. J Mol Diagn. 2010;12(2):226–37.
57. Baro C, Espinet B, Salido M, Garcia M, Sanchez B, Florensa L, et al. Cryptic IGH/BCL2 rearrangements with variant FISH patterns in follicular lymphoma. Leuk Res. 2011;35(2):256–9.
58. Shin HJ, Thorson P, Gu J, Katz RL. Detection of a subset of CD30+ anaplastic large cell lymphoma by interphase fluorescence in situ hybridization. Diagn Cytopathol. 2003;29(2):61–6.
59. Rambaldi A, Carlotti E, Oldani E, Della Starza I, Baccarani M, Cortelazzo S, et al. Quantitative PCR of bone marrow BCL2/IgH+ cells at diagnosis predicts treatment response and long-term outcome in follicular non-Hodgkin lymphoma. Blood. 2005;105(9):3428–33.
60. Treon SP, Cao Y, Xu L, Yang G, Liu X, Hunter ZR. Somatic mutations in MYD88 and CXCR4 are determinants of clinical presentation and overall survival in Waldenström macroglobulinemia. Blood. 2014;123(18):2791–6.
61. Scott DW, Mottok A, Ennishi D, Wright GW, Farinha P, Ben-Neriah S, et al. Prognostic Significance of Diffuse Large B-Cell Lymphoma Cell of Origin Determined by Digital Gene Expression in Formalin-Fixed Paraffin-Embedded Tissue Biopsies. J Clin Oncol. 2015;33(26):2848–56.
62. Landsburg DJ, Falkiewicz MK, Petrich AM, Chu BA, Behdad A, Li S, et al. Sole rearrangement but not amplification of MYC is associated with a poor prognosis in patients with diffuse large B cell lymphoma and B cell lymphoma unclassifiable. Br J Haematol. 2016;175(4):631–40.
63. Li S, Desai P, Lin P, Yin CC, Tang G, Wang XJ, et al. MYC/BCL6 double-hit lymphoma (DHL): a tumour associated with an aggressive clinical course and poor prognosis. Histopathology. 2016;68(7):1090–8.

64. Li S, Lin P, Young KH, Kanagal-Shamanna R, Yin CC, Medeiros LJMYC. BCL2 double-hit high-grade B-cell lymphoma. Adv Anat Pathol. 2013;20(5):315–26.
65. Stein EM, DiNardo CD, Pollyea DA, Fathi AT, Roboz GJ, Altman JK, et al. Enasidenib in mutant IDH2 relapsed or refractory acute myeloid leukemia. Blood. 2017;130(6):722–31.
66. Levis M. Midostaurin approved for FLT3-mutated AML. Blood. 2017;129(26):3403–6.
67. Woyach JA, Ruppert AS, Guinn D, Lehman A, Blachly JS, Lozanski A, et al. BTK C481S-mediated resistance to ibrutinib in chronic lymphocytic leukemia. J Clin Oncol. 2017;35(13):1437–43.
68. Gulley ML, Tang W. Laboratory assays for Epstein-Barr virus-related disease. J Mol Diagn. 2008;10(4):279–92.
69. Semenova T, Lupo J, Alain S, Perrin-Confort G, Grossi L, Dimier J, et al. Multicenter evaluation of whole-blood Epstein-Barr viral load standardization using the WHO international standard. J Clin Microbiol. 2016;54(7):1746–50.

Part II
Laboratory Processing: Practical Considerations

Chapter 2
The Cytology Specimen and Preparations: Advantages and Limitations

Gilda da Cunha Santos and Mauro Ajaj Saieg

Abbreviations

CB	Cell block
DNA	Deoxyribonucleic acid
FFPE	Formalin fixed paraffin embedded
FISH	Fluorescence *in situ* hybridization
FNA	Fine-needle aspiration
H&E	Hematoxylin and eosin
ICC	Immunocytochemistry
LBC	Liquid-based cytology
LCM	Laser capture microdissection
NGS	Next-generation sequencing
ROSE	Rapid on-site evaluation

G. da Cunha Santos (✉)
Department of Laboratory Medicine, University of Toronto,
Toronto, ON, Canada

M. A. Saieg
Head, Cytopathology, AC Camargo Cancer Center,
São Paulo, SP, Brazil

S. Roy-Chowdhuri et al. (eds.), *Molecular Diagnostics in Cytopathology*, https://doi.org/10.1007/978-3-319-97397-5_2

Key Terminology

Biomarker	According to the NIH biomarker definition working group, a biomarker is any objectively measurable characteristic that can be used as an indicator of normal biological processes, pathogenic processes, or a pharmacological response to a therapeutic intervention
Cell block	A cytologic preparation obtained by concentrating and fixing (most commonly in formalin) cytology specimens followed by paraffin embedding, thereby mimicking a histologic tissue block
Core-needle biopsy	A biopsy obtained by the use of a needle usually with caliber larger than 18 gauge
Cytospins	Preparations produced from cytocentrifugation of cytology specimens and concentration of cells onto a glass slide
Fresh samples	Samples obtained directly from patients without any fixatives
Liquid-based preparations	Automatically produced preparations from cytology specimens fixed in alcohol-based proprietary solutions, with automated machine-based processing, resulting in a thin-layer slide preparation
Microdissection	Dissection of specific areas of a slide with collection of the cells of interest. Can be performed manually or with the aid of laser (laser capture microdissection)

Smears	The preparation produced by the act of smearing or spreading the material obtained from fine-needle aspirations or exfoliative cytology onto a slide

Key Points

- Cytology samples should be used judiciously in order to maximize their use for molecular analysis
- FFPE cell blocks have an advantage for molecular testing due to their similarities to histological tissue blocks; however, they may be limited by DNA degradation caused by formalin fixation. Cytology specimens collected in alcohol-based fixatives may yield better-quality nucleic acids
- A variety of cytologic preparations can be routinely used for molecular studies, and this can augment the number of samples available for molecular testing
- Rapid on-site assessment is a useful tool to ensure adequate material is present and to check tumor fraction
- Cytologic smears and cytospins are well-suited for FISH studies, and unlike FFPE sections, are not subjected to nuclear truncation artifact
- The main limitation of wide adoption of cytology specimens in molecular analysis is due to the need for additional test validation

Molecular pathology has evolved in recent years and is now part of routine clinical laboratory analysis, with wide applications from detection of microorganisms to discovery of diagnostic biomarkers, with impact on personalized medicine and targeted therapy. In oncologic pathology in particular, it plays a vital role in guiding clinical management and determining patient's overall response to therapy and prognosis.

Among the specimens available for molecular analysis, cytology samples provide a versatile option, with several advantages over histology specimens (core-needle/surgical biopsies) as outlined below. Therefore, it is extremely important for the practicing cytopathologist to be aware of the advantages (and limitations) of cytology specimens for molecular analysis, as well as optimize pre-analytical factors for achieving reliable results.

Overall molecular biomarkers are assessed using three main technologies: immunocytochemistry (ICC) for protein products, fluorescence *in situ* hybridization (FISH) for chromosomal abnormalities, and mutation analysis for gene alterations. Due to the fact that protocols for molecular analysis of histology specimens are usually validated using FFPE tissue blocks, FFPE cell blocks are usually preferred and most commonly used among cytologic preparations, due to seamless transition of the protocols originally designed for histology samples. However, all the other cytologic preparations have already been validated and are currently widely used. The current chapter envisions, therefore, to list the main advantages and limitations of cytology specimens for molecular tests as compared to surgical biopsies, discuss the appropriate handling of these samples, describe the main differences among the various specimen preparations, and discuss ways to minimize their limitations in order to achieve an optimal analysis using these types of preparations.

Advantages of Cytology Samples

Cytology and histology samples (small biopsies and surgical specimens) are received for processing either fresh or in a fixative solution. The main differences between these specimens for molecular testing are related to sample handling and processing and their effect on the nucleic acids and proteins.

For histology specimens, hematoxylin and eosin (H&E)-stained tissue sections obtained from formalin-fixed paraffin-embedded (FFPE) blocks are used for morphological evaluation during diagnostic work-up. Although other fixatives are available, 10% formalin has been widely adopted as a universal tissue fixative for producing paraffin blocks. FFPE tissue blocks have the advantage of yielding serial sections that can be used for ancillary studies, including a variety of molecular tests, and have been traditionally used for long-term storage. However, the detrimental effects of formalin fixation leading to DNA fragmentation and sequencing artifacts have been well described [1–6].

Cytology specimens, on the other hand, have the advantage of immediate and rapid fixation, as many of these samples are received fresh, frequently with a preliminary assessment performed by a cytopathologist or cytotechnologist at the time of the procedure, ensuring adequate material is obtained. Furthermore, due to their minimal volume, there is no delay for the penetration of the fixative solution. Since multiple cytologic preparations can be produced from fresh samples, usually more than one type is available for molecular testing.

For cytology samples, in addition to the H&E-stained slides from cell blocks, Papanicolaou- and Romanowsky-stained direct smears or cytospin slides or Papanicolaou-stained liquid-based cytology slides can be also produced from fresh or fixed material. Therefore, many non-formalin fixatives and multiple types of preparations are routinely used for diagnostic assessment and are often suitable for molecular tests and most frequently provide higher-quality nucleic acids than their formalin-fixed counterparts [2, 7].

Cytology samples are obtained by minimally invasive procedures, which are better tolerated and usually the method of choice for critically ill, advanced stage cancer patients [8]. In addition, fine-needle aspiration specimens show high proportion of neoplastic cells with lower numbers of nonneoplastic stromal and inflammatory cells.

For fluorescence *in situ* hybridization (FISH) assays in particular, cytologic preparations such as direct smears and cytospin slides provide an advantage over FFPE sections as they are not subject to nuclear truncation artifact [9].

In summary, since for histology samples only FFPE tissue blocks are routinely available, judicious use of the tissue sections for morphological examination and ancillary diagnostic tests is required to save material for molecular tests. In contrast, for cytology, fresh samples are frequently available and can be utilized to produce a variety of substrates that offer therefore high versatility for molecular studies. Familiarity with handling and processing protocols for different cytologic preparations, their advantages and limitations, and the fixatives and transport media routinely used can help to overcome the self-imposed limited material of cytology samples and safeguard an accurate analysis (Table 2.1).

Limitations of Cytology Samples: What to Expect and how to Minimize Them

The main limitations of cytological samples are related to (1) the multitude of cytologic substrates and fixatives that require additional test validation as the majority of molecular assays are developed on FFPE tissue blocks, (2) the limited cellularity and the nucleic acid yield especially when the neoplastic cells are present on a single smear or concentrated in small areas of the slide, (3) when the specimen has low tumor content with large amount of nonneoplastic cells, and (4) medicolegal issues if smears or cytospin slides are used for testing and the slide has to be sacrificed without an archival slide for future morphological review.

Some of these limitations can, however, be solved using the following strategies: (1) samples can be enriched for tumor by microdissection of tumor-rich areas to optimize low tumor fraction samples for molecular testing (discussed further in Chap. 8); (2) digital images or scanned slides (whole slide imaging) can be used as archival records to circumvent

TABLE 2.1 Comparison of cytology and histology samples for molecular analysis

Overall features	Cytology samples	Histology samples
Influence from fixatives	Minimal; usually received fresh or fixed in ethanol Immediately fixed Fast fixation	Formalin causes severe DNA degradation and may hamper RNA yield Prolonged exposure to fixatives
Types of preparations	Multiple, often many can be obtained from the same sample	Limited, usually FFPE tissue or snap frozen
Quantity of tumor cells	Physical enrichment "per se" High tumor/stromal cell ratio	Depends on the area, may carry lots of stroma or "non-tumoral areas"
Nuclear truncation artifact for FISH assays	Avoided	Present
Validation	Except for FFPE cell blocks, non-formalin-fixed preparations need extensive validation	Widely validated, most platforms designed for FFPE material
Archived material	Need digital images or WSI if sacrificed, might be the only material available	Option to obtain extra sections for ancillary tests

FFPE formalin-fixed paraffin-embedded material, *WSI* whole slide imaging

legal requirements of slide retention; and (3) various cytologic preparations can be employed for different assays, such as cell blocks for ICC and direct smears for mutation analysis.

Transport Media and Fixatives

A multitude of transport media and fixatives are routinely used to preserve cytology specimens from the time of collection to sample processing and have been employed to achieve optimal morphological details for diagnostic purposes and prevent protein and nucleic acid degradation for molecular assays. Some transport media can also serve as fixatives. In overall, cytology samples are collected and transported until processing usually using one or more of the following: (1) fresh (no fixative), (2) ethanol, (3) air-dry fixation, (4) spray fixation, (5) alcohol-based preservative solutions, (6) formalin, (7) sterile saline, (8) phosphate-buffered saline (PBS), and (9) Roswell Park Memorial Institute (RPMI) medium. The choices might have effects on downstream analysis. For example, for biomarkers assessed by ICC, validation and protocol optimization must be performed when using alcohol-fixed cytology specimens since the results might differ from those obtained from FFPE samples [10].

The type of transport media or fixative is closely linked to the type of sampling method, the cytologic preparation produced and/or algorithm used for sample triage. Regardless of the differences in sample preparation, the different non-formalin fixatives used for cytology samples provide superior results in terms of DNA quality when compared to formalin-fixed material [11]. In general, cytologic preparations (except for cell blocks) usually preclude formalin fixation, thus avoiding fragmentation issues and base-pair changes associated with this fixative [6]. Alcohol-based preserving solutions used for LBC showed different results for DNA yield. Samples collected in CytoLyt (Hologic, Bedford, Massachusetts) gave fivefold higher DNA yield than those in CytoRich Red (Fisher Scientific UK Ltd., Loughborough, Leicestershire, England) [12]. Spray or ethanol-fixed Papanicolaou-stained slides provided the best results in terms of yield and fragment length compared to LBC and air-dried slides [12].

Cytologic Preparations

Routinely several cytologic preparations are produced from a single cytology specimen. Therefore, multiple options are available for the different molecular techniques with protocol optimization and validation required for each of the cytologic preparation employed (Fig. 2.1).

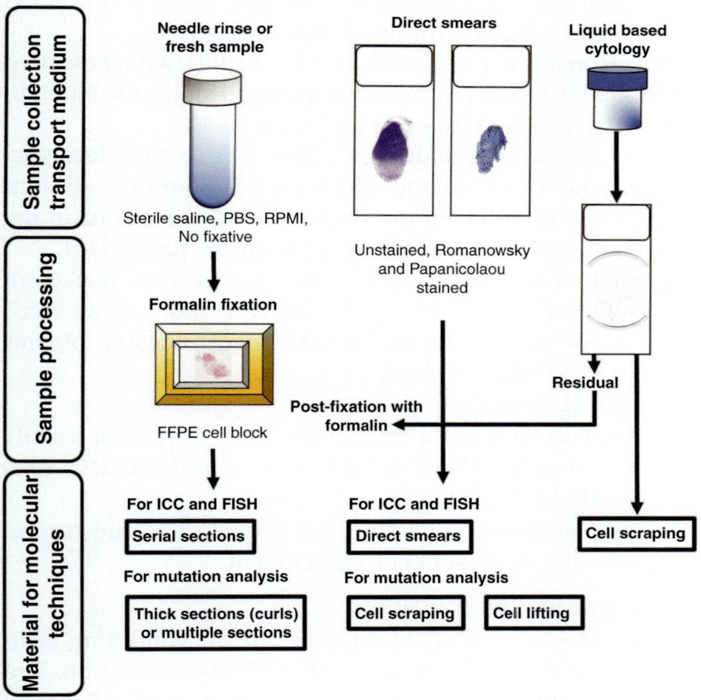

FIGURE 2.1 Diagram of main cytologic preparations with emphasis on sample collection and transport medium, sample processing, and the material required for molecular techniques. PBS, phosphate-buffered saline; RPMI, Roswell Park Memorial Institute; FFPE, formalin fixed paraffin embedded; ICC, immunocytochemistry; FISH, fluorescence *in situ* hybridization

Direct Smears

- Smears are the cornerstone of cytology, inexpensive and efficient for morphological analysis. Cost-effective method to address sample eligibility.
- Smears usually depict high tumor purity. This ensures a confident molecular analysis of the area of interest, even when there is low DNA yield.
- Romanowsky- or Papanicolaou-stained as well as unstained slides are adequate for molecular testing.
- For Romanowsky-stained smears, cellularity assessment can be performed on non-coverslipped slides for immediate selection and triage to molecular assays.
- Diff-Quik-stained slides are equivalent to cell block sections and Papanicolaou slides for NGS testing, without relevant variations in the total number of reads or in the percentage of reads aligning to the target region [13].
- Digital slides (whole slide scanning or digital images of specific areas) may be needed prior to slides being sacrificed for testing to circumvent medicolegal problems related to slide retention.
- For FISH analysis:
  - Nuclear truncation artifact avoided, a problem usually encountered when sections from paraffin blocks (cell blocks) are used.
  - Adhesive-coated or positive charged slides are recommended to prevent cell detachment.
- For gene mutation analysis:
  - Macrodissection (cell scraping) or the cell-lifting technique should be performed for DNA extraction. The latter employs the Pinpoint solution of the Pinpoint Slide DNA Isolation System (Zymo Research). For low cellularity smears, laser capture microdissection (LCM) can be used to enrich tumor cell content targeting specific areas with high tumor cellularity.

- The enrichment of tumor cells is required for specimens with an estimated tumor fraction below a threshold dictated by the analytical sensitivity of the molecular assay employed.

- Nucleic acids extracted from smears show comparable or even superior results to those observed in formalin-fixed paraffin-embedded (FFPE) cell blocks due to non-formalin fixation.

Cell Blocks

- Most common source for molecular analysis among cytologic preparations.
- A variety of fixatives and preparation methods can be employed. Variation in acquisition, preparation, and processing of tumor material due to different clinical and laboratory practices might have minimal impact on test results [14].
- Generated from specimens fixed in formalin- or ethanol- and alcohol-based preserving solutions (CytoLyt and CytoRich red), with post-fixation in formalin.
- Similar processing protocol to histological specimens: Easily validated for clinical use.
- Long-term storage cell preservation.
- Multiple serial sections can be obtained from CBs for several different assays.
- Techniques for cell enrichment such as LCM can be used for samples with low cellularity.
- Special attention to formalin-induced errors that might limit an unbiased and exploratory sequencing analysis (higher chance of errors).
- For ICC:
  - Multiple external controls can be placed on the same tested section which cannot be performed for the other cytologic preparations.

- For FISH analysis:
  - A corresponding H&E-stained slide usually used to circle areas with high tumor cellularity or specific areas for scoring.
  - Non-fluorescence-based assays such as chromogenic *in situ* hybridization (CISH) and silver *in situ* hybridization (SISH) can be performed.
- For mutation analysis:
  - Microdissection of multiple unstained slides with regular thickness (4μ) or thick (>10μ) unstained sections ("curls") can be used for DNA extraction.
- For PCR-based assays, test failure is similar to that of histology specimens, regardless of the type of fixative used (alcohol or formalin) [15].

Liquid-Based Cytology (LBC)

- Valid alternative to conventional smears, limiting sampling artifacts as the automated process for producing LBC slides leads to minimal contamination by blood, inflammation, and cellular debris.
- Macrodissection (cell scraping) or the cell-lifting technique used for DNA extraction and digital slides (whole slide scanning or digital images of specific areas) required for slides to be sacrificed for testing, similar to smears.
- The residual cell suspension (cellularity can be macroscopically assessed by the cloudiness of the fluid) after LBC slides are produced can be submitted to formalin fixation to produce cell block slides that can be used for additional molecular tests or other ancillary techniques.

The residual LBC sample can also be sent directly for molecular testing although the residual solution may not be sufficient for testing and can be stored just for a short period of time [16]. However, multiple FNA passes and changes in workflow for sample processing can yield adequate material for analysis in the majority of cases [17, 18].

Cytospin Preparations

- Stained and unstained slides are adequate for testing.
- Underutilized preparation for mutation analysis. Most frequently used for FISH analysis.
- For FISH analysis:
  - Facilitates analysis due to the nature of the specimen: avoidance of nuclear truncation artifact.
  - Widely used and well validated in the literature, especially for study of lymphomas.
- Macrodissection (cell scraping) or the cell-lifting technique used for DNA extraction similarly to smears.
- Scalpel-blade cell scraping provide higher DNA yield than the cell lifting [19].
- Concentration of the cells in a small area in the center of the slide makes the analysis faster.
- Option to produce multiple slides from one sample and archive them for future studies.
- Archived cytospins could be used as a source of DNA, with results comparable to archived smears [7, 20].

Other Preparations for Storage and Future Molecular Analysis (Cryopreservation and FTA Cards)

Cryopreservation

- Biobanking of fresh cells has the advantage of not being fixed or processed.
- "In natura" DNA can be harvested from the cells, whenever needed.
- Lack of morphological assessment (exact percentage of tumor cells might not be accurately determined—A cytospin can be run with an aliquot of the material for cellularity assessment).
- Demands more sophisticated infrastructure, such as −70 °C freezers; might be costly and not readily available.

FTA Cards

- Cheap, convenient to extract and store. Fast turnaround time for targeted panels.
- Suitable for most PCR-based technologies and NGS. Easy to transport and a viable solution for remote or underdeveloped centers.
- Lack of morphological assessment (similar to frozen material, a cytospin can be produced at the time of collection for cellularity assessment).
- Not widely validated, and therefore, needs multicenter studies.
- Robust studies on RNA extraction are not yet available.

Conclusions

As the use of minimally invasive sampling procedures expands and medicine progresses to personalized therapies, more information will be needed from limited specimens for the management of patients who might require collection of tumor material for repetitive biomarker testing on resistant, recurrent, or metastatic tumors. A rationale use of different cytologic preparations and methods aiming to increase nucleic acid quality and yield, as described in this chapter, is a sine qua non condition for a steady incorporation of cytology as a valid source of molecular material.

References

1. Do H, Dobrovic A. Sequence artifacts in DNA from formalin-fixed tissues: causes and strategies for minimization. Clin Chem. 2015;61(1):64–71.
2. Roy-Chowdhuri S, Chen H, Singh RR, Krishnamurthy S, Patel KP, Routbort MJ, et al. Concurrent fine needle aspirations and core needle biopsies: a comparative study of substrates for next-generation sequencing in solid organ malignancies. Mod Pathol. 2017;30(4):499–508.

3. Spencer DH, Sehn JK, Abel HJ, Watson MA, Pfeifer JD, Duncavage EJ. Comparison of clinical targeted next-generation sequence data from formalin-fixed and fresh-frozen tissue specimens. J Mol Diagn. 2013;15(5):623–33.
4. Srinivasan M, Sedmak D, Jewell S. Effect of fixatives and tissue processing on the content and integrity of nucleic acids. Am J Pathol. 2002;161(6):1961–71.
5. Stigt JA, 'tHart NA, Knol AJ, Uil SM, Groen HJ. Pyrosequencing analysis of EGFR and KRAS mutations in EUS and EBUS-derived cytologic samples of adenocarcinomas of the lung. J Thorac Oncol. 2013;8(8):1012–8.
6. Williams C, Pontén F, Moberg C, Söderkvist P, Uhlén M, Pontén J, et al. A high frequency of sequence alterations is due to formalin fixation of archival specimens. Am J Pathol. 1999;155(5):1467–71.
7. Saieg MA, Geddie WR, Boerner SL, Bailey D, Crump M, da Cunha Santos G. EZH2 and CD79B mutational status over time in B-cell non-Hodgkin lymphomas detected by high-throughput sequencing using minimal samples. Cancer Cytopathol. 2013;121(7):377–86.
8. Eapen GA, Shah AM, Lei X, Jimenez CA, Morice RC, Yarmus L, et al.; American College of Chest Physicians Quality Improvement Registry, Education, and Evaluation (AQuIRE) Participants. Complications, consequences, and practice patterns of endobronchial ultrasound-guided transbronchial needle aspiration: results of the AQuIRE registry. Chest. 2013;143(4):1044–53.
9. Jain D, Mathur SR, Iyer VK. Cell blocks in cytopathology: a review of preparative methods, utility in diagnosis and role in ancillary studies. Cytopathology. 2014;25(6):356–71.
10. Sauter JL, Grogg KL, Vrana JA, Law ME, Halvorson JL, Henry MR. Young investigator challenge: validation and optimization of immunohistochemistry protocols for use on cellient cell block specimens. Cancer Cytopathol. 2016;124(2):89–100.
11. da Cunha Santos G. Standardizing preanalytical variables for molecular cytopathology. Cancer Cytopathol. 2013;121(7):341–3.
12. Dejmek A, Zendehrokh N, Tomaszewska M, Edsjö A. Preparation of DNA from cytological material: effects of fixation, staining, and mounting medium on DNA yield and quality. Cancer Cytopathol. 2013;121(7):344–53.
13. Baum JE, Zhang P, Hoda RS, Geraghty B, Rennert H, Narula N, Fernandes HD. Accuracy of next-generation sequencing for the identification of clinically relevant variants in cytology smears in lung adenocarcinoma. Cancer Cytopathol. 2017;125(6):398–406.

14. da Cunha Santos G, Saieg MA, Troncone G, Zeppa P. Cytological preparations for molecular analysis: a review of technical procedures, advantages and limitations for referring samples for testing. Cytopathology. 2018;29(2):125–32.
15. Shiau CJ, Babwah JP, da Cunha Santos G, Sykes JR, Boerner SL, Geddie WR, et al. Sample features associated with success rates in population-based EGFR mutation testing. J Thorac Oncol. 2014;9(7):947–56.
16. Bellevicine C, Malapelle U, Vigliar E, de Luca C, Troncone G. Epidermal growth factor receptor test performed on liquid-based cytology lung samples: experience of an academic referral center. Acta Cytol. 2014;58(6):589–94.
17. Krane JF, Cibas ES, Alexander EK, Paschke R, Eszlinger M. Molecular analysis of residual ThinPrep material from thyroid FNAs increases diagnostic sensitivity. Cancer Cytopathol. 2015;123(6):356–61.
18. Tian SK, Killian JK, Rekhtman N, Benayed R, Middha S, Ladanyi M, et al. Optimizing workflows and processing of cytologic samples for comprehensive analysis by next-generation sequencing: Memorial Sloan Kettering Cancer Center experience. Archives of Pathology & Laboratory Medicine. 2016;140(11):1200–205.
19. Roy-Chowdhuri S, Chow CW, Kane MK, Yao H, Wistuba II, Krishnamurthy S, et al. Optimizing the DNA yield for molecular analysis from cytologic preparations. Cancer Cytopathol. 2016;124(4):254–60.
20. Santos Gda C, Saieg MA, Ko HM, Geddie WR, Boerner SL, Craddock KJ, et al. Multiplex sequencing for EZH2, CD79B, and MYD88 mutations using archival cytospin preparations from B-cell non-Hodgkin lymphoma aspirates previously tested for MYC rearrangement and IGH/BCL2 translocation. Cancer Cytopathol. 2015;123(7):413–20.

Chapter 3
Sample Acquisition and Test Requisition

Ross A. Miller and Ashwyna Sunassee

Abbreviations

CNB	Core-needle biopsy
EBUS	Endobronchial ultrasound
EUS	Endoscopic ultrasound
FNA	Fine-needle aspiration
ROSE	Rapid on-site evaluation

Key Points

- Cytopathology specimens are acquired in different ways depending on the site of interest
- Exfoliative cytopathology refers to specimens that are spontaneously shed or can be brushed off, for example, cervical smears and body fluids

R. A. Miller
Memorial Pathology Consultants, P.A., Kingwood, TX, USA

A. Sunassee (✉)
Department of Pathology and Genomic Medicine, Houston Methodist Hospital, Houston, TX, USA

S. Roy-Chowdhuri et al. (eds.), *Molecular Diagnostics in Cytopathology*, https://doi.org/10.1007/978-3-319-97397-5_3

- Fine-needle aspiration is a minimally invasive way of acquiring specimen that is not amenable to exfoliation
- The FNA technique is critical to obtain optimal material for diagnosis and ancillary testing
- Rapid on-site evaluation is frequently utilized and is a useful adjunct to ensure adequacy and proper triage
- A well-formatted test requisition form with essential components ensures that the cytopathology specimen is well triaged and processed

Part 1: Sample Acquisition

Sample Types

Cytopathologic specimen acquisition refers to how cellular material is collected or obtained for cytopathologic examination. Acquisition can be broadly categorized as either *exfoliative* or *aspirational* (Fig. 3.1). Exfoliative cytopathology refers to the collection of cellular material that has been spontaneously shed or manually detached (i.e., scraped or brushed off a surface), whereas aspirational cytopathology refers to specimen collection by actively procuring material from an area of interest within the body not amenable by exfoliation (e.g., using a needle in a back and forth fashion with intentional forward cutting motion to obtain material from within the tissue). Regardless of the acquisition method, ancillary studies may be desired (to supplement the diagnosis) or required for diagnostic purposes and therapeutic selection.

Exfoliative cytopathology refers to collected cellular material that has been spontaneously shed or manually detached from a body surface. Examples of spontaneous exfoliation

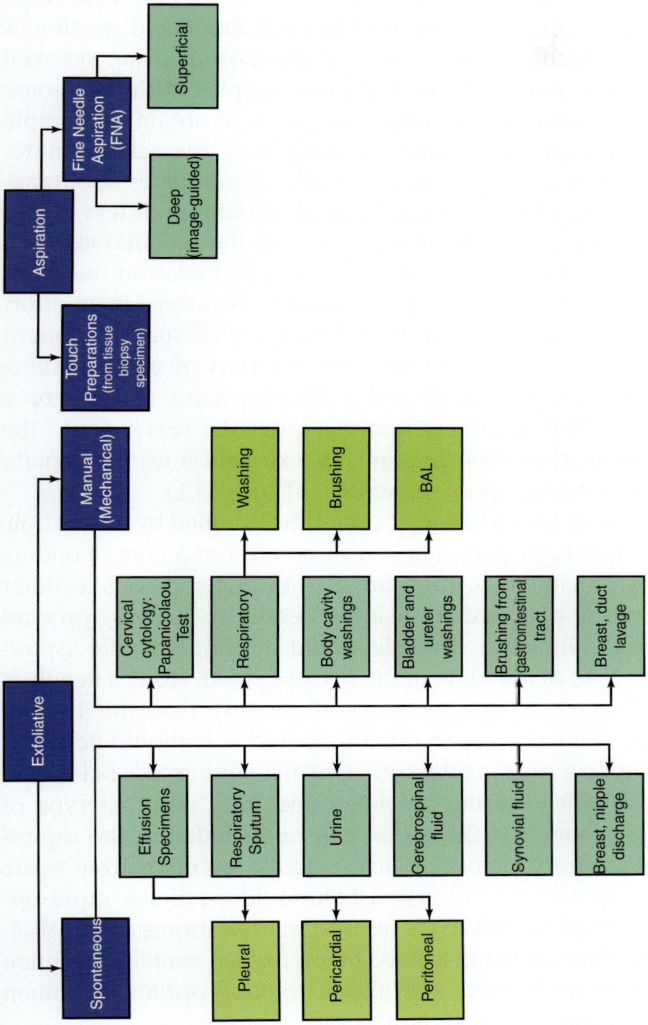

FIGURE 3.1 Various types and methods of cytopathologic material acquisition [1–5]

specimens include fluid collection from body cavity effusions. Effusions (i.e., excess fluid accumulation) can occur within pleural, pericardial, or peritoneal cavities and indicate some pathologic process. Other spontaneous exfoliated specimens include sputum, voided urine, catheterized urine, synovial joint fluid, and cerebrospinal fluid samples. Although some degree of intervention may be acquired to obtain the sample (i.e., thoracentesis, lumbar puncture, etc.), the cellular material present in the sample typically accumulates spontaneously in the obtained fluid. Manual exfoliation differs in that mechanical manipulation is used to exfoliate cellular material from a body surface. Mechanical manipulation methods include brushing, scraping, or irrigating a surface in an effort to dislodge cellular material. Examples of such specimens include brushing specimens (from a variety of sites), washing samples, and the modern-day Papanicolaou test where a brush is used to collect material from the cervix (note the original method was spontaneous exfoliation using a pipette to collect vaginal pool secretions [6]) (Fig. 3.1).

When an area of interest cannot be sampled by exfoliation, aspirational cytopathology (with or without a corresponding biopsy specimen) is often utilized. In this approach, cellular material is obtained by using a needle to actively procure material. One such example would be a fine-needle aspiration (FNA) of a nodule in the thyroid gland. Here, a needle is directly placed into the area of interest (i.e., the thyroid lesion) in an attempt to procure material. It should be noted that appropriate technique (further discussed below) is essential for ensuring specimen adequacy. Another type of cytopathology specimen that can be included in the aspirational category includes touch preparations made from tissue biopsy specimens (discussed below). Many times, rapid on-site evaluation (ROSE) is utilized in aspirational cytopathology (ROSE further discussed below) which enables specimen adequacy evaluation and allows for appropriate specimen triage during the procedure.

Fine-Needle Aspiration Procedure

The term fine-needle aspiration (FNA) is somewhat of a misnomer in that procured material is not acquired by *aspiration*; rather, it is the back and forth *cutting* action of the needle that facilitates the movement of material into the bore of the needle. Proper technique is essential in order to maximize the amount of procured material. Simply placing a needle in an intended target, generating negative pressure, and "wiggling" the needle back and forth will almost invariable result in localized hemorrhage and suboptimal cellular collection. In many instances, the pathologist is not the one performing the FNA procedure. However, the pathologist may be in the position to provide feedback or make suggestions on how the proceduralist could potentially increase yield, particularly when ROSE (discussed below) is being performed.

After it has been determined that an FNA is warranted and the patient has been consented, the patient should be positioned accordingly, the area prepped, and the target lesion immobilized (as much as possible). The needle can then be placed into the lesion for sampling. Needle location can be verified by image guidance such as ultrasound; however, imaging assistance is generally not needed for superficial palpable lesions. For deep-seated lesions, the use of CT- or MRI-guided imaging is usually utilized. It should be noted that placing the needle along the long axis can help facilitate more cellular procurement of material [7] during the procedure. After the needle has been placed into the lesion, a vacuum can be generated by pulling back on the plunger of the syringe that the needle is attached to (*see* Fig. 3.2 for an example of devices that can assist with providing negative pressure). This negative pressure should be maintained throughout the procedure and released *before* the needle is removed. After negative pressure has been generated, the needle should be moved in a back and forth fashion at a rate of 2–3 times per second with intentional forward

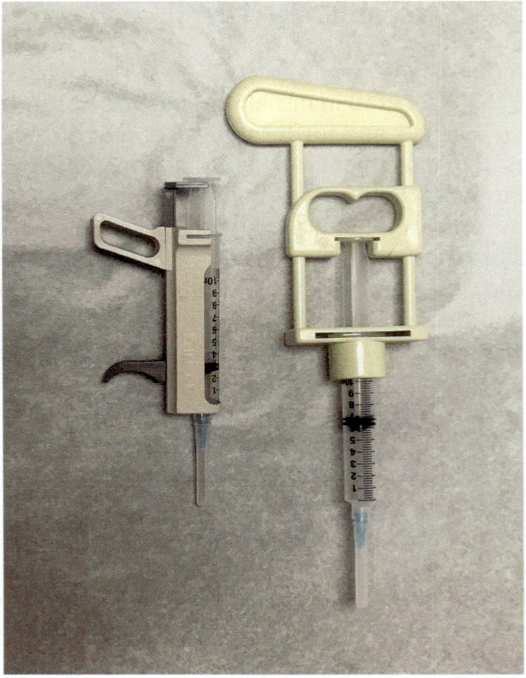

FIGURE 3.2 Devices that can help provide negative pressure during the fine-needle aspiration (FNA) procedure

cutting motion while maintaining the tip of the needle in the lesion. It is the cutting motion of the needle that procures material; negative pressure (aspiration) is simply added to help facilitate the movement of material into the bore of the needle. The length of time the needle is in the lesion is referred to as the "dwell time"; the dwell time should not exceed 20 s [8] and should be limited to 2–5 s in vascular lesions or tissues [9]. Excessive dwell times can result in blood clotting within the bore of needle. The cells of interest can become entrapped in the clotted material obscuring cytomorphologic details (Fig. 3.3). If interpretation is hindered due to clotted material, one can attempt to salvage this

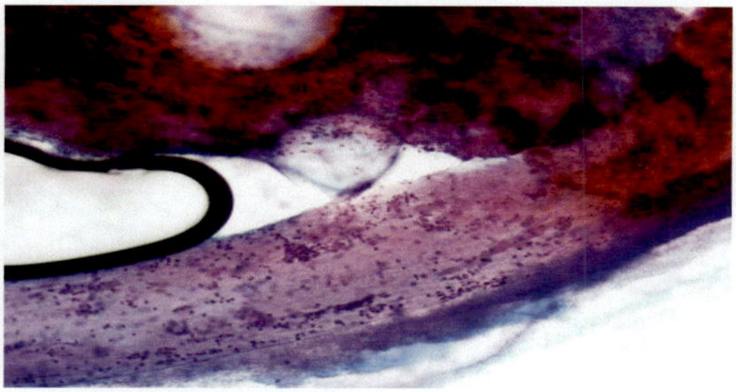

FIGURE 3.3 Excessive dwell time during a fine-needle aspiration can lead to clotted blood entrapping cellular material of interest which obscures cytomorphologic features

material during ROSE by picking the clotted material off the slide with a sterile needle and placing it in liquid media for cell block preparation.

As mentioned earlier, negative pressure should be discontinued before removing the needle; continued negative pressure can result in procured material becoming trapped in the syringe making it irretrievable. Using a “fanning” technique with the needle [8], that is, slightly redirecting the needle trajectory with each back and forth movement, can help facilitate sampling a larger area of the lesion (see Fig. 3.4 for an outline of FNA technique). The trajectory should only be changed when the needle tip is in a superficial location as moving the needle when it is placed deep in the lesion can result in tissue tearing and excessive bleeding. Localized bleeding and hemorrhage can compromise the specimen quality as the material procured will become more hemodilute. Needle selection is also an important consideration. Larger bore needles often result in more bleeding where thinner needles can minimize bleeding. As such, 25 and 27 gauge needles are typically preferred for vascular lesions or tissues [9, 10]. Larger bore needles (23 gauge) may help procure material from sclerotic nonvascular lesions.

It should be mentioned that not all performed FNA need accompanying negative pressure. The same procedure

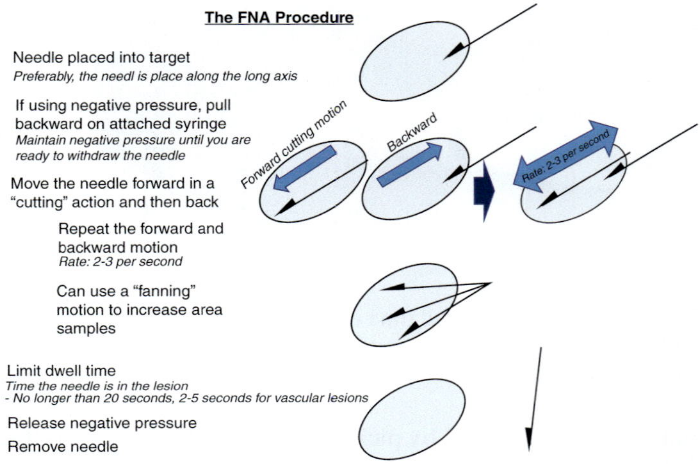

Figure 3.4 The fine-needle aspiration procedure illustrating the different steps involved and the correct technique for obtaining an adequate sample

described above can be used without applying suction, known as the *French technique* or *capillary action needle biopsy*. The choice of technique to use is generally based on operator preference, as both techniques can procure adequate material [11, 12]. One theoretical advance of using the *French technique* is a reduction of trauma to the targeted area and potentially less bleeding as the negative pressure component is being eliminated from the procedure. Conversely, a potential disadvantage is in the setting of cystic lesions as cyst fluid present cannot be readily drained. Again, when selecting which procedure to utilize, lesion location, lesion characteristics, and comfort/familiarity of the technique should all be taken into consideration. Some prefer simply using a needle when performing the *French technique* and then attaching to a syringe (with the plunger pulled backward a few cc's) after removing the needle from the biopsy target in order to express the material out of the bore of the needle. Another approach is to attach the needle to a syringe (again, with the

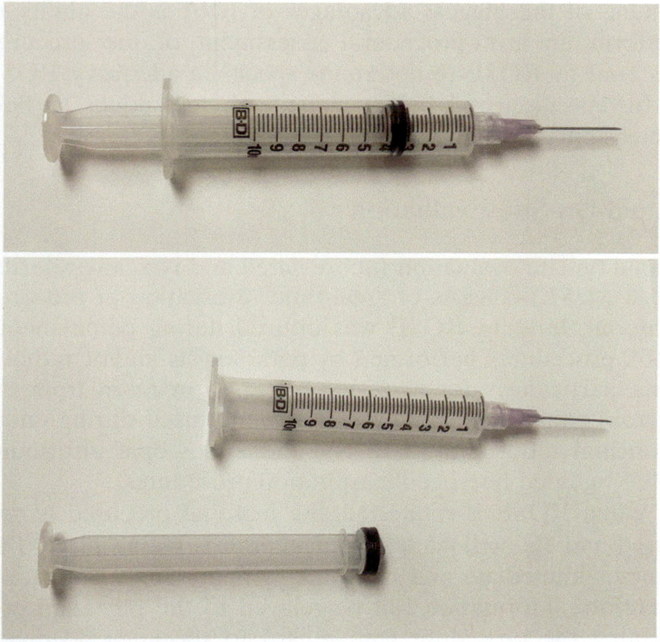

FIGURE 3.5 Needle and syringe set up for the *French technique*. Note: the plunger has been pulled backward a few cc's. Alternatively, the plunger can be removed completely. The needle and syringe can be held like a pencil when performing the procedure

plunger pulled back a few cc's or completely removed, Fig. 3.5) and then perform the procedure. The needle and syringe can be held as a pencil when performing the procedure which can potentially give one more control. Second, the needle is already attached to the syringe for material expulsion after the needle is removed from the target. And third, if the lesion is cystic, a syringe is already attached to the needle should fluid need to be drained. A good resource to learn optimal FNA techniques is the video series by Britt-Marie Ljung, M.D. (http://www.papsociety.org/fna.html) [13].

One of the biggest advantages of FNA is the ability to perform an intra-procedural assessment of the procured material by ROSE to determine specimen adequacy. ROSE is further discussed below along with techniques to help increase diagnostic yields.

Rapid On-Site Evaluation

Rapid on-site evaluation (abbreviated and typically referred to as *ROSE*) consists of "real-time" evaluation of procured material. Initially, ROSE was utilized during percutaneous FNA procedures performed by pathologists and/or radiologists, particularly for assessing material procured from the thyroid gland. ROSE is now commonly used during endobronchial ultrasound (EBUS)- and endoscopic ultrasound (EUS)-guided fine-needle aspiration procedures.

When ROSE is requested, the material procured is prepared and stained, while the procedure is taking place. This enables immediate and real-time cytopathologic evaluation; therefore, information can be relayed to the physician performing the procedure with regard to specimen adequacy. Additionally, preliminary diagnostic information can be given, and the specimen can be appropriately triaged for potential ancillary tests (i.e., flow cytometry, microbiology studies, molecular studies, immunohistochemical studies, etc.).

Procured material can be evaluated by Romanowsky stain preparations (such as the Diff-Quik stain) or by a rapid Papanicolaou stain. The Diff-Quik stain is a proprietary rapid differential stain of the Romanowsky family that gives a similar optical quality to the Wright-Giemsa stain which can performed in under a minute. Slides should be allowed to dry completely before staining. Depending on one's preference, other smears prepared from the pass can be alcohol fixed and later stained with the Papanicolaou stain. To stain with Diff-Quik, the air-dried slides are typically stained as follows: 10 dips in fixative, 10 dips in xanthene dye, and 10–20 dips in thiazine dye, followed by a rinse in tap water (Fig. 3.6a, b). This can be performed rapidly at the bedside or in the operating room.

Alternatively, a rapid Pap stain can be utilized or simultaneously performed with the Diff-Quik stain. The staining time typically takes between 90 and 130 s, which is slower than Diff-Quik but faster than the traditional Papanicolaou staining procedure. The rapid Papanicolaou stain requires the use of a hood as xylene is one of the solutions used. Hence, it may not be feasible for bedside use. A modified ultrafast

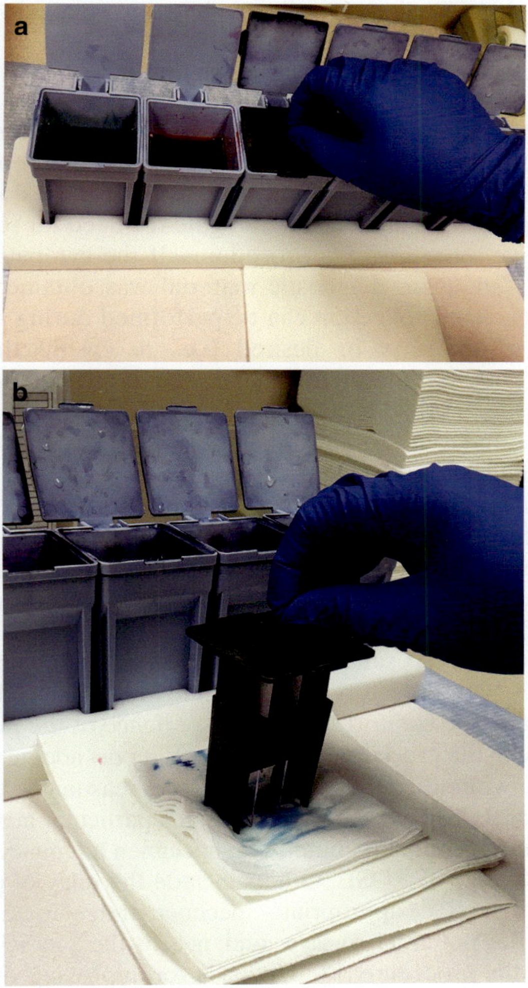

FIGURE 3.6 (**a**) Stain set up for Diff-Quik stain (**b**) Multiple slides can be stained at a time using a slide holder

Papanicolaou (MUPF) stain requires air-dried smears; these are placed in normal saline for 30 s followed by 6 dips in tap water, 30 s in Harris hematoxylin, 6 dips in tap water, 15 dips in EA-36, 6 dips in 95% alcohol, 6 dips in 100% isopropyl alcohol, and 10 slow dips in xylene. The rapid Pap staining process is more complex than the Romanowsky stain; however, nuclear detail is typically much better assessed with the Papanicolaou stain.

If the cytopathologist determines that the sample is inadequate, the physician performing the procedure can modify the FNA technique (by using or discontinuing use of negative pressure, altering the puncture site, changing the depth and/or angle of puncture) [14]. These measures can be done during the procedure in efforts to mitigate the need for repeat or alternative more invasive procedures. If the cytopathologist confirms adequate diagnostic material was obtained, additional specimen collection can be performed during the procedure if necessary or desired (i.e., to ensure thorough sampling of the intended target or for ancillary studies as appropriate) [15].

Many studies have shown the use of ROSE improves diagnostic yield, aids in clinical decision-making [16], and reduces the number of passes performed during the procedure [14], all of which are theoretical advantages of ROSE. Some studies have concluded that ROSE does not improve diagnostic yield [14, 17] and, given the added cost, ROSE is not always warranted [18, 19]. It is important to point out that molecular testing success of FNA samples is directly dependent on specimen adequacy. Various factors can contribute to specimen adequacy, particularly the comfort level and experience of the physician performing the procedure. Some centers report adequacy rates of >90% without ROSE [20]; as such, it is reasonable to tailor the use of ROSE based on the needs of a particular hospital or institution. It should be noted that specimen adequacy is only one advantage of ROSE. Others include the relay of preliminary information, appropriate specimen triage for ancillary studies, the potential to give guidance to the physician performing the procedure (i.e., feedback for improving yield; see the above section on FNA procedure), the ability to stop sampling when appropriate material has been obtained (opposed to doing a set number of passes), and building a relationship between the cytopathologist and proceduralist (which may potentially enhance patient care).

Like with any procedure, there are some challenges that exist for ROSE. Some hospitals or institutions may not have ROSE readily accessible. Perhaps the biggest challenge from a cytopathology management standpoint is the amount of time ROSE can potentially take. The average amount of time per site sampled can range from 12 to 22 min, and often, more than one site is sampled [21, 22]. In addition, current Medicare compensation rates are insufficient to cover the costs pathology incurs when performing ROSE [18]. Telecytopathology can be employed as a potential time-efficient technique in busy cytopathology laboratories. Setup requires a microscope connected to a high-resolution digital camera, video software, secure intranet, access, and appropriate validation (Fig. 3.7). A trained person, such as a cytotechnologist can prepare the

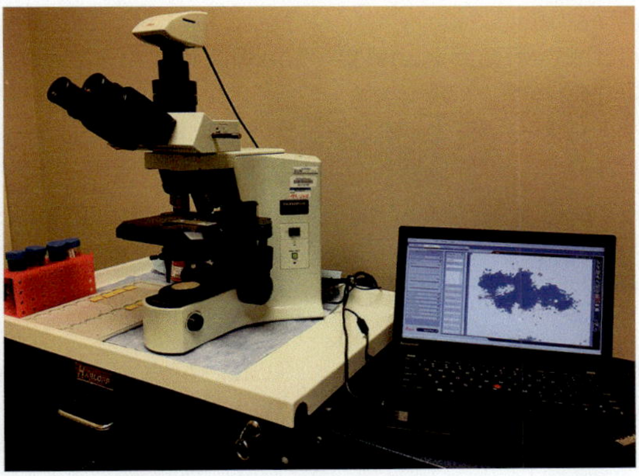

FIGURE 3.7 Setup for telecytopathology illustrating a microscope connected to a high-resolution digital camera equipped with appropriate video software and secure intranet access. A trained person, such as a cytotechnologist, can prepare the slides and relay the live images to a pathologist who may be present at a different location

slides and relay the live images to a pathologist at a different location [23, 24].

Given the numerous potential advantages of ROSE (Table 3.1) [25], particularly with regard to specimen triage,

Table 3.1 Advantages and disadvantages of ROSE [25]

Summary of the advantages and disadvantages of ROSE	
Advantages	**Disadvantages**
Reduces the need for additional sampling (core-needle biopsies) with a lower risk of procedure complications	Need for an experienced on-site cytopathologist (experience and familiarity with results)
Cost-effective (fewer ancillary techniques)	Equivocal on-site diagnosis may prematurely end a procedure
Improves the adequacy rate	Need for extra time from the cytopathologist
Decreases the number of passes needed for an adequate sample	Financial under compensation of pathologist's time
Assists further diagnostic triage (assess whether extra material is needed, decide how to preserve material for further ancillary studies)	Need for optimal staining quality
Stores fresh cells when needed, optimization of storing material for molecular analysis	Extended time for procedure, as well as extended anesthesia time (higher doses of narcotics)
Improves overall diagnostic yield	Relies solely on morphology (thus a need for an experienced cytopathologist)
Improves diagnostic yield of cystic lesions	Need for optimal clinical-pathologist communication
Improves sensitivity	

Abbreviation: *ROSE* rapid on-site evaluation

many cytopathologists advocate for implementing ROSE whenever appropriate and feasible.

Touch Preparations

The core-needle biopsy (CNB) is often used as a minimally invasive technique to sample tissue without the need for a more invasive procedure (surgical excision or resection). Although the CNB specimen is typically considered a histology specimen (opposed to a cytopathology specimen), often a cytopathology specimen is prepared from the CNB in the form of a touch preparation for rapid on-site adequacy assessment. Traditionally, if material representative of the targeted lesion is seen on the touch preparation, the procedure is stopped, and the specimen is considered adequate for diagnosis. Conversely, if material representative of the targeted lesion is absent, the biopsy is considered inadequate, and additional biopsies are obtained in an effort to procure diagnostic material. However, in the current era of molecular diagnostics and the increasing need for adequate tissue to perform molecular testing for targeted therapeutic selection, the presence or absence of lesional material alone is insufficient for *adequacy* determination. When doing an adequacy assessment, the pathologist needs to be aware of the purpose of the specimen adequacy. As such, it is essential to know the intent of the biopsy (i.e., why it is being performed and what information is being sought after). A specimen may be "adequate" from a diagnosis standpoint (presence of tumor) but, however, inadequate for desired ancillary testing which may have been the sole intent of the biopsy.

Traditionally, CNB was performed purely for diagnostic purposes (i.e., in order to determine the pathologic process). However, in the molecular diagnostic era, CNB is frequently performed for diagnostic purposes *and* ancillary testing (i.e., immunohistochemical and/or molecular studies to determine if targeted therapy is warranted). In some instances, CNB is obtained solely for ancillary testing purposes (for instance, in cases where the diagnosis has already been established and additional tissue is needed for ancillary testing to guide clinical management). Mishandling the specimen can result in unnecessary repeat procedures which are both costly and increase the overall risk of harm to the patient. As such, it is advised to treat each malignant sample as if ancillary testing will be needed and performed at some point in time, even if ancillary testing is not requested at the time of the procedure. Anticipating potential ancillary testing can help mitigate the need for repeat procedures for additional tissue acquisition.

The advantage and disadvantage of the touch preparation are at odds with each other, particularly, when ancillary testing is desired. Using touch preparations for specimen adequacy, assessment can be quite useful and is generally accurate (accuracy reports around 90%) [26, 27]. The major disadvantage of the touch preparation is its potential effect on the cellularity of the CNB. For example, if the majority of malignant cells are "touched" off when making the touch preparation, there may be insufficient material on the tissue specimen to perform desired ancillary tests. This can be problematic as, in this setting, the specimen is typically determined to be *adequate* during the on-site adequacy assessment; however, the material on the biopsy is insufficient for ancillary testing. One could argue that sufficient material is present on the cytopathology touch preparation specimen, which could be a potential substrate for molecular testing; however, due to ease of assay validation, a large fraction of laboratories prefer formalin-fixed paraffin-embedded material for molecular testing (even though cytopathology specimens are sufficient and may provide better testing material than biopsy samples [28–31], please refer to Chap. 4 for more information on specimen selection). This "loss" of material on the CNB specimen has been demonstrated as lower CNB DNA content [32] and decreased cellularity [33], particularly in cases where more *aggressive* touch preparation methods were employed [32].

Potential ways to maximize the amount of material present on CNB specimens when adequacy assessment is desired include FNA of the intended target with ROSE (FNA and

ROSE discussed below) followed by CNB [34] or performing very light touch imprints on the CNB while limiting "dragging" of the core across the slide if an initial FNA is not performed [32]. In the ideal situation, the former is done (FNA with ROSE followed by CNB) in order to maximize the amount of material present for potential ancillary tests. There may be certain situations where an initial FNA is not ideal (i.e., very small lesions and/or the fear that the FNA will result in extensive localized bleeding limiting or precluding targeting of the CNB) [33]. Sometimes, the CNB tissue is extremely friable and does not hold together. Even a light touch imprint may result in a significant loss of tissue from the biopsy specimen leaving small tissue fragments on the cytopathology slide. These small tissue fragments are generally poorly visualized on cytological examination as they are often multiple cell layers thick. One way to potentially salvage this material is to manually "pick" it off the touch preparation slide using a sterile needle and placing it in liquid media that can be used for a cell block preparation (and potential ancillary testing). Regardless of the situation, care and "intra-procedural trouble shooting" should be implemented in efforts to facilitate diagnosis and conserve as much material as possible for potential ancillary studies.

Part 2: Test Requisition

An appropriate requisition form must accompany all cytopathology samples received, and the requisition must be completed by the physician sending the specimen or by an authorized/designated person (i.e., nurse or physician assistant working with the physician sending the sample). As stated by the CLIA '88 guidelines, requisition forms must be retained for at least 2 years. The requisition form must contain certain informational elements; additional elements can be added as to tailor the requisition to ones' particular preferences (Fig. 3.8). Required elements include the patient's name or other unique identifier, the patient's age or date of

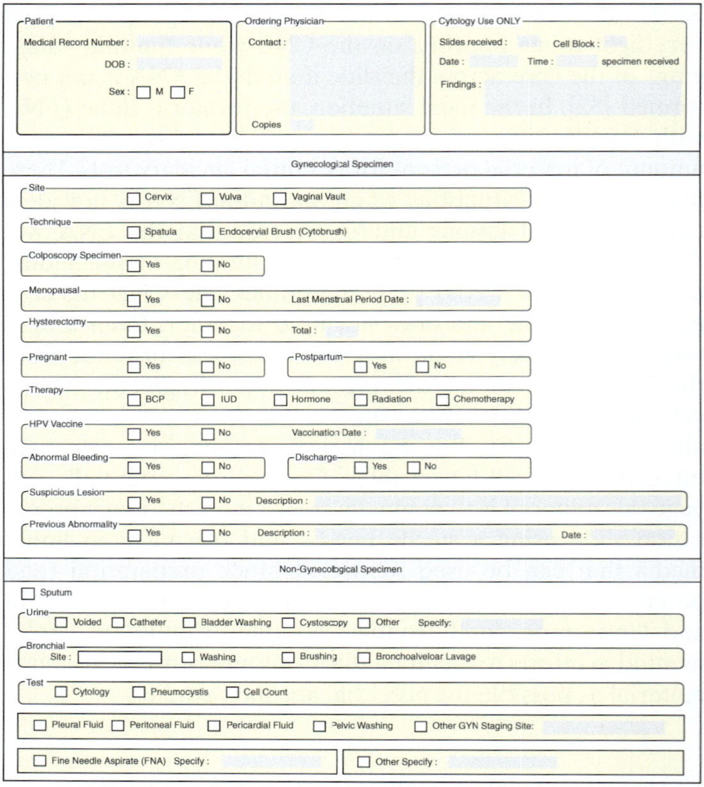
Patient
Medical Record Number :
DOB :
Sex : ☐ M ☐ F

Ordering Physician
Contact :
Copies

Cytology Use ONLY
Slides received : Cell Block :
Date : Time : specimen received
Findings :

Gynecological Specimen

Site: ☐ Cervix ☐ Vulva ☐ Vaginal Vault
Technique: ☐ Spatula ☐ Endocervial Brush (Cytobrush)
Colposcopy Specimen: ☐ Yes ☐ No
Menopausal: ☐ Yes ☐ No Last Menstrual Period Date :
Hysterectomy: ☐ Yes ☐ No Total :
Pregnant: ☐ Yes ☐ No
Postpartum: ☐ Yes ☐ No
Therapy: ☐ BCP ☐ IUD ☐ Hormone ☐ Radiation ☐ Chemotherapy
HPV Vaccine: ☐ Yes ☐ No Vaccination Date :
Abnormal Bleeding: ☐ Yes ☐ No
Discharge: ☐ Yes ☐ No
Suspicious Lesion: ☐ Yes ☐ No Description :
Previous Abnormality: ☐ Yes ☐ No Description : Date :

Non-Gynecological Specimen

☐ Sputum
Urine: ☐ Voided ☐ Catheter ☐ Bladder Washing ☐ Cystoscopy ☐ Other Specify:
Bronchial: Site : ☐ Washing ☐ Brushing ☐ Bronchoalveloar Lavage
Test: ☐ Cytology ☐ Pneumocystis ☐ Cell Count
☐ Pleural Fluid ☐ Peritoneal Fluid ☐ Pericardial Fluid ☐ Pelvic Washing ☐ Other GYN Staging Site:
☐ Fine Needle Aspirate (FNA) Specify :
☐ Other Specify :

Figure 3.8 Sample test requisition form containing the appropriate required informational elements such as the patient's unique identifier, the patient's date of birth and gender, the contact information of the ordering/authorized provider, the date of specimen collection, the test to be performed, and the source of the specimen

birth, the patient's gender, the name and address of the ordering/authorized provider, the date of specimen collection, the test to be performed, and the source of the specimen [35]. Gynecological specimens should include the last menstrual period (LMP) and any patient history of abnormal Papanicolaou tests, treatments, and/or biopsies [8]. The patient's name/unique identifier and date of birth are especially important to assure the correct specimen is being matched with the correct patient. Age and gender provide demographic information, which can be particularly helpful as certain conditions are more common in certain patient populations. This information also has utility when during case sign out, for example, reporting endometrial cells in a Papanicolaou test in women over 45 years of age. The additional information required in gynecology specimens such as LMP, abnormal history, and/or treatment may alert the pathologist to prudently seek out any abnormality and may explain the pathology being seen. Documentation of the specimen source is vitally important with regard to knowing which part of the body the material was collected from and for determination of specimen adequacy. The various types of cytopathology specimens were discussed earlier in the chapter. Knowing the site and method used to obtain the specimen is required to determine if sampling is adequate and to avoid misinterpretation. For example, a bronchial washing mislabeled as a bronchoalveolar lavage (BAL) may be inadvertently called inadequate due to lack of alveolar macrophages.

When a cytopathology sample and appropriate requisition is received, the next step in the pre-analytic phase is to determine the type of material received and what types of preparations can (and should) be made. Received material can include smeared slides (fixed and/or air-dried), a brush, material placed in various fixatives, material placed in media for flow cytometric studies, or fluid obtained directly from a particular site (fluid from an effusion, CSF, urine, etc.). Tailoring a requisition form so the specimen is appropriately processed is essential in order to avoid pre-analytic error (e.g., having information regarding the desire for microbiology studies or flow cytometry).

With the exception of received smears, various preparations can be made from received specimens (smears prepared from a brush, cytospins, ThinPrep or SurePath preparations, and/or cell block preparations). The type of preparation is often determined by specimen type, personal preferences, and potential/desired ancillary testing; particulars of specimen preparations for molecular testing purposes are further discussed elsewhere in this text.

References

1. Light RW. Useful tests on the pleural fluid in the management of patients with pleural effusions. Curr Opin Pulm Med. 1999;5:245–9.
2. Friedman MA, Slater E. Malignant pleural effusions. Cancer Treat Rev. 1978;5:49–66.
3. Meyers DG, Meyers RE, Prendergast TW. The usefulness of diagnostic tests on pericardial fluid. Chest. 1997;111:1213–21.
4. Sahn SA. Plueral effusions in lung cancer. Clin Chest Med. 1982;3:443–52.
5. Ben-Horin S, Shinfeld A, Kachel E, et al. The composition of normal pericardial fluid and its implications for diagnosing pericardial effusions. Am J Med. 2005;118:636–40.
6. Papanicolaou GN. New cancer diagnosis. In: Proceeding of the third race Betterment conference. 1928; p. 528–34.
7. Kreula J, Brondestaom S, Virkkunun P. Sample size in fine needle aspiration biopsy. Br J Surg. 1989;76(12):1270–2.
8. Ly A. Fine-needle aspiration biopsy technique and specimen handling. In: Cibas ES, Ducatman BS, editors. Cytology: diagnostic principles and clinical correlates. 4th ed. Philadelphia: Elsevier Saunders; 2014. p. 221–32.
9. Pitman MB, Abele J, Ali SZ, et al. Techniques for thyroid FNA: a synopsis of the National Cancer Institute Thyroid fine-needle aspiration state of the science conference. Diagn Cytopathol. 2008;36(6):407–24.
10. Guidelines of the Papanicolaou Society of Cytopathology for fine-needle aspiration procedure and reporting. The Papanicolaou society of cytopathology task force on standards of practice. Diagn Cytopathol. 1997;17(4):239–47.
11. Mair S, Dunbar F, Becker PJ, Du Plessis W. Fine needle cytology – is aspiration suction necessary? A study of 100 masses in various sites. Acta Cytol. 1989;33(6):809–13.
12. Kamal MM, Arjune DG, Kulkarni HR. Comparative study of fine needle aspiration and fine needle capillary sampling of thyroid lesions. Acta Cytol. 2002;46(1):30–4.

13. Papanicolaou Society of Cytopathology. Optimal FNA techniques video series by Britt-Marie Ljung, M.D. http://www.papsociety.org/fna.html.
14. Sehgal IS, Dhooria S, Aggarwal AN, Agarwal R. Impact of rapid on-site cytological evaluation (ROSE) on the diagnostic yield of transbronchial needle aspiration during mediastinal lymph node sampling: systematic review and meta-analysis. Chest. 2018;153(4):929–38.
15. Yarmus L, Van Der Kloot T, Lechtzin N, et al. A randomized prospective trial of the utility of rapid on-site evaluation of transbronchial needle aspiration. J Bronchol Intervent Pulmonol. 2011;18(2):121–7.
16. Yasukufu K, Chiyo M, Sekine Y, Chhajed PN, Shibuya K, Iizasa T, et al. Real-time endobronchial ultrasound-guided transbronchial needle aspiration of mediastinal and hilar lymph nodes. Chest. 2004;126:122–8.
17. Joseph M, Jones T, Lutterbie Y, et al. Rapid on-site pathologic evaluation does not increase the efficacy of endobronchial ultrasonographic biopsy for mediastinal staging. Ann Thorac Surg. 2013;96:403–10. 10.
18. Layfield LJ, Bentz JS, Gopez EV. Immediate on-site interpretation of fine-needle: aspiration smears: a cost and compensation analysis. Cancer. 2001;93(5):319–22.
19. Schmidt RL, Walker BS, Cohen MB. When is rapid on-site evaluation cost-effective for fine-needle aspiration biopsy Schmitt F, ed. PLoS One. 2015;10(8):e0135466.
20. Iglesias-Garcia J, Dominguez-Munoz JE, Abdulkader I, Larino-Noia J, Eugenyeva E, Lozano-Leon A, Forteza-Vila J. Influence of on-site cytopathology evaluation on the diagnostic accuracy of endoscopic ultrasound-guided fine needle aspiration (EUS-FNA) of solid pancreatic masses. Am J Gastroenterol. 2011;106:1705–10.
21. Eedes CR, Wang HH. Cost-effectiveness of immediate specimen adequacy assessment of thyroid fine-needle aspirations. Am J Clin Pathol. 2004;121(1):64–9.
22. Miller RA, Wright AM, Satrum LS, Mody DR, Schwartz MR, Thrall MJ. Utilization, review and reimbursement of cytology services in endobronchial ultrasound-guided procedures: challenge and opportunity. JASC. 2016;5:139–44.
23. Thrall M, Pantanowitz L, Khalbuss W. Telecytology: clinical applications, current challenges, and future benefits. J Pathol Inform [serial online]. 2011;2:51.

24. Khurana KK. Telecytology and its evolving role in cytopathology. Diagn Cytopathol. 2012;40:498–502.
25. da Cunha Santos G, Ko HM, Saieg MA, Geddie WR. "The petals and thorns" of ROSE (rapid on-site evaluation). Cancer Cytopathol. 2013;121(1):4–8.
26. Appelbaum L, Kane RA, Kruskal JB, et al. Focal hepatic lesions: US-guided biopsy–lessons from review of cytologic and pathologic examination results. Radiology. 2009;250:453–8.
27. Liao WY, Jerng JS, Chen KY, et al. Value of imprint cytology for ultrasound-guided transthoracic core biopsy. Eur Respir J. 2004;24:905–9.
28. Williams C, Ponten F, Moberg C, et al. A high frequency of sequence alterations is due to formalin fixation of archival specimens. Am J Pathol. 1999;155(5):1467–71.
29. Chowdhuri SR, Chen H, Staerkel G, Stewart JM. Concurrent fine needle aspirations and core needle biopsies: a comparative study of substrates for next-generation sequencing in solid organ malignancies. Mod Pathol. 2017;30(4):499–508.
30. Killian JK, Walker RL, Suuriniemi M, et al. Archival fine-needle aspiration cytopathology (FNAC) samples: untapped resource for clinical molecular profiling. J Mol Diagn. 2010;12(6):739–45.
31. Gailey MP, Stence AA, Jensen CS, Ma D. Multiplatform comparison of molecular oncology tests performed on cytology specimens and formalin-fixed, paraffin-embedded tissue. Cancer Cytopathol. 2015;123(1):30–9.
32. Rekhtman N, Kazi S, Yao J, et al. Depletion of core needle biopsy cellularity and DNA content as a result of vigorous touch preparations. Arch Pathol Lab Med. 2015;139(7):907–12.
33. Tong LCB, Rudomina D, Rekhtman N, Lin O. Impact of touch preparations on core needle biopsies. Cancer Cytopathol. 2014;122(11):851–4.
34. Cobb CJ. FNA or core needle biopsy? Why not both? CAP Today [serial online] 2007, p. 107.
35. Cibas ES, Ducatman BS. Cytology: diagnostic principles and clinical correlates. Philadelphia: Saunders/Elsevier; 2014.

Chapter 4
Pre-analytic Workflow and Specimen Evaluation

John M. Stewart

Abbreviations

CNB	Core-needle biopsy
DQ	Diff-Quik
EBUS-TBNA	Endobronchial ultrasound-guided transbronchial needle aspiration
EHR	Electronic health record
FFPE	Formalin-fixed paraffin embedded
FISH	Fluorescence *in situ* hybridization
FNA	Fine-needle aspiration
IHC	Immunohistochemistry
LBC	Liquid-based cytology preparation (e.g., ThinPrep, SurePath)
NGS	Next-generation sequencing
Pap	Papanicolaou
PCR	Polymerase chain reaction
TQL	Tissue qualification laboratory

J. M. Stewart
MD Anderson Cancer Center, The University of Texas, Houston, TX, USA
e-mail: jostewart@mdanderson.org

S. Roy-Chowdhuri et al. (eds.), *Molecular Diagnostics in Cytopathology*, https://doi.org/10.1007/978-3-319-97397-5_4

Key Terminology

Analytic threshold	Minimal input requirement for successful testing as determined by laboratory validation
Input DNA	Minimum amount of DNA needed to obtain a result by PCR or NGS
Pre-analytical workflow	Includes the processing and handling of samples and clinical requests for testing, evaluating samples for adequacy for testing, and preparing samples for testing
Tumor fraction	Percentage of tumor cells in a sample. The analytic threshold for T% is defined as the minimum amount of tumor DNA that can be reliably detected in a background of wild-type DNA. Calculated by the total number of tumor cells divided by the total number of nucleated cells. Also referred to as tumor cellularity and tumor proportion
Tumor mapping	Process by which areas of relative tumor enrichment on smears or paraffin sections are marked for extraction (by macrodissection or microdissection) and processing

Key Points

- An optimal pre-analytic workflow requires a proactive adaptation to the demands of molecular pathology and takes into account the strengths and weaknesses of one's practice environment
- Pre-analytic evaluation requires an understanding of the platforms used for testing and their analytic requirements

- Adequately assessing cellularity/input DNA, tumor fraction, and tumor mapping is not difficult but does require attention to detail and some self-training
- In-house validation is needed when using nontraditional substrates
- Communication with the clinical team is especially important with marginally adequate samples at risk for a false-negative result and when triaging of multi-test requests is needed because of limited sample

A Workflow Adaptation to the Molecular World

Clinically requested molecular testing for prognostic and therapeutic information has changed the practice of pathology across most institutions. Ten years ago, the number of tests for solid tumors was relatively small and the sporadic molecular test requests received, usually via email or phone, were generally handled by the pathologist who had signed out the case. As the number of tests expanded and the clinical requests for testing exploded, it became painfully clear that this *reactive* approach to testing was grossly inefficient and inconsistent. Therefore, for the good of patient care, a *proactive* approach is needed to anticipate the possibility of receiving a request for testing.

The best pre-analytical workflow depends on the particular strengths and limitations of the practice environment (e.g., frequency of requests for testing, availability of in-house molecular testing, ability to use non-FFPE substrates, staffing, clerical and informatics infrastructure, etc.). One would therefore expect a wide variety of healthy workflow adaptations to molecular testing. Although the approach outlined below is our particular adaptation and appropriate for a large tertiary care cancer center, elements discussed herein may be of general interest or applicability.

Conservation

The first and most fundamental adaptation has been a change in mindset. It used to be that whenever we received an FNA or biopsy, we would attempt to make a definitive diagnosis and subtype every tumor, however many immunostains were needed. More recently, the most important clinical question is sometimes less about a highly specific diagnosis and more about the mutational status of the tumor. In fact, sometimes the diagnosis is already well established and the FNA/biopsy is performed specifically to acquire tissue for molecular testing. So it is important now to firmly understand the clinical context of the biopsy, anticipate the need for current or future molecular testing, and conserve the FNA/biopsy as much as possible.

Diagnostic Reports

The second adaptation has been in our pathology reports. Several years ago, we would spend an inordinate amount of time and energy chasing down recent and archival cases for re-review just to find a block or smear adequate for testing. With a small change in reporting, we have spared ourselves this aggravation. Our surgical pathology reports now contain a biomarker field, in which the best blocks (primary and metastatic tumor and normal control when appropriate) are identified. Our FNA reports now contain a field to indicate the number of smears suitable for PCR and FISH testing and the quality of the cell block for testing (see Fig. 4.1).

Streamlining Pre-analytic Evaluation

The third adaptation has been in clerical, laboratory, and informatics infrastructure. Upon finalization of the surgical pathology report, the paraffin blocks designated in the biomarker field are sequestered in a separate laboratory, known

a

Biomarker testing

Tumor block:	D3
Non-neoplastic antral mucosa block:	D34
Liver metastasis block:	E1

****

b

SR: 6 S, 2 CB
MDL CB: 300+
MDL Pap: 2 S
MDL DQ: No
FISH DQ: 2 S

FIGURE 4.1 Examples of biomarker fields in (**a**) surgical pathology and (**b**) cytopathology reports. The biomarker field appears at the bottom of the surgical pathology report and indicates primary tumor, metastatic tumor, and block for use as normal control. Limited or insufficient tumor is reported as such. A biomarker field also appears at the bottom of the cytopathology report and indicates the number of smears (SR) and cell block sections (CB) retained in file. The tumor cellularity of the cell block is reported as 300+ (high), 50–300 (medium), or < 50 (low). The number of Pap- and DQ-stained smears suitable for PCR/NGS testing (MDL Pap/DQ) and the number of DQ-stained smears suitable for FISH (FISH DQ) are reported. This reporting informs not only the pathologist evaluating a future clinical request for testing but also the clinician who may want to order testing

as the Tissue Qualification Laboratory (TQL) and staffed by experienced histotechnologists who function apart from the main histology laboratory. This ensures that blocks are not lost and are always available for quick access. Our clinical service is no longer disrupted by fielding clinicians' phone and email requests for testing, since these are routinely made in the electronic health record (EHR) as order sets, which preserve the documentation needed for billing purposes. The tracking of order sets provides metrics, such as turnaround time to lab, to identify problems and improve efficiency. We also now have a clerical office of pathology expeditors who organize and manage these clinical requests from the EHR, gather relevant in-house case materials for the pathologist's review, and interface with the TQL histology laboratory, referring hospitals, and the molecular laboratory on problematic cases.

Ensuring Quality and Uniformity of Pre-analytic Evaluation

The fourth adaptation has been the development of a clinical service for pathologists to perform pre-analytic assessments of cases for testing. The number of pathologists who rotate on this TQL service is limited in order to maximize the quality and uniformity of these pre-analytic evaluations. Although a focused accountant mentality in evaluating tumor fractions and a diligence in pursuing alternative material for testing are the only essential qualifications, it helps that several of these pathologists also sign out the molecular results of solid tumors and can therefore inform the group of recurring problems and new developments in the molecular lab.

Hierarchy of Testing and Communication

The clinician often specifies which sample is to be used for testing. Whenever this is unsuitable, alternative or supplemental concurrent or archival material is queried within the context of the requested tests and in communication with the clinical team. Historically, testing histologic samples is preferred, but when a core biopsy is insufficient or only partly adequate, the concurrent FNA and/or effusion are pulled for evaluation. Sometimes slides from the concurrently acquired FNA and core biopsy are combined for PCR/NGS mutational analysis, as long as they were obtained from the same site during the same procedure. For a significant subset of requests, cytology samples are the only material available for testing. Cell block sections are preferred when the tumor fraction is high and tumor mapping is not required. Since our molecular lab accommodates smears as well as cell blocks, smears are used in about half of our cytology cases used for molecular testing, especially when tumor mapping is needed or when the smears are cellular but the cell block is sparse. Because the use of non-FFPE substrates has not yet been widely adopted, it is important to know the capabilities of the molecular laboratory used by one's practice.

Sample Preparation

The final adaptation to consider is how the potential need for molecular testing may impact routine sample preparation [1–3]. The optimal sample preparation will depend on the practice environment. Are resources available for immediate assessment? Are the proceduralists cooperative? Does the molecular lab process smears and liquid-based preparations? The strengths and weaknesses of the various preparations commonly used in cytology are outlined in Table 4.1 and discussed in more detail below.

TABLE 4.1 Strengths and weaknesses of various preparations used in cytopathology used for ancillary studies

	IHC	**FISH**	**PCR/NGS**	**Adequacy guaranteed by ROSE**
Smear – DQ	No	Good	Better for low T%	Yes
Smear – Pap	Limited	Limited	Better for low T%	Yes
LBC	Limited	Good	Good	No
Cell block	Good	Good	Good	No
CNB	Good	Good	Good	No

Input Requirements of Testing

IHC Studies

Although in general there is no specific cut-off for the minimum number of cells necessary for IHC assays, the interpretation of some antibodies recommends that the FFPE sample contains at least 100 tumor cells [4]. Most immunoperoxidase stains perform as well on FNA cell block preparations as on core-needle biopsy samples, but validation may be needed, since there is some variation in cell block preparation methodologies and a recent study reported suboptimal staining with methanol-fixed (Cellient in PreservCyt) cell blocks [5–7].

Immunoperoxidase staining of direct smears or liquid-based cytology (LBC) preparations requires validation [5]. In our laboratory, when necessary we will use direct ethanol-fixed Pap-stained direct smears or cytospins for diagnostic immunoperoxidase stains with the understanding that an absence of staining must be interpreted cautiously. Negative stain results can be better interpreted when performed as part of a diagnostic panel and/or when internal positive controls are present [8]. Immunoperoxidase stains on direct smears for prognostic/therapeutic marker testing need to be used with some caution as some biomarkers have shown suboptimal results with validation studies (e.g., BRAF V600E VE1 clone) [9, 10].

There are three pre-analytic requirements for using Pap-stained direct smears or LBCs. The first is that tumor must be readily identified from background normal. This can be an issue in some effusions with a low tumor burden and reactive cellular elements, and it is equally problematic in cell block sections. The second is that the tumor cells must be intact and show no air-drying artifact, as can be seen in some touch preparations and sometimes also in FNAs when there has been a delay to fixation for whatever reason. The third is that the slide must have been properly smeared such that tumor is not excessively three-dimensional, so that reagents are able to penetrate and wash off the sample adequately (not an issue with LBCs). When using smears or LBCs of low tumor cellularity, it is always prudent to etch the back of the smear with a diamond-tipped pen to easily identify the cells of interest post-staining, since there can be loss of material in the process of immunoperoxidase staining.

FISH Studies

The minimum number of cells required for FISH studies depends on the specific assay (see Chap. 7 for more details). Whether the substrate is CNB, cell block, direct smear, or LBC, the tumor should be within an area about the size of a nickel (2 cm diameter) to conserve expensive reagents and the tumor cells need to be distinguishable from background benign cellular elements under fluorescent illumination. For FNA cell blocks and core biopsies, an H&E-stained section is marked to locate areas of tumor and submitted with unstained sections. For previously stained smears, the back of the glass slide is etched with a diamond-tipped pen to demarcate the area of interest.

DQ-stained direct smears perform as well or better than FFPE sections [11–13]. The advantage of DQ-stained smears over FFPE is the larger nuclear size as well as the presence of the entire nucleus. An important requirement for using smears is a well-prepared monolayer, since nuclear overlap and three-dimensional clusters obscure interpretation under fluorescence. For this reason, LBCs also work very well. More than one FISH test can be performed on a single smear provided there is enough separation between the areas marked for testing. (A single good DQ smear should be adequate for both PCR/NGS and FISH tests, by scraping parts of the smear for PCR and then submitting the rest of the slide for FISH.) Pap-stained smears can be used for FISH assays, but in our experience, we have found them to be less reliable due to the difficulty in washing out all of the interfering hematoxylin, and consequently they are attempted only as a last resort. Unstained cytospin slides and liquid-based preparations are also suitable [14].

PCR/NGS Studies

Unlike IHC and FISH testing, in which test results are visually tied to cellular morphology, PCR/NGS is a black box in which the test results are divorced from morphology in the process of harvesting DNA. Therefore, the pre-analytic evaluation is crucial for reliable PCR/NGS testing.

PCR/NGS testing has two input requirements – amount of DNA and tumor fraction. A minimum amount of DNA is needed to obtain a result and a minimum tumor fraction is needed to detect a mutation against the background of wild-type signal. It is obvious when insufficient DNA is tested, since there is no result (uninformative). However, an insufficient tumor fraction is undetectable and can lead to false-negative results (misinformative) (see Fig. 4.2).

The analytic thresholds for input DNA and tumor fraction differ considerably, depending on the method of analysis (see Table 4.2), and generally follow manufacturers' recommendations with confirmation during validation testing. The amount of input DNA has been shown to have some flexibility with adequate validation [15].

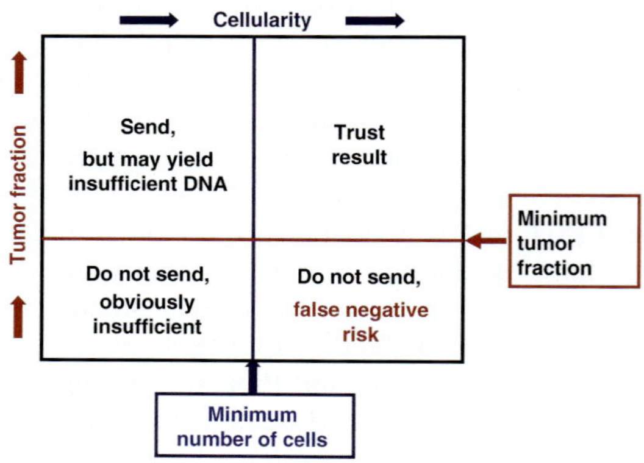

FIGURE 4.2 Graph of input cellularity vs. tumor fraction. Analytic thresholds vary considerably by assay and are validated in the molecular lab. Samples to the left of the blue line will result in no amplification (uninformative results). Samples below the red line will return wild-type data (potentially misinformative results)

TABLE 4.2 Examples of PCR/NGS tests with analytic thresholds

DNA requirements of PCR/NGS assays			
Method	**DNA**	**Total DNA**	**% tumor**
Pyrosequencing	2 ul DNA (at ~5 ng/ul)	10 ng	20%
Sanger sequencing	2 ul DNA (at ~5 ng/ul) *per exon*	10 ng *per exon*	40%
Ion Torrent™ NGS (50 gene panel)	10 ng DNA (>0.85 ng/ul)	10 ng	20%
Oncomine Ion Proton™ NGS (143 gene panel)	20 ng (>0.85 ng/ul)	20 ng	20%
Ion Proton™ NGS (409 gene panel)	30 ul (at 2 ng/ul)	60 ng	20%

Therefore, a proper pre-analytic evaluation of a biopsy requires knowing not just which test is requested but also which analytic method will be used and the tumor fraction needs to be scrutinized and, if necessary, adjusted by tumor mapping. It is also important to know what substrates the molecular lab will accept, since the use of smears and LBCs requires internal validation in the molecular laboratory and has not yet been widely adopted.

Input DNA

We know the minimum DNA input requirement (usually expressed in micrograms or nanograms), but what does that look like in terms of cells? A normal diploid human cell contains approximately 6–7 picograms of DNA [16]. If we assume an extraction efficiency of roughly 15%, then 1000 cells should yield approximately 1 ng DNA. What do 1000 cells look like on a smear or FFPE section? Surprisingly little.

A useful exercise to train one's eye is to count cells on a smear using a graticule (see Fig. 4.3). Sample an area under high magnification (×400), and use the graticule to quickly estimate the number of cells in the field. Note that the same

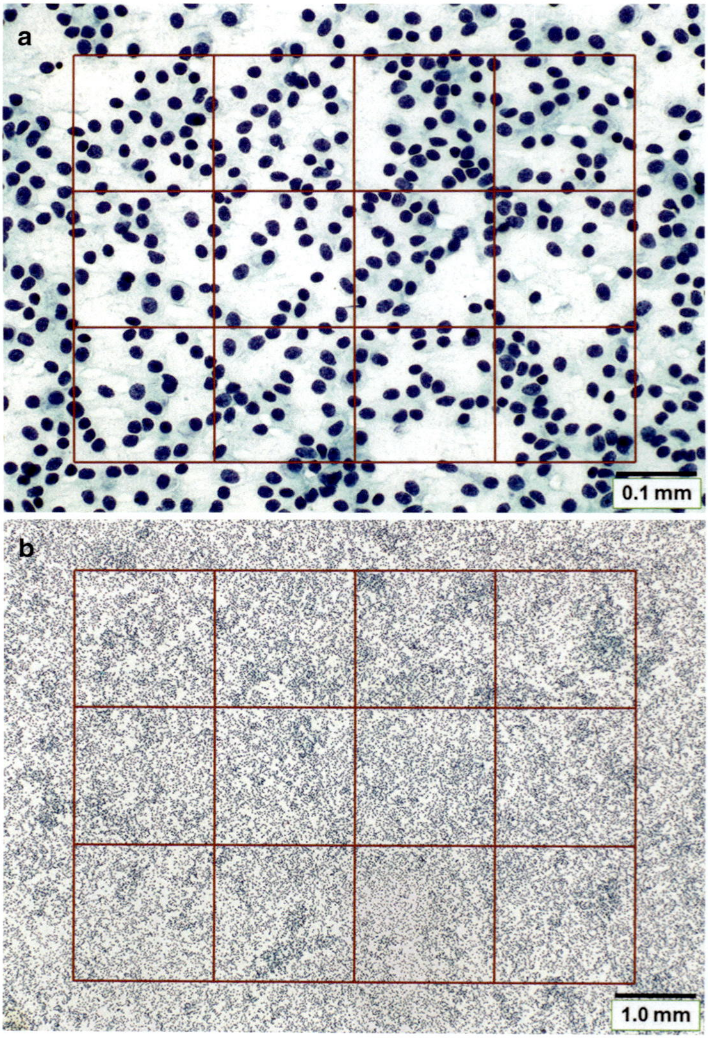

FIGURE 4.3 Counting cells with a graticule. Neuroendocrine tumor, Pap-stained smear of FNA, at 400× (**a**) and 40× (**b**) with simulated graticule. A quick review of a representative high power field (**a**) demonstrates approximately 20 cells per box or 240 cells in larger rectangle. Therefore, the corresponding low power field (**b**) contains approximately 24,000 cells (or 24 ng DNA) in the larger rectangle

distribution of cells under low magnification (×40) will contain 100-fold more cells. Of course, the goal is not to submit the minimum number of cells for mutational studies; however, it helps to be aware of how many cells are present, especially in samples of marginal cellularity or when a single case has to be partitioned among multiple tests.

Tumor necrosis is an interesting variable. Although the DNA obtained from tumor necrosis is often too degraded to be useful in conventional sequencing, this DNA degradation seems to have little effect in NGS [17]. Consequently, samples with insufficient viable tumor but abundant tumor necrosis may sometimes be adequate for NGS.

Tumor Fraction

Tumor fraction (T%) is the percentage of tumor cells in a sample. The analytic threshold for T% is defined as the minimum relative amount of tumor DNA that can be reliably detected in a background of wild-type DNA. This threshold is determined by the laboratory and varies by analytic sensitivity of an assay. For instance, in our laboratory, the required tumor fraction is ≥40% for Sanger sequencing but ≥20% by NGS. Therefore, a sample cannot be adequately evaluated for molecular testing unless the assay to be used and its analytic thresholds are known.

Very high or very low tumor fractions are easily evaluated, but most samples fall between the extremes and these require greater scrutiny. Generally, pathologists who guesstimate at low power grossly overestimate tumor fraction. Figure 4.4 illustrates this point. This case was submitted to the molecular laboratory as 50% tumor for *EGFR* Sanger sequencing. But to a practiced observer, this sample is guaranteed to produce a wild-type *EGFR* result and could possibly be a false-negative result.

Reliably estimating tumor fraction requires some self-training. Several inter-observer studies have shown the variability in tumor fraction assessment among pathologists [18, 19]. A graticule is helpful. In my personal experience at our institution, pathologists are reasonably good at estimating relative areas of tumor, but inexperienced pathologists fail to account for the difference in size of non-tumor cells or, alternatively, the difference in cell densities between areas of tumor and non-tumor. This is especially important in cytology

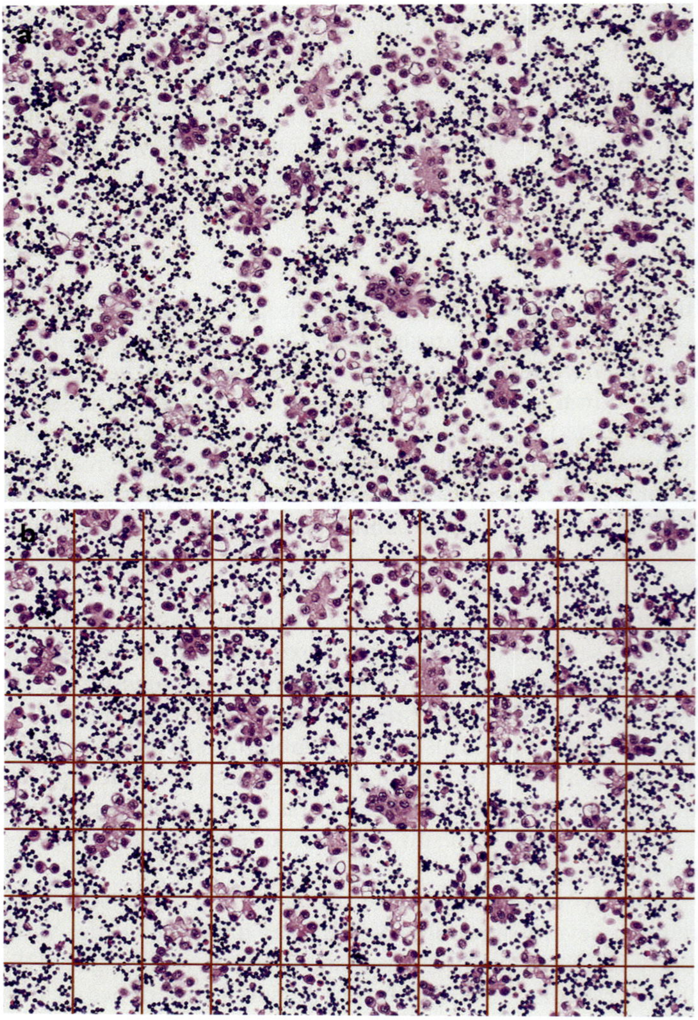

samples, many of which originate in effusions or lymph node aspirations.

Two methods for estimating T% are outlined below:

1. At low power, estimate the areas of tumor and non-tumor and then account for the density of cells within each area (at high power), and divide the percentage of tumor area accordingly. For example, an FNA preparation from a nodal metastasis of a typical lung adenocarcinoma will require dividing by 3 or 4. A similar sample with large tumor cells (see Fig. 4.5) would require a higher factor, whereas an effusion containing a background of mostly histiocytes and mesothelial cells would require a lower factor. This method works best for samples containing cohesive clusters and in core biopsies with distinct areas of tumor and non-tumor (Fig. 4.4).
2. For discohesive tumor on smears, or highly infiltrating tumor on biopsies, go to high power and estimate the number of non-tumor cells per tumor cell (Fig. 4.5).

The key points to whatever method is employed for estimating tumor fraction are to be very attentive to the non-tumoral cell component and not to presume based on a low power impression. Samples with lower tumor fraction obviously require more scrutiny.

FIGURE 4.4 Specimen submitted to the molecular laboratory with an overestimated tumor fraction (estimated at 50%). (**a**) H&E-stained cell block section from a pleural effusion with abundant metastatic lung adenocarcinoma. *EGFR* Sanger sequencing, which requires 40% tumor fraction, was requested. The area occupied by tumor relative to the lymphoid background is around 40–50%, but consider how many more lymphocytes are present in the same unit area. This is more obvious when using a graticule. (**b**) Same field with simulated graticule. The area occupied by tumor, when the tumor is of this size and in this background, can be divided by 3–4, which gives a rapid approximation of 10–17% tumor fraction, far below the analytic threshold. Not surprisingly, Sanger sequencing showed only wild-type *EGFR*

Tumor Mapping

Amount of input DNA and tumor fraction are independent variables as far as the mechanics of testing is concerned, but they are not independent in the pre-analytic evaluation of the

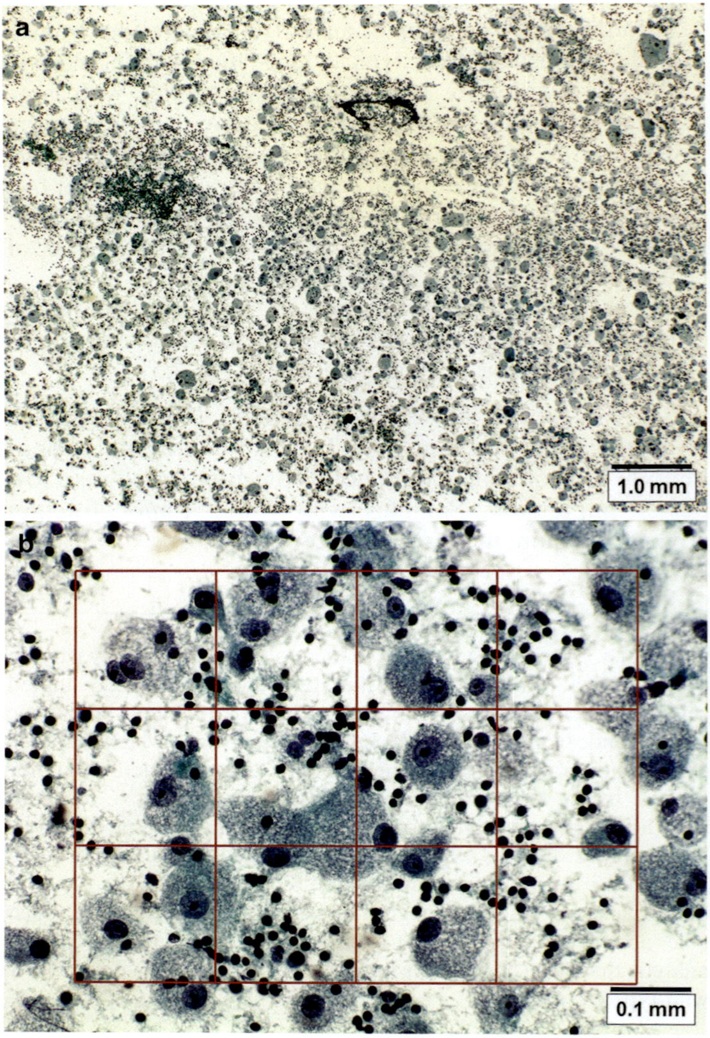

histologic section or cytologic preparation. Both variables must be considered, but tumor fraction is the more important, assuming a wrong answer (false negative) is worse than no answer. Tumor mapping is the process by which areas of relative tumor enrichment are marked for extraction (by macro–/microdissection) and processing. Tumor mapping decreases the amount of DNA tested but increases the tumor fraction of the tested DNA (see Fig. 4.6).

In tumor mapping smears, areas of tumor enrichment are circled and the back of the slide is etched with a diamond-tipped pen. Since the sample is spread out over a very large area, tumor fragments can be more cleanly mapped on smears than cell block sections. Consequently, the use of smears is particularly advantageous in samples with inherently low tumor fractions. Because of parallax, it's best to first circle the back of the slide before etching. (In difficult cases with small circles and high non-tumor content, this requires reviewing and marking the slide with the coverslip side down.) (See Fig. 4.7) Cell blocks can be problematic and require reviewing H&Es of the first and last sections to ensure integrity of the mapped areas. This is also true for core biopsies with low tumor content.

Sometimes when no alternative material is available, a questionably adequate sample has to be submitted for mutational studies. Under these circumstances, it is best to notify the clinical team of the increased risk of false-negative results.

Figure 4.5 Ratio of non-tumor to tumor cells at high power. Melanoma metastatic to lymph node, EBUS-TBNA, Pap-stained smear, at 40× (**a**) and at 400× with simulated graticule (**b**); the NGS requested has a 20% tumor fraction threshold. The low power impression suggests adequacy for mutational analysis, but note the large size disparity between tumor cells and lymphocytes. At high power, one can quickly determine that there are more than four lymphocytes per melanoma cell, and therefore the tumor fraction is less than 20%. The sample is not adequate for the requested NGS testing

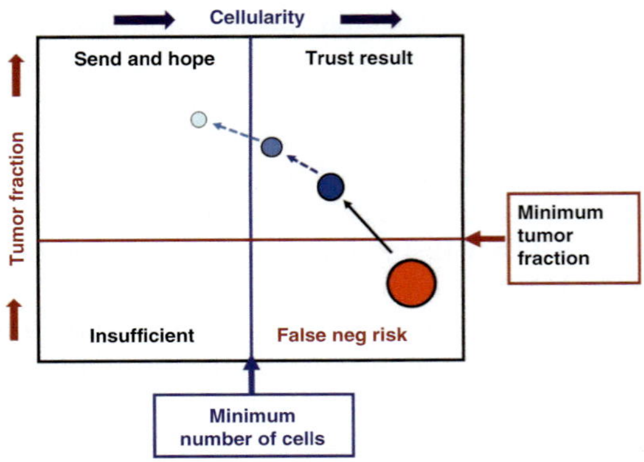

FIGURE 4.6 Tumor mapping schematic. Reliable test results are ensured by enhancing the tumor fraction at the expense of input DNA. Tumor mapping requires a clear understanding of the analytic thresholds of the assay to be used and a facility with evaluating cellularity and tumor fractions

How to Handle Numerous Tests Requested with Limited Material?

Not infrequently, we encounter an order set that includes IHC, FISH, and NGS testing on FNA/CNB limited by low cellular yield or low tumor fraction. These limited samples are adequate for some but not all of the tests. In these circumstances, it is best to discuss the problem with the clinical team, to communicate what is and is not feasible, and to ask the clinician to prioritize tests. Since mutational information can lose its clinical relevance (e.g., primary tumor vs. recurrence post-therapy), testing of alternative archival samples should only be performed after consultation with the clinical team.

Summary

An important adaptation to the molecular world for any cytopathology practice is developing a pre-analytic workflow suitable to the particulars of the practice environment. The competing priorities are efficiency and quality, while also

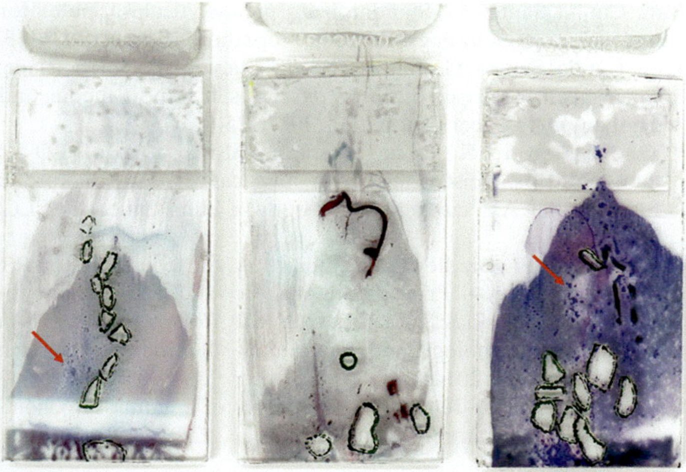

FIGURE 4.7 Example of a difficult tumor mapping. This is an EBUS-TBNA lymph node case of metastatic adenocarcinoma with very high lymphoid content. The cell block tumor fraction was <2%. Areas of tumor enrichment are marked (with green ink here) under the microscope with the coverslip side down. The trail from the diamond-tipped pen can be faintly seen. The slides were returned to cytopathology after macro-dissection. The red arrows point to areas with macroscopically visible specks of tumor, each of which contains at least 1000 tumor cells

minimizing the disruption to routine services. The cytopathologist's pre-analytic evaluation of the sample is essential for reliable test results, particularly for PCR/NGS. Although not technically challenging, this pre-analytic evaluation does require attention to detail, thoroughness, and some self-training. Difficult cases due to sample limitations require judgment and communication with the clinical team.

References

1. Bellevicine C, Malapelle U, Vigliar E, Pisapia P, Vita G, Troncone G. How to prepare cytological samples for molecular testing. J Clin Pathol. 2017;70(10):819–26.

2. da Cunha Santos G. Standardizing preanalytical variables for molecular cytopathology. Cancer Cytopathol. 2013;121(7):341–3.
3. da Cunha Santos G, Saieg MA. Preanalytic specimen triage: smears, cell blocks, cytospin preparations, transport media, and cytobanking. Cancer Cytopathol. 2017;125(S6):455–64.
4. Tsao MS, Kerr K, Dacic S, et al. IASLC atlas of PD-L1 immunohistochemistry testing in lung cancer. 1st ed. Aurora: International Association for the Study of Lung Cancer: IASLC; 2017.
5. Fitzgibbons PL, Bradley LA, Fatheree LA, Alsabeh R, Fulton RS, Goldsmith JD, et al. Principles of analytic validation of immunohistochemical assays: guideline from the College of American Pathologists Pathology and Laboratory Quality Center. Arch Pathol Lab Med. 2014;138(11):1432–43.
6. Maxwell P, Salto-Tellez M. Validation of immunocytochemistry as a morphomolecular technique. Cancer Cytopathol. 2016;124(8):540–5.
7. Sauter JL, Grogg KL, Vrana JA, Law ME, Halvorson JL, Henry MR. Young investigator challenge: validation and optimization of immunohistochemistry protocols for use on cellient cell block specimens. Cancer Cytopathol. 2016;124(2):89–100.
8. Gong Y, Symmans WF, Krishnamurthy S, Patel S, Sneige N. Optimal fixation conditions for immunocytochemical analysis of estrogen receptor in cytologic specimens of breast carcinoma. Cancer. 2004;102(1):34–40.
9. Smith AL, Williams MD, Stewart J, Wang WL, Krishnamurthy S, Cabanillas ME, et al. Utility of the BRAF p.V600E immunoperoxidase stain in FNA direct smears and cell block preparations from patients with thyroid carcinoma. Cancer Cytopathol. 2018;126(6):406–13.
10. Wobker SE, Kim LT, Hackman TG, Dodd LG. Use of BRAF v600e immunocytochemistry on FNA direct smears of papillary thyroid carcinoma. Cancer Cytopathol. 2015;123(9):531–9.
11. Betz BL, Dixon CA, Weigelin HC, Knoepp SM, Roh MH. The use of stained cytologic direct smears for ALK gene rearrangement analysis of lung adenocarcinoma. Cancer Cytopathol. 2013;121(9):489–99.
12. Knoepp SM, Roh MH. Ancillary techniques on direct-smear aspirate slides: a significant evolution for cytopathology techniques. Cancer Cytopathol. 2013;121(3):120–8.

13. Roh MH. The utilization of cytologic fine-needle aspirates of lung cancer for molecular diagnostic testing. J Pathol Translat Med. 2015;49(4):300–9.
14. Minca EC, Lanigan CP, Reynolds JP, Wang Z, Ma PC, Cicenia J, et al. ALK status testing in non-small-cell lung carcinoma by FISH on ThinPrep slides with cytology material. J Thoracic Oncol. 2014;9(4):464–8.
15. Goswami RS, Luthra R, Singh RR, Patel KP, Routbort MJ, Aldape KD, et al. Identification of factors affecting the success of next-generation sequencing testing in solid tumors. Am J Clin Pathol. 2016;145(2):222–37.
16. Ranek L. Cytophotometric studies of the DNA, nucleic acid and protein content of human liver cell nuclei. Acta Cytologica. 1976;20(2):151–7.
17. Chen H, Luthra R, Goswami RS, Singh RR, Roy-Chowdhuri S. Analysis of pre-analytic factors affecting the success of clinical next-generation sequencing of solid organ malignancies. Cancers. 2015;7(3):1699–715.
18. Viray H, Li K, Long TA, Vasalos P, Bridge JA, Jennings LJ, et al. A prospective, multi-institutional diagnostic trial to determine pathologist accuracy in estimation of percentage of malignant cells. Arch Pathol Lab Med. 2013;137(11):1545–9.
19. Smits AJ, Kummer JA, de Bruin PC, Bol M, van den Tweel JG, Seldenrijk KA, et al. The estimation of tumor cell percentage for molecular testing by pathologists is not accurate. Modern Pathol. 2014;27(2):168–74.

Chapter 5
DNA-Based Sequencing Assays

Pasquale Pisapia, Miriam Cieri, Francesco Pepe, Umberto Malapelle, and Giancarlo Troncone

Abbreviations

BRAF	v-raf murine sarcoma viral oncogene homolog B
DNA	Deoxyribonucleic acid
EGFR	Epidermal growth factor receptor
IVD	In vitro diagnostic
KIT	KIT proto-oncogene receptor tyrosine kinase
KRAS	Kirsten rat sarcoma viral oncogene homolog
LDT	Laboratory developed tests
LOD	Limit of detection
NGS	Next-generation sequencing
NRAS	Neuroblastoma RAS viral oncogene
PDGFRA	Platelet-derived growth factor receptor A
PPA	Positive percentage agreement
PPV	Positive predictive value
RT-PCR	Real-time polymerase chain reaction
TAT	Turnaround time

P. Pisapia · M. Cieri · F. Pepe · U. Malapelle · G. Troncone (✉)
Department of Public Health, University of Naples "Federico II", Naples, Italy
e-mail: francesco.pepe4@unina.it; umberto.malapelle@unina.it; giancarlo.troncone@unina.it

S. Roy-Chowdhuri et al. (eds.), *Molecular Diagnostics in Cytopathology*, https://doi.org/10.1007/978-3-319-97397-5_5

Key Terminology

DNA library	Collection of DNA fragments that are captured, barcoded, and clonally amplified, prior to sequencing on NGS platforms.
Gene panel	Representative gene regions covered by a sequencing assay.
Laboratory developed tests	Test designed, developed, and adapted in-house after validation.
Limit of detection	Corresponds to the analytical sensitivity of a given NGS assay, reflecting the lowest amount of analyte which can be reliably detected.
Molecular cytopathology	Discipline of cytopathology based on the integration of morphologic changes with the genomic alterations/molecular features underlying the development, progression, and prognosis of neoplastic diseases.
Next-generation sequencing	High-throughput molecular platform that allows sequencing multiple gene sequences in parallel and interrogating various genetic alterations for multiple patients in a single run.
Personalized medicine	Cancer therapy based on the specific molecular alterations of a patient's tumor.
Pyrosequencing	"sequencing by synthesis"-based technology, in which the sequential incorporation of nucleotides is identified by the

	detection of a released pyrophosphate.
Reads	DNA fragments that are sequenced by a NGS platform during a run.
Real-Time PCR	PCR-based assay that detects and quantifies in "real time" the amplification of a given DNA target using specific fluorescent probes.
Reference range	The interval between the upper and lower concentrations of analyte in the sample for which a suitable level of precision, accuracy, and linearity has been demonstrated
Sanger sequencing	Standard sequencing technology based on the incorporation of chain-terminating dideoxynucleotides (usually fluorochrome labeled) during the process of sequencing by DNA polymerase.
Turnaround time	Time required to analyze a sample and deliver a test result from when the sample is accessioned in the laboratory.
Validation	Procedure that defines the performance parameters of an assay, such as sensitivity, specificity, accuracy, precision, detection limit, range, and limits of quantitation of a novel methodology prior to clinical implementation.

Key Points

- Molecular cytopathology plays a key role in clinical diagnostics, prognostication, and the selection of patients for targeted treatment
- Modern cytopathologists need to be familiar with molecular techniques to appropriately triage specimens for molecular testing
- In comparison to histologic material, cytology specimens often provide better-quality DNA
- Most DNA-based assays including NGS can be successfully applied to cytology specimens
- In order to improve NGS laboratory workflow, it is important to create a gene panel to cover relevant hotspot targets with a defined cost
- In-house validation of each new diagnostic methodology implemented in routine practice is required, even when commercially available and validated for in vitro diagnostic use

In the last 10 years, the landscape of *Personalized Medicine* has included the contribution of *Molecular Cytopathology*, in particular for advanced stage patients with solid tumors. Since these patients are not candidates for surgical resection, a concurrent histology specimen is not always available [1, 2]. Therefore, in order to be a knowledgeable partner in diagnostic and predictive approaches to cancer therapy, the modern cytopathologist needs to be familiar with the basic principles and some of the more advanced molecular techniques used in clinical practice [3, 4].

Cytology samples (Fig. 5.1) provide high-quality DNA, sufficient for a wide array of DNA-based sequencing assays, including next-generation sequencing (NGS) [5]. This novel high-throughput technology represents an evolution of conventional DNA sequencing methodologies, such as Sanger sequencing and pyrosequencing.

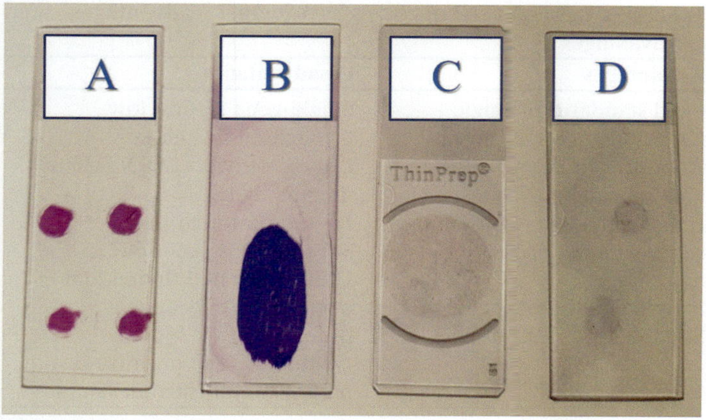

FIGURE 5.1 Examples of different cytologic preparations commonly used for molecular assays: (**A**) cell block; (**B**) direct smear; (**C**) liquid-based cytology; (**D**) cytospin

Sanger sequencing has long been the gold standard for the identification of point mutations, deletions, and small insertions [6, 7]. In this method, a chemically modified nucleotide (dideoxynucleotide) terminates the extension of the DNA strand at the point of incorporation. This results in a mixture of DNA fragments of varying lengths. Each dideoxynucleotide, (A, T, C, or G) is labeled with a different fluorescent dye (dye terminator). The newly synthesized and labeled DNA fragments are sequentially separated by size through capillary gel electrophoresis. The fluorescence is detected by an automated sequence analyzer, and the order of nucleotides (base calling) in the target DNA is visualized as a sequence electropherogram [7, 8]. Although Sanger sequencing was the method first employed in most clinical pathology laboratories, its low sensitivity (around 20% of mutant alleles) limits its application in low tumor content samples, in which the tumor often constitutes a minority of the mixed cell population present. Thus, Sanger sequencing frequently requires tumor enrichment by microdissection prior to analysis to avoid false-negative results [9]. Although low throughput,

TABLE 5.1 Sanger sequencing: principal advantages and disadvantages

Advantages	Disadvantages
Gold standard for single nucleotide polymorphisms	Single-gene testing, low-throughput technique
Robust technology featuring high specificity	Low sensitivity (LOD 5–20% mutant allele)
Enables the detection of both common and uncommon gene mutations	High turnaround time
Simple data interpretation	Several steps post PCR
Suitable on FFPE samples	Unincorporated fluorescent nucleotides may appear very prominent (dye blobs)
	Generates false-negative results on low tumor fraction samples

Sanger sequencing is a robust technology, suitable for analyzing complex genomic regions featuring combined deletion and insertions (Table 5.1).

Pyrosequencing is another method of DNA sequencing by synthesis and is a valid alternative to Sanger sequencing. It relies on the detection of a pyrophosphate released during the DNA polymerase reaction with an enzymatic cascade resulting in the production of visible light [10]. This is converted in analog signal as a peak in a pyrogram. Pyrosequencing provides higher sensitivity (around 5% of mutated allele) than Sanger sequencing, but its error rate (1.07%) is not negligible [11]. When a heterozygous mutation is identified by direct sequencing or by pyrosequencing, both mutant and wild-type alleles are seen on the sequencing electropherograms and on the pyrograms, respectively [10, 11].

With the increase in the number of predictive and prognostic biomarker testing needed for patient management, there is a growing need for high-throughput sequencing technology with the capability of evaluating multiple genes simultaneously. A suitable and flexible multigene testing approach to evaluating known somatic point mutations is by the Sequenom MassARRAY®. This genotyping platform is based on the matrix-assisted laser desorption/ionization time-of-flight (MALDI-TOF) mass spectrometry and can provide customized genotyping assays to analyze allele-specific primer extension products [12]. The basic principle underlying this assay is that mutant and wild-type alleles for a given point mutation produce single-allele base extension reaction products of a mass that is specific to the sequence of the product. Mutation calls are based on the mass differences between the wild-type product and the mutant products as resolved by MALDI-TOF mass spectrometry [12].

Compared to conventional sequencing technologies, next-generation sequencing (NGS) offers high analytic sensitivity together with a high clinical sensitivity. Analytic sensitivity (also known as allelic fraction) is defined as the ability of a mutational assay to identify an alteration in a background of wild-type alleles. Clinical sensitivity covers the spectrum of possible alterations that can be identified by any given assay [13]. NGS exploits a massively parallel sequencing technology, which increases sequencing throughput from hundreds of thousands to millions of sequences (reads) and enables simultaneous analyses of different gene targets for multiple patients in each run [14, 15]. The balance between analytic and clinical sensitivity seen in NGS, together with the minimal amounts of input DNA required, makes this technology ideal for application in cytology samples. The increasing use of NGS in combination with advanced tumor sampling techniques using novel bronchoscopic/endoscopic approaches makes the practice of cytopathology an attractive field in the realm of molecular medicine [16, 17]. A key advantage of NGS over more targeted sequencing technologies is the opportunity to evaluate biomarkers in novel genes of potential clinical interest, in addition to standard of care testing, and thereby facilitate enrollment of patients in clinical trials [18–20].

The principal advantages and limitations of NGS are listed in Table 5.2 [5, 15, 18–24].

A variety of NGS platforms are available for clinical use. Despite the availability of different platforms, the NGS workflow is characterized by four principal steps: (1) DNA library generation, (2) single fragment clonal amplification, (3) massive parallel sequencing, and (4) data analysis [16, 21, 25] (Fig. 5.2).

TABLE 5.2 Next-generation sequencing: principal advantages and disadvantages

Advantages	Disadvantages
Suitable on paucicellular samples	Extensive in-house validation
High throughput	Need of orthogonal techniques to validate the assay and refine borderline results
Open and flexible technology	Challenges in bioinformatics interpretation
Analysis for multiple patients simultaneously in a single run	Validation for different sample preparation
Evaluation of mutational assessment for prediction, prognostic, and clinical trials purposes	Short average read lengths
Wide reference range	Costs and reimbursement
Shorter turnaround time and improved laboratory cost-effectiveness	
Choice of panel	

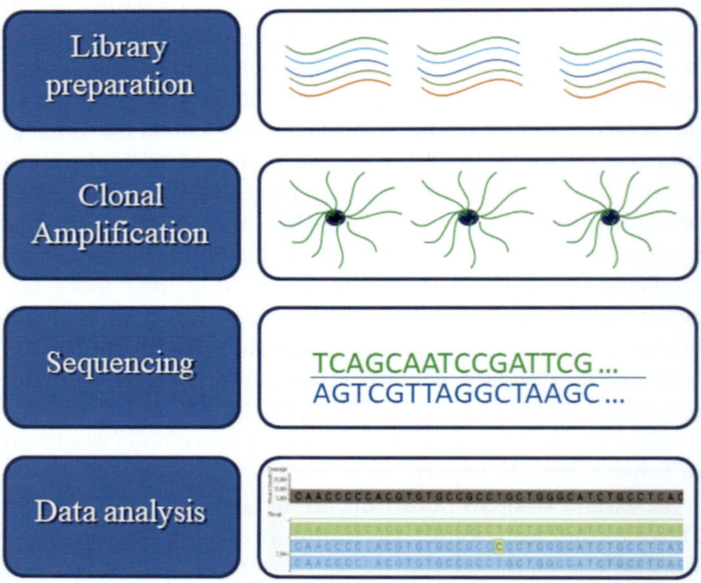

FIGURE 5.2 Schematic representation of the four steps of the NGS workflow, including DNA library preparation, single fragment clonal amplification, massive parallel sequencing, and data analysis

The DNA input required to generate the library is dependent on the target gene selection. The Illumina(TM) platforms (San Diego, CA, USA) utilize a hybridization-based capture system and require a DNA input ranging from 50 to 250 ng and 24–72 h for processing the sequencing data [22]. Recent advances in library preparation have enabled a reduction in the required input DNA, and Illumina validated protocols can be optimized to analyze 10–100 ng of DNA [26]. Alternatively, the IonTorrent platforms(TM) (Life Technologies, Carlsbad, CA, USA) utilize an amplicon-based technology. Multiple primer pairs are employed to select target gene regions by PCR, which requires as little as 10 ng (or even less) DNA input and only 1–3 h to generate the sequence results [23]. Another NGS platform, the GeneReader NGS System(TM) (Qiagen, Hilden, Germany), more recently became available. This platform requires at least 40 ng of DNA, adopts a hybridization-based library preparation methodology, and requires a relatively long analysis time (approximately 30 h) [27].

Clonal amplification is the second step in the NGS workflow. To enhance the chemical signal in the subsequent sequencing reaction, each single fragment of the library needs to be clonally expanded in hundreds of thousands of copies [15]. On the Illumina platform, clonal amplification takes place on a solid support of a flat glass microfluidic channel (flow cell) by the so-called bridge amplification [22], whereas the Ion Torrent and GeneReader platforms carry out clonal amplification by emulsion PCR on beads [5, 21, 27].

The third step in the NGS workflow is the massive parallel sequencing with generation of hundreds of thousands to millions of reads in parallel for each run [14, 27]. The differences among the most commonly adopted platforms are highlighted in Table 5.3. Despite the differences in DNA input requirements, the run times, read lengths, and costs per sample, the two most popular bench-top sequencing platforms (Illumina and Ion Torrent) produce comparable results [16].

Finally, sequencing data are analyzed by using a combination of software pipelines (Fig. 5.3) [27, 28]. This process requires four major steps: base calling, read alignment, variant identification, and variant annotation [29, 30].

TABLE 5.3 Difference between the commonly used NGS platforms in clinical laboratories

	Ion Torrent PGM	Illumina	GeneReader
Input [DNA] ng to generate library	10 or less	10–100	40
DNA library generation	Amplicon-based system	Hybridization-based capture system	Hybridization-based capture system
Clonal amplification	Emulsion PCR	Bridge PCR	Emulsion PCR
Sequencing signal	pH change	Reversible dye terminators	Reversible dye terminators

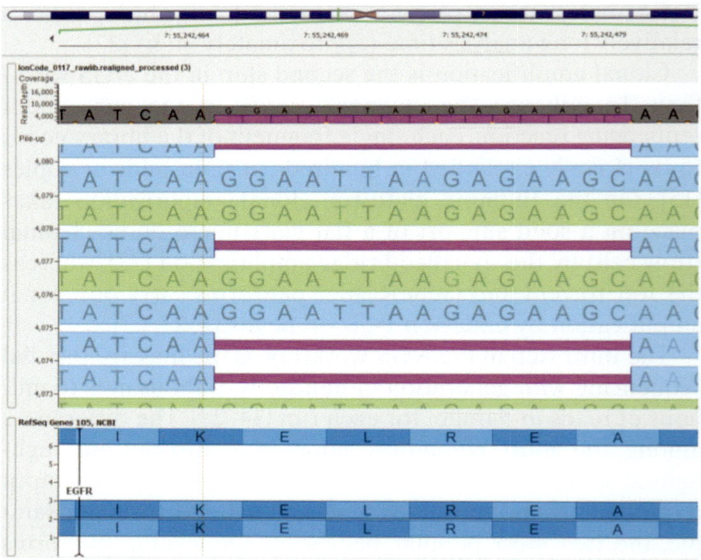

FIGURE 5.3 *EGFR* mutation analysis by NGS. Read alignment visualization of Golden Helix GenomeBrowse v.2.0.7 (Bozeman, MT, USA) software showing an epidermal growth factor receptor (EGFR) exon 19 deletion (p.E746_A750delELREA)

The combination of informatics tools used for processing, aligning, and detecting variants in NGS data is commonly referred to as the bioinformatics pipeline. This process requires careful optimization at the time of validation to ensure that a variant call is effectively present in the sequence as well as continued quality control, as bioinformatics is constantly evolving. The necessity of validation of NGS technologies prior to clinical implementation cannot be overemphasized. Validation includes the identification of positive percentage agreement (PPA) and positive predictive value (PPV), the reproducibility of variant detection, the determination of the reference range, limits of detection (LOD), clinical and analytical sensitivity and specificity, and if appropriate, the validation of bioinformatics pipelines, and other parameters [31].

NGS is a powerful and versatile technique. A variety of gene panels is commercially available and can be classified in four distinct groups, as summarized in Table 5.4 [31, 32].

The versatility of NGS lies in its ability to use custom panels to improve analytical performance and laboratory cost-effectiveness [3, 33]. Although it is widely held that NGS is an expensive technique, our experience with the commercially

TABLE 5.4 Examples of gene panels

Panels covering up to 10–15 actionable genes	Clinically relevant genes (narrow panels), these panels represent a viable alternative to RT-PCR assays
Panels covering up to 50 genes	Target both actionable and potentially clinically relevant genes, the assessment of which may affect eligibility for clinical trials
Panels covering up to 150 genes	Extensively targeting the common and uncommon driver genes of specific cancer type
Panels covering up to 400 genes	Essentially cover most of the known cancer-related genes. Such panels are also used to assess the so-called tumor mutational burden which may affect eligibility for cancer immunotherapy

available AmpliSeq Colon and Lung Cancer Panel, which covers 22 genes involved in colon and lung cancer, showed that the consumable cost is only €196 ($238) per sample [25]. Moreover, the cost per sample could be even reduced to €98 ($119) by the use of a narrow gene panel targeting 568 clinically relevant mutations in 6 genes (*EGFR*, *KRAS*, *NRAS*, *BRAF*, *KIT*, and *PDGFRA*) [33].

In summary, NGS-based assays on routine cytology samples have the potential to improve patient care through diagnostic, prognostic, and predictive biomarker assessment. The basic principles of NGS described in this chapter underscore the need of a new generation of molecular cytopathologists [34–36].

References

1. Clark DP. Seize the opportunity: underutilization of fine-needle aspiration biopsy to inform targeted cancer therapy decisions. Cancer. 2009;117:289–97.
2. Bellevicine C, Malapelle U, Vigliar E, et al. How to prepare cytological samples for molecular testing. J Clin Pathol. 2017;70:819–26.
3. Schmitt FC, Longatto-Filho A, Valent A, et al. Molecular techniques in cytopathology practice. J Clin Pathol. 2008;61:258–67.
4. Bellevicine C, Vita GD, Malapelle U, et al. Applications and limitations of oncogene mutation testing in clinical cytopathology. Semin Diagn Pathol. 2013;30:284–97.
5. Malapelle U, Mayo-de-Las-Casas C, Molina-Vila MA, et al. Consistency and reproducibility of next-generation sequencing and other multigene mutational assays: a worldwide ring trial study on quantitative cytological molecular reference specimens. Cancer. 2017;125:615–26.
6. McCourt CM, McArt DG, Mills K, et al. Validation of next generation sequencing technologies in comparison to current diagnostic gold standards for BRAF, EGFR and KRAS mutational analysis. PLoS One. 2013;8:e69604.
7. Sanger F, Nicklen S, Coulson AR. DNA sequencing with chain-terminating inhibitors. Proc Natl Acad Sci USA. 1977;74:5463–7.

8. Smith LM, Sanders JZ, Kaiser RJ, et al. Fluorescence detection in automated DNA sequence analysis. Nature. 1986;321:674–9.
9. Aisner DL, Rumery MD, Merrick DT, et al. Do more with less: tips and techniques for maximizing small biopsy and cytology specimens for molecular and ancillary testing: the University of Colorado experience. Arch Pathol Lab Med. 2016;140:1206–20.
10. Ronaghi M, Uhlén M, Nyrén P. A sequencing method based on real-time pyrophosphate. Science. 1998;363:281, 365.
11. Gilles A, Meglécz E, Pech N, et al. Accuracy and quality assessment of 454 GS-FLX Titanium pyrosequencing. BMC Genomics. 2011;12:245.
12. Alì G, Proietti A, Pelliccioni S, et al. ALK rearrangement in a large series of consecutive non-small cell lung cancers: comparison between a new immunohistochemical approach and fluorescence in situ hybridization for the screening of patients eligible for crizotinib treatment. Arch Pathol Lab Med. 2014;138:1449–58.
13. Aisner DL, Sams SB. The role of cytology specimens in molecular testing of solid tumors: techniques, limitations, and opportunities. Diagn Cytopathol. 2012;40:511–24.
14. Bentley DR, Balasubramanian S, Swerdlow HP, et al. Accurate whole human genome sequencing using reversible terminator chemistry. Nature. 2008;456:53–9.
15. Rothberg JM, Hinz W, Rearick TM, et al. An integrated semiconductor device enabling non-optical genome sequencing. Nature. 2011;475:348–52.
16. Vigliar E, Malapelle U, de Luca C, et al. Challenges and opportunities of next-generation sequencing: a cytopathologist's perspective. Cytopathology. 2015;26:271–83.
17. Roy-Chowdhuri S, Stewart J. Preanalytic variables in cytology: lessons learned from next-generation sequencing-the MD Anderson experience. Arch Pathol Lab Med. 2016;140:1191–9. [Epub ahead of print].
18. Rizzo JM, Buck MJ. Key principles and clinical applications of "next-generation" DNA sequencing. Cancer Prev Res (Phila). 2012;5:887–900.
19. Malapelle U, Vigliar E, Sgariglia R, et al. Ion Torrent next-generation sequencing for routine identification of clinically relevant mutations in colorectal cancer patients. J Clin Pathol. 2015;68:64–8.

20. Malapelle U, Pisapia P, Sgariglia R, et al. Less frequently mutated genes in colorectal cancer: evidences from next-generation sequencing of 653 routine cases. J Clin Pathol. 2016;69:767–71.
21. Li J, Batcha AM, Grüning B, et al. An NGS workflow blueprint for DNA sequencing data and its application in individualized molecular oncology. Cancer Inform. 2016;14:87–107.
22. Mardis ER. Next-generation sequencing platforms. Ann Rev Anal Chem (Palo Alto Calif). 2013;6:287–303.
23. Beadling C, Neff TL, Heinrich MC, et al. Combining highly multiplexed PCR with semiconductor-based sequencing for rapid cancer genotyping. J Mol Diagn. 2013;15:171–6.
24. Rothberg JM, Leamon JH. The development and impact of 454 sequencing. Nat Biotechnol. 2008;26:1117–24.
25. Clinical and Laboratory Standards Institute. Nucleic acid sequencing methods in diagnostic laboratory medicine; approved guideline, CLSI document MM09-A2. 2nd ed. Wayne: Clinical and Laboratory Standards Institute; 2014.
26. Middleton G, Crack LR, Popat S, et al. The National Lung Matrix Trial: translating the biology of stratification in advanced non-small-cell lung cancer. Ann Oncol. 2015;26:2464–9.
27. Koitzsch U, Heydt C, Attig H, et al. Use of the GeneReader NGS System in a clinical pathology laboratory: a comparative study. J Clin Pathol. 2017;70:725–8.
28. Scarpa A, Sikora K, Fassan M, et al. Molecular typing of lung adenocarcinoma on cytological samples using a multigene next generation sequencing panel. PLoS One. 2013;8:e80478.
29. Gargis AS, Kalman L, Bick DP, et al. Good laboratory practice for clinical next-generation sequencing informatics pipelines. Nat Biotechnol. 2015;33:689–93.
30. Roy-Chowdhuri S, Roy S, Monaco SE, et al. Big data from small samples: informatics of next-generation sequencing in cytopathology. Cancer Cytopathol. 2017;125:236–44.
31. Jennings LJ, Arcila ME, Corless C, et al. Guidelines for validation of next-generation sequencing-based oncology panels: a joint consensus recommendation of the Association for Molecular Pathology and College of American Pathologists. J Mol Diagn. 2017;19:341–65.
32. Hynes SO, Pang B, James JA, et al. Tissue-based next generation sequencing: application in a universal healthcare system. Br J Cancer. 2017;116:553–60.
33. Malapelle U, Mayo de-Las-Casas C, Rocco D, et al. Development of a gene panel for next-generation sequencing of clinically rel-

evant mutations in cell-free DNA from cancer patients. Br J Cancer. 2017;116:802–10.
34. Fassan M. Molecular diagnostics in pathology: time for a next-generation pathologist? Arch Pathol Lab Med. 2018;142:313–20.
35. Salto-Tellez M. More than a decade of molecular diagnostic cytopathology leading diagnostic and therapeutic decision-making. Arch Pathol Lab Med. 2018;142:443–45.
36. Moore DA, Young CA, Morris HT, et al. Time for change: a new training programme for morpho-molecular pathologists? J Clin Pathol. 2018;71:285–90.

Chapter 6
RNA-Based Assays

Umberto Malapelle, Pasquale Pisapia, Miriam Cieri, Francesco Pepe, and Giancarlo Troncone

Abbreviations

ALK	Anaplastic lymphoma kinase or ALK receptor tyrosine kinase
BRAF	v-Raf murine sarcoma oncogene homolog B
DNA	Deoxyribonucleic acid
EGFR	Epidermal growth factor receptor
IVD	In vitro diagnostic
LOD	Limit of detection
MET	MET proto-oncogene, receptor tyrosine kinase
NGS	Next-generation sequencing
NRG1	Neuregulin 1
NTRK	Neurotrophic tyrosine kinase, receptor
RET	Proto-oncogene tyrosine-protein kinase receptor ret
ROS1	ROS proto-oncogene 1, receptor tyrosine kinase
RNA	Ribonucleic acid
RT-PCR	Reverse transcription-polymerase chain reaction
TAT	Turnaround time

U. Malapelle · P. Pisapia · M. Cieri · F. Pepe · G. Troncone (✉)
Department of Public Health, University of Naples "Federico II", Naples, Italy
e-mail: umberto.malapelle@unina.it; francesco.pepe4@unina.it; giancarlo.troncone@unina.it

S. Roy-Chowdhuri et al. (eds.), *Molecular Diagnostics in Cytopathology*, https://doi.org/10.1007/978-3-319-97397-5_6

Key Terminology

Exome	The entire set of exons within a genome
Gene expression	Evaluation of a specific or a group of mRNA levels
Gene panel	Representative gene regions covered by a sequencing assay
Limit of detection	Corresponds to the analytical sensitivity of a given NGS assay, reflecting the lowest amount of analyte which can be reliably detected.
Molecular cytopathology	Discipline of cytopathology based on the integration of morphologic changes with the genomic alterations/molecular features underlying the development, progression, and prognosis of neoplastic diseases
Next-generation sequencing	High-throughput molecular platform that allows sequencing multiple gene sequences in parallel and interrogating various genetic alterations for multiple patients in a single run
Personalized medicine	Cancer therapy based on the specific molecular alterations of a patient's tumor
Reads	cDNA fragments that are sequenced by a NGS platform during a run
Real-time PCR	PCR-based assay that detects and quantifies in "real time" the amplification of a given target using specific fluorescent probes

Reference range	The interval between the upper and lower concentrations of analyte in the sample for which a suitable level of precision, accuracy, and linearity has been demonstrated
RNA library	Collection of cDNA fragments that are captured, barcoded, and clonally amplified, prior to sequencing on NGS platforms
Transcriptome	Set of all RNA molecules in one cell or in a cell population
Turnaround time	Time required to analyze a sample and deliver a test result from when the sample is accessioned in the laboratory

Key Points

- Cytology specimens can be used for RNA-based molecular testing
- Non-formalin-fixed cytology specimens may yield better-quality albeit lower-quantity RNA, in comparison to formalin-fixed paraffin-embedded histological material
- High-throughput technologies, such as next-generation sequencing (NGS) and multiplex digital color-coded barcode technology, have improved the scope of RNA-based assays and can be successfully applied to cytology specimens

Cytology has an expanded role in patient care through the application of molecular diagnostics and guiding targeted therapy for management of patients [1–6]. One such example is the diagnosis of non-small cell lung cancer (NCSLC) and the pivotal role played by cytology in guiding targeted treatment [7]. In NSCLC, predictive biomarker testing is primarily DNA-based molecular testing from neoplastic cells; however, frequently cytology samples are also used for RNA-based detection of actionable gene fusions [8, 9]. These are chimeric genes resulting from fusion of two previously independent genes, occurring within the same chromosome or between different chromosomes [4, 6, 8, 10]. In NSCLC, several gene fusions (e.g., *ALK*, *ROS1*, *RET*, and *NTRK*) are evaluated to select patients for approved treatments or for enrollment into preclinical and clinical trials [8]. Detection of gene fusions is also utilized to refine the cytologic diagnosis of indeterminate thyroid nodules. In particular, the detection of *PAX8/PPARG* and *RET/PTC* gene fusions, associated with follicular thyroid carcinomas (FTCs) and papillary thyroid carcinomas (PTCs), respectively, can improve the cytologic diagnosis of these entities [4]. Another important application of RNA-based assays is the detection of splice variants, arising out of an alternative splicing point that can lead to different biological properties [11]. Some splice variants, such as *MET* splicing variants leading to exon 14 skipping, represent a potential target for cancer therapy in NSCLC patients [12].

Both gene fusions and splice variants can be detected, using RNA extracted from cytology samples, by a wide range of RNA-based molecular techniques, including reverse transcription-polymerase chain reaction (RT-PCR), real-time RT-PCR (quantitative reverse transcription-polymerase chain reaction [qRT-PCR]) assays, and microarrays [13]. More recently, high-throughput technologies such as next-generation sequencing (NGS) and multiplex digital color-coded barcode technology have improved the scope of RNA-based assays [14, 15]. In this chapter, we discuss the pros and cons of both conventional techniques and novel approaches of RNA-based molecular assays, with a focus on their application in cytology samples.

RNA Quality and Quantity: Pre-analytic Specimen Requirements

The RNA quality and quantity is strongly impacted by a number of pre-analytic variables, including the cytology specimen preparation type, the volume of tissue available, the specimen processing (e.g., fixation), and storage conditions [8, 9, 16]. For instance, non-cross-linking alcoholic reagents used as a fixative often yield superior results because they cause minimal chemical change and usually provide higher-quality nucleic acids for molecular testing than formalin-fixed paraffin-embedded (FFPE) sections [17]. Further, liquid-based cytology (LBC), such as PreservCyt and CytoLyt (Hologic Inc., Marlborough, Massachusetts, USA) which are methanol-based, has been shown to have optimal RNA integrity, suitable for nucleic acid isolation and subsequent analysis by RT-PCR, whereas CytoRich Red (Thermo Fisher Scientific, Waltham, Massachusetts, USA) containing formaldehyde can cause RNA degradation and modification by cross-linking of cytosine residues [16, 18]. Cryopreservation of cells in vials containing RNAlater (Applied Biosystems/Ambion, Dallas, TX) is considered the optimal storage method for maximizing RNA integrity (high-quality RNA) [16]. A detailed study evaluating the effect of ischemic time, by assessing the RNA preservation of FNA specimens obtained from fresh tumor resections, showed that the time interval from surgical resection to FNA collection should be kept under 6 h, while the time interval from FNA collection to freezing should not exceed an hour. However, the amount of time each sample remained frozen in liquid nitrogen did not impact RNA quality [19].

The initial evaluation of RNA quality and quantity is crucial prior to its application in any RNA-based assay [15, 16]. Earlier protocols have utilized denaturing agarose gel stained with ethidium bromide to qualify the extracted RNA; this procedure allows the visualization of two bands containing the ribosomal RNA (rRNA), 28S and 18S [17, 20]. The extracted RNA quality is considered good when the 28S rRNA band has an intensity that is twice that of the 18S rRNA band [21]. More recent procedures rely on spectrophotometer assays; these are based on UV-light absorption of diluted nucleic acid samples read at 260 and 280 nm [16]. A linear correlation between the nucleic acid concentration and absorbance (A) can predict the DNA or RNA quantity in the solution. Pure RNA has an A260/A280 ratio of 2.1 [16]. Currently, fluorimetric assays that utilize the binding of fluorescent dyes to nucleic acids to measure changes in fluorescence levels represent an alternative to spectrophotometric methods [16]. Fluorescence-based quantification is more sensitive and accurate than spectrophotometric methods [16]. A recently developed approach is based on the use of microfluidic chambers, combining capillary electrophoresis with fluorescence [22]. This technology yields both quantitative (concentration in ng/μl) and qualitative data (RNA integrity number, RIN). The RNA quality is estimated in a range of 1–10, with 10 being the highest quality with the least amount of degradation [22] (Fig. 6.1). The RIN evaluation strongly impacts the downstream molecular application. As shown in a study by Ladd et al., cytology samples scoring a RIN < 5 can be used in RNA-based assays requiring <250 bp amplicons, whereas RIN of 5–8 can allow the sample to be used in assays requiring up to 400 bp amplicons. Samples with RIN > 8, demonstrating well-preserved higher-molecular weight RNA, can be exploited for microarray gene expression analysis [19].

RNA extraction is typically performed using commercially available kits, capable of separating RNA (total or specific form) from DNA and protein, for an efficient reverse transcription [13, 23–25]. Since cytology samples are often limited in cellularity, it is critical to expedite RNA extraction after specimen collection to minimize the ischemic time and RNA degradation and better preserve RNA quality by collecting the cytology sample in a dedicated buffer [13, 16, 23–25]. Genomic DNA (gDNA) elimination by an efficient deoxyribonuclease step is also critical.

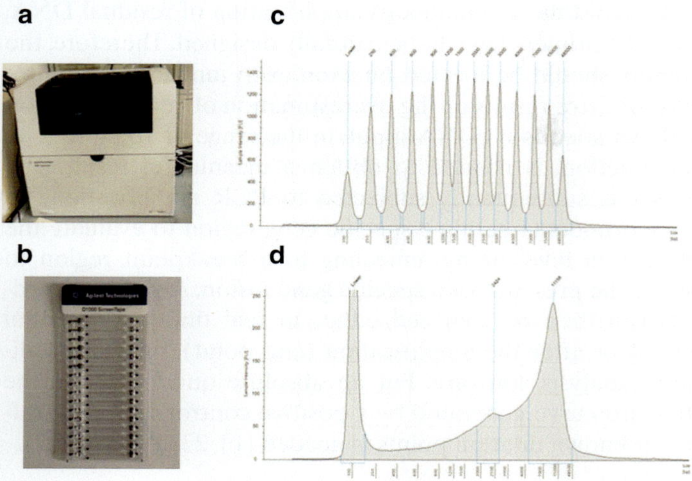

Figure 6.1 (**a**) RNA quantity and quality evaluation of a routine cytology sample using TapeStation 4200 microfluidic platform; (**b**) example of an RNA high-sensitivity cartridge; (**c**) a pool of artificial fragmented cDNA was used as a size and concentration ladder; (**d**) example of a pherogram showing a peak of RNA extracted from cytology sample

RT-PCR and qRT-PCR

Reverse transcription-polymerase chain reaction (RT-PCR) represents a versatile molecular technique that can be applied to improve the sensitivity and accuracy of cytologic diagnosis, as well as to predict responses to molecularly targeted drugs [17]. Moreover, quantitative RT-PCR (qRT-PCR) allows real-time evaluation of gene expression in a quantitative manner (relative or absolute) [13, 23–25]. The qRT-PCR workflow analysis is characterized by three main steps:

- Reverse transcription of RNA to complementary DNA (cDNA)
- cDNA PCR amplification
- Data analysis

To avoid the simultaneous amplification of residual DNA, RT-PCR primers have to be carefully designed. Therefore, the primers should be located on exon/exon junctions to reduce false-positive results or the overestimation of gene expression [26]. An adequate cDNA input, in the range of 10 pg to 1 µg per reaction, is needed to obtain a meaningful result. The cDNA is subsequently subjected to PCR amplification, by using primers targeting a specific gene region to evaluate the expression level or by annealing to a breakpoint region to define the presence of a specific gene fusion. Amplified products can then be analyzed either in real time (exponential phase) or after the amplification (end point), by using dedicated analysis software. For an absolute quantification, the standard curve generated by a positive control sample at different known dilution points is needed [13, 23–25] (Fig. 6.2).

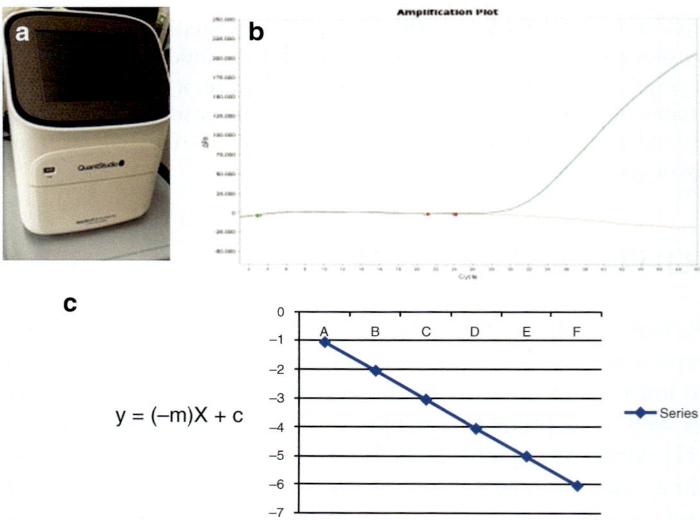

FIGURE 6.2 (**a**) Example of a QuantStudio 5 instrument used for RT-PCR; (**b**) RT-PCR amplification plot from a TaqMan probe-based assay; (**c**) a standard curve generated from a positive control sample at different dilution points is used to obtain absolute quantitative information

In routine practice, qRT-PCR offers an alternative approach to detecting gene fusions in cytology specimens using an integrated approach, which includes immunocytochemistry (ICC) and fluorescence *in situ* hybridization (FISH) [13, 23–25, 27]. For instance, RT-PCR with specific fusion primers for *ALK* rearrangements can be reliably carried out using the RNA extracted from fresh pleural fluid samples. In fact, fresh, unfixed cells may be readily processed for immediate nucleic acid extraction to obtain high-integrity RNA and minimize RNA degradation [8]. *ALK* RT-PCR can also be applied on RNA directly extracted from archival cytology slides [8]. Mitiushkina et al. and more recently Oktay and colleagues obtained a 100% success rate for assessment of *ALK* translocations using archival cytologic slides [28, 29]. In their study, Oktay et al. report a successful result even when the microdissection was limited to as few as 50 cells obtained from a cancer cell-rich microscopic field, thereby leaving sufficient diagnostic material for the archival slide [28]. RT-PCR has also been successfully implemented in thyroid cytologic smears. Ferraz et al. demonstrated the feasibility of detecting *PAX8/PPARG* and *RET/PTC* rearrangements using qRT-PCR using RNA extracted from air-dried FNA smears [30].

While qRT-PCR enables the precise identification of the rearrangement variants in the samples, it can analyze only known variants; next-generation technologies overcome this limitation, allowing the identification of even novel variants.

Next-Generation RNA Sequencing

In addition to evaluation of DNA alterations (e.g., point mutations, insertion/deletion), the comprehensive molecular assessment of cancer biomarkers also requires extended molecular testing for gene fusions and rearrangements [31–33]. NGS is a modern testing approach to detecting transcriptome alterations, with a broad reference range and high throughput that can be easily applied to the RNA extracted from routine cytology samples [8, 16]. In contrast to RT-PCR, NGS offers an extensive cDNA analysis including evaluation start sites of genes, 5′ and 3′ ends, splicing patterns, and other post-transcriptional modifications [34].

Different NGS platforms (e.g., Illumina or Thermo Fisher) can be used for RNA sequencing (Table 6.1). In general NGS using an Ion Torrent sequencer (Thermo Fisher Scientific, Waltham, MA) requires less RNA input than Illumina (Illumina, San Diego, CA) RNA-based sequencing. cDNA sequencing is analyzed by comparing "reads" sequence with a reference genome or a reference transcript [34].

The advantages and disadvantages of next-generation RNA sequencing are illustrated in Table 6.1.

The main steps of next-generation RNA sequencing are cDNA library preparation, template preparation, sequencing, and data analysis [31, 32]. Briefly, the cDNA fragments library is generated after the reverse transcription step; patient barcodes and platform adapters are attached to cDNA fragments ends [33–35]; each molecule is sequenced in

Table 6.1 Next-generation RNA sequencing advantages and disadvantages

Advantages
High resolution (single base)
Analysis of complex transcriptome
Detection of alterations in transcript regions
Low background noise
Large dynamic range of expression levels (ability to distinguish allelic expression and different isoforms)
Low amount of RNA required
Disadvantages
High costs
High bioinformatics requirements for data analysis and interpretation

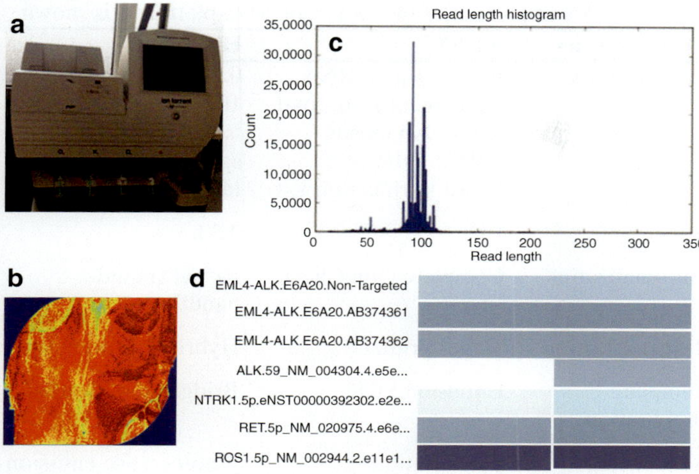

FIGURE 6.3 (**a**) Ion Torrent Personal Genome Machine (Thermo Fisher) used for next-generation RNA sequencing; (**b**) example of an Ion Torrent 316 loaded chip; (**c**) a read length histogram generated by an NGS fusion panel assay used to detect gene fusions in *ALK*, *ROS1*, *RET*, and *NTRK* genes was reported; (**d**) an example of *ALK* fusion, analyzed by using Ion Reporter Software

a high-throughput manner to obtain short sequences from one end (single-end sequencing) or both ends (pair-end sequencing) depending on the NGS technology (Fig. 6.3).

During the library preparation, when the starting material is represented by short RNA molecules such as microRNAs (miRNAs), it can be directly fractioned in small fragments and sequenced after the barcode ligation [36, 37]. Template preparation and sequencing steps are subject to the same variables that affect DNA sequencing and are related to the specific NGS platform used [6, 33–35] (Table 6.2). Sequencing data interpretation is often challenging, especially in context of small RNA molecules analysis. In fact, short high-quality reads may be difficult to map on standard reference sequence unless using specific bioinformatics tools. Exon site splicing may be identified by the presence of GT-AG dinucleotides while poly(A) tails may identify the 3′ end of a sequence [31, 32].

TABLE 6.2 A comparison of two different NGS platforms is shown

Characteristics	Ion S5	HiSeq
Input mRNA	100 ng–1 μg mRNA enrichment from total RNA Dynabeads mRNA DIRECT Micro Purification Kit	0.1–1 ug total RNA or 10–100 ng previously isolated mRNA (from species with poly(A) tails)
Bench time	1 h	4.5 h
Automatization	Complete (Ion Chef)	Partial (liquid-handling robots)
Target selection	Target primer	Hybrid capture
Template preparation	Emulsion PCR	Bridge amplification
Sequencing	pH variation	Fluorescence emission
TAT	2 days	4 days

Abbreviations: *TAT* turnaround time

However, in general for most cases, the vendor-supplied bioinformatics pipeline is adequately robust and sensitive for routine clinical use, without the need for a stand-alone dedicated bioinformatics infrastructure.

Next-generation RNA sequencing has immense potential in terms of sensitivity and throughput. NGS assays, based on small gene panels, may be designed to detect gene fusions with high sensitivity from scant cytology samples featuring a limited population of neoplastic cells. In setting of a lung carcinoma FNA, a sensitive NGS assay can represent a single assay alternative to RT-PCR or FISH assays for detection of *ALK*, *RET*, and *ROS-1* gene fusions [6, 33–35].

Different approaches can be adopted to generate sequencing library from cytology samples. While Velizheva et al. prepared distinct DNA and RNA libraries for separate downstream sequencing [38], Guseva et al. applied an alternative total nucleic acid extraction approach for both DNA-based and RNA-based applications based on a single smear [39]. Total nucleic acid, representing a pool of mixed

DNA and RNA, was extracted from smears with a minimal tumor content of 20%. The DNA-based application offers simultaneous detection of hotspot mutations in a large number of actionable or clinically relevant genes such as *EGFR*, *BRAF*, *KRAS*, *NRAS*, *HRAS*, and *PIK3CA*, while the RNA-based applications allow the detection and identification of *ALK*, *ROS1*, and *RET* fusions. This combined DNA- and RNA-based NGS analysis is based on the innovative anchored multiplex PCR (AMP) library preparation that can be successfully combined with Illumina and Ion Torrent. A minimum of 5 reads with ≥3 unique sequencing start sites that cross the breakpoints was used as the cutoff value for strong evidence of fusions by Guseva et al. [39, 40].

More recently, Etheridge et al. described a modified protocol for preparation of small RNA libraries for NGS analysis, optimized for use with low-input RNA, making the RNA-based test ideal for scant cellularity samples [37].

Multiplex Digital Color-Coded Barcode Technology

It is widely held that the gold standard technique to comprehensively evaluate simultaneous gene expression is still represented by microarray techniques, an approach based on fluorescent probes attached to solid surfaces such as glass or chip forming a matrix [41]. However, this technology is most commonly used in a research setting, while applications in clinical diagnostics are limited due to multiple issues related to spot identification, signal normalization, background signal, and the need for high-quality/high-quantity RNA. In reality, RNA recovered from routine cytology and small biopsies samples is often unsuitable for RNA-based gene array methodology [16]. To overcome these limitations and to encourage the implementation of gene expression analysis assays in clinical practice, new platforms based on innovative technologies are emerging. In particular, the nCounter platform (NanoString, Seattle, WA) based on multiplex digital color-coded barcode technology represents a fascinating option to evaluate both gene expression and fusion/translocation detection. Moreover, the nCounter platform can yield quantitative information because of the direct visualization and digital count of nucleic acids labeled by color barcodes [10, 15, 27, 42].

The nCounter system is able to detect gene fusions from low amounts of RNA. Each target of interest is detected by a unique pair of capture and reporter probes, the sequences of which are adjacent and complementary to a particular messenger RNA. The capture probe is biotinylated, whereas the reporter probe is linked to a digital color barcode. After this step, each pair of probes is hybridized in a multiplex reaction with the targeted messenger RNA; these complexes are then immobilized and elongated to allow the detection and counting of specific fluorescence barcodes. This methodology enables the simultaneous detection of *ALK*, *ROS1*, and other NSCLC fusion genes (*RET*, *NRG1*, and *BRAF*) and *MET*-skipping transcript and can be accomplished in a relatively short turnaround time (3 working days) (Fig. 6.4).

The main steps of nCounter workflow are:

- The RNA hybridization with probe pairs (reporter probe and capture probe), which are designed to be adjacent to one another along the target sequence of a transcript.
- Following hybridization of capture and reporter probes with mRNA molecules in a 1:1 ratio, a stable tripartite structure is formed and the excess probes are washed away.
- The tripartite structure is bound to the surface of the sample cartridge that is coated with streptavidin, and reporters are aligned by an electric current and immobilized for data collection.
- The sample cartridge is scanned by the digital analyzer, and each fluorescent barcode is counted and tabulated according to the gene identity.

One of the advantages of applying nCounter to a routine clinical setting is the relative low amount of input RNA

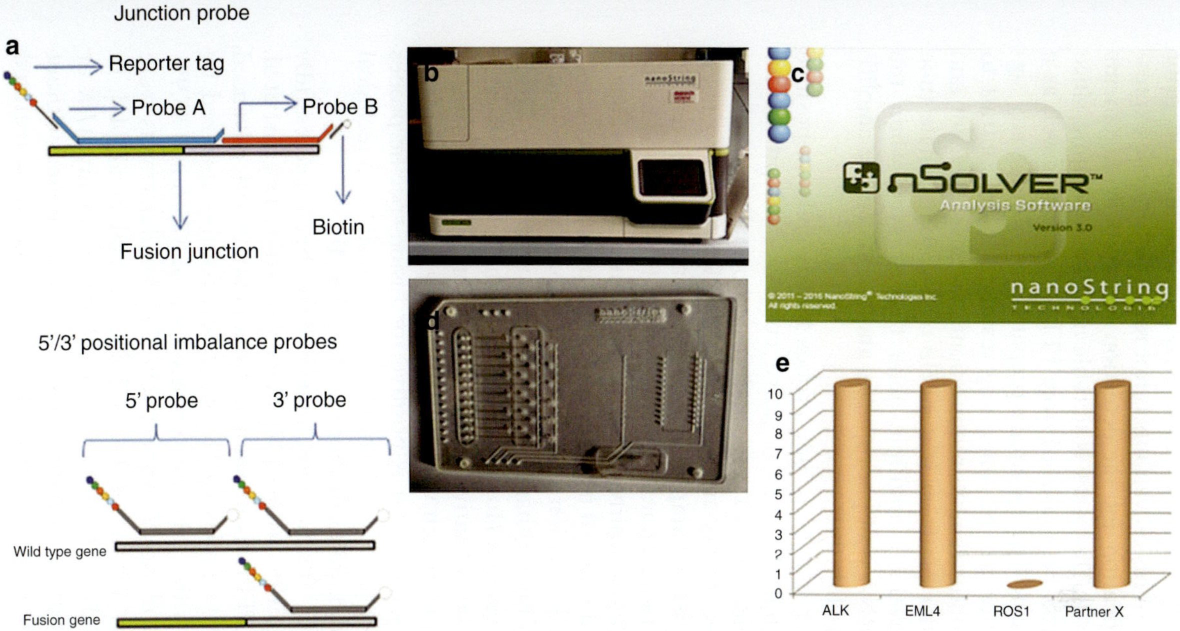

Figure 6.4 (**a**) The digital color-coded barcode technology detects gene fusion transcripts either by specific capture and reporter probes or by quantification of *ALK* 5′ and 3′ expression levels; (**b**) nCounter Sprint (NanoString) platform used to detect gene expression and fusion/translocation detection; (**c**) data analysis for nCounter is performed using the nSolver software; (**d**) example of a cartridge used to load hybridize RNA; (**e**) graphical representation of results: a histogram is produced if a gene fusion is detected

required (25–250 ng of total RNA). In addition, a prior knowledge of fusion variants is not required for gene expression identification and the detection of gene rearrangements [10, 15, 27, 42]. This assay is suitable in a clinical setting, since the RNA can be extracted from FFPE samples as well as a variety of cytology specimen preparations without any significant difference in generating results [16]. In contrast to NGS, nCounter sample requirements are less stringent and the nCounter platform is a viable option for a single tube assay to evaluate multiple gene fusions even when the extracted RNA is of poor quality and target capture amplification fails [40].

nCounter panels include probes for six spike-in positive controls, eight spike-in negative controls, and probes for housekeeping genes. These are done to normalize samples, to evaluate the quality and quantity of the RNA, and to assess the feasibility of sample analysis [10]. Data analysis usually includes a two-step normalization procedure, which is based on the spike-in positive controls and housekeeping genes, a background removal based on the spike-in negative controls, and fusion prediction that is based on both the 30:50 ratio (positive, if higher than a pre-specified threshold) and fusion probe expressions. However, if only a high 30:50 ratio is present, it may be indicative of a fusion transcript from a novel or a rare variant, which would be missed by the specific fusion probes. A sample that is positive for fusion-specific probes but negative for the 30:50 ratio may be a result of a technical artifact and requires further investigation [10].

nCounter fusion gene assays have been successfully applied on FFPE tissues [27]. In a recent study, Reguart et al. tested 108 FFPE tissue samples from patients with advanced NSCLC; 98 samples (91%) were successfully analyzed by nCounter, with FISH concordance rates of 87.5% and 85.9% for *ALK* and *ROS1*, respectively [27]. Similar results were reported by Lira et al. [42, 43] and Sunami et al. [44]. In another study, nCounter analysis did not reveal any *ALK* or *ROS1* alterations in pure squamous cell carcinoma without an adenocarcinoma component [45]. Fang et al. demonstrated that patient-derived xenografts can also be used to detect *ALK* rearrangements and to assess crizotinib response using nCounter technology [46].

Although the literature investigating the feasibility of NanoString system to analyze RNA from lung cytologic smears is very limited, the application of NanoString assays is feasible in lung cytology. In a methodological proof-of-concept study on RNA extracted from 12 archival routine stained cytologic smears of NSCLC processed using the nCounter 48 gene panel, most samples (92%) were successfully analyzed [15]. The sample requirements were >30% neoplastic cells and at least 100 or more preserved cells, and the RNA input in these specimens ranged from 3.24 to 12.96 ng/μl [15]. These results are in concordance with data from a recent study by Ali et al. using a novel assay, the RealQuant lung fusion genes kit in lung cytology samples, that demonstrated concordance with FISH of 97.7%, 100%, and 100%, for *ALK*, *ROS1,* and *RET*, respectively [10].

Final Consideration

The implementation of new-generation technologies, such as NGS and multiplex digital color-coded barcode technology, allows maximizing the yield of molecular tests on small routine cytology samples, through integrated analysis of DNA and RNA for better diagnostic and therapeutic strategies.

References

1. Malapelle U, Mayo-de-Las-Casas C, Molina-Vila MA, Rosell R, Savic S, Bihl M, et al., Molecular Cytopathology Meeting Group. Consistency and reproducibility of next-generation sequencing and other multigene mutational assays: a worldwide ring trial study on quantitative cytological molecular reference specimens. Cancer Cytopathol. 2017;125:615–26.

2. Clark DP. Seize the opportunity: underutilization of fine-needle aspiration biopsy to inform targeted cancer therapy decisions. Cancer. 2009;117:289–97.
3. Schmitt FC, Longatto-Filho A, Valent A, et al. Molecular techniques in cytopathology practice. J Clin Pathol. 2008;61:258–67.
4. Bellevicine C, Sgariglia R, Malapelle U, Vigliar E, Nacchio M, Ciancia G, et al. Young investigator challenge: can the ion AmpliSeq Cancer Hotspot Panel v2 be used for next-generation sequencing of thyroid FNA samples? Cancer Cytopathol. 2016;124:776–84.
5. Aisner DL, Sams SB. The role of cytology specimens in molecular testing of solid tumors: techniques, limitations, and opportunities. Diagn Cytopathol. 2012;40:511–24.
6. Weinreb I, Bishop JA, Chiosea SI, Seethala RR, Perez-Ordonez B, Zhang L, et al. Recurrent RET gene rearrangements in intraductal carcinomas of salivary gland. Am J Surg Pathol. 2018;42:442–52.
7. Dietel M, Bubendorf L, Dingemans AM, Dooms C, Elmberger G, García RC, et al. Diagnostic procedures for non-small-cell lung cancer (NSCLC): recommendations of the European Expert Group. Thorax. 2016;71:177–84.
8. Pisapia P, Lozano MD, Vigliar E, Bellevicine C, Pepe F, Malapelle U, Troncone G. ALK and ROS1 testing on lung cancer cytologic samples: perspectives. Cancer Cytopathol. 2017;125:817–30.
9. Aisner DL, Rumery MD, Merrick DT, et al. Do more with less: tips and techniques for maximizing small biopsy and cytology specimens for molecular and ancillary testing: the University of Colorado experience. Arch Pathol Lab Med. 2016;140:1206–20.
10. Alì G, Bruno R, Savino M, Giannini R, Pelliccioni S, Menghi M, et al. Analysis of fusion genes by nanoString system: a role in lung cytology? Arch Pathol Lab Med. 2018;142:480–9.
11. Tazi J, Bakkour N, Stamm S. Alternative splicing and disease. Biochim Biophys Acta. 2009;1792:14–26.
12. Awad MM, Oxnard GR, Jackman DM, Savukoski DO, Hall D, Shivdasani P, et al. MET exon 14 mutations in non-small-cell lung cancer are associated with advanced age and stage-dependent MET genomic amplification and c-met overexpression. J Clin Oncol. 2016;34:721–30.
13. Fink L, Seeger W, Ermert L, Hänze J, Stahl U, Grimminger F, et al. Real-time quantitative RT-PCR after laser-assisted cell picking. Nat Med. 1998;4:1329–33.

14. Malapelle U, Mayo de-Las-Casas C, Rocco D, Garzon M, Pisapia P, Jordana-Ariza N, et al. Development of a gene panel for next-generation sequencing of clinically relevant mutations in cell-free DNA from cancer patients. Br J Cancer. 2017;116:802–10.
15. Sgariglia R, Pisapia P, Nacchio M, De Luca C, Pepe F, Russo M, et al. Multiplex digital colour-coded barcode technology on RNA extracted from routine cytological samples of patients with non-small cell lung cancer: pilot study. J Clin Pathol. 2017;70:803–6.
16. Bellevicine C, Malapelle U, Vigliar E, Pisapia P, Vita G, Troncone G. How to prepare cytological samples for molecular testing. J Clin Pathol. 2017;70:819–26.
17. Bridge JA. Reverse transcription-polymerase chain reaction molecular testing of cytology specimens: pre-analytic and analytic factors. Cancer. 2017;125:11–9.
18. Dejmek A, Zendehrokh N, Tomaszewska M, Edsjö A. Preparation of DNA from cytological material: effects of fixation, staining, and mounting medium on DNA yield and quality. Cancer Cytopathol. 2013;121:344–53.
19. Ladd AC, O'Sullivan-Mejia E, Lea T, Perry J, Dumur CI, Dragoescu E, et al. Preservation of fine-needle aspiration specimens for future use inRNA-based molecular testing. Cancer Cytopathol. 2011;119:102–10.
20. Imbeaud S, Graudens E, Boulanger V, Barlet X, Zaborski P, Eveno E, et al. Towards standardization of RNA quality assessment using user-independent classifiers of microcapillary electrophoresis traces. Nucleic Acids Res. 2005;33:e56.
21. Skrypina NA, Timofeeva AV, Khaspekov GL, Savochkina LP, Beabealashvilli RS. Total RNA suitable for molecular biology analysis. J Biotechnol. 2003;105:1–9.
22. Wilkes TM, Devonshire AS, Ellison SL, Foy CA. Evaluation of a novel approach for the measurement of RNA quality. BMC Res Notes. 2010;3:89.
23. Zhang Y, Ni M, Liu N, Zhou Y, Chen X, Ding YB, et al. Expression and function of Pdcd4 in mouse endometrium during early pregnancy. Reproduction. 2018. pii: REP-17-0787.
24. Attri KS, Mehla K, Shukla SK, Singh PK. Microscale gene expression analysis of tumor-associated macrophages. Sci Rep. 2018;8:2408.
25. Wang J, Yao A, Wang JY, Sung CC, Fink LM, Hardin JW, Hauer-Jensen M. cDNA cloning and sequencing, gene expression, and

immunolocalization of thrombomodulin in the Sprague-Dawley rat. DNA Res. 1999;6:57–62.
26. Ruiz-Villalba A, van Pelt-Verkuil E, Gunst QD, Ruijter JM, van den Hoff MJ. Amplification of nonspecific products in quantitative polymerase chain reactions (qPCR). Biomol Detect Quantif. 2017;14:7–18.
27. Reguart N, Teixidó C, Giménez-Capitán A, Paré L, Galván P, Viteri S, et al. Identification of ALK, ROS1, and RET fusions by a multiplexed mRNA-based assay in formalin-fixed, paraffin-embedded samples from advanced non-small-cell lung Cancer patients. Clin Chem. 2017;63:751–60.
28. Oktay MH, Adler E, Hakima L, Grunblatt E, Pieri E, Seymour A, et al. The application of molecular diagnostics to stained cytology smears. J Mol Diagn. 2016;18:407–15.
29. Mitiushkina NV, Iyevleva AG, Poltoratskiy AN, Ivantsov AO, Togo AV, Polyakov IS, et al. Detection of EGFR mutations and EML4-ALK rearrangements in lung adenocarcinomas using archived cytological slides. Cancer Cytopathol. 2013;121:370–6.
30. Ferraz C, Rehfeld C, Krogdahl A, Precht Jensen EM, Bösenberg E, Narz F, et al. Detection of PAX8/PPARG and RET/PTC rearrangements is feasible in routine air-dried fine needle aspiration smears. Thyroid. 2012;22:1025–30.
31. Jennings LJ, Arcila ME, Corless C, et al. Guidelines for validation of next-generation sequencing-based oncology panels: a joint consensus recommendation of the Association for Molecular Pathology and College of American Pathologists. J Mol Diagn. 2017;19:341–65.
32. Clinical and Laboratory Standards Institute. Nucleic acid sequencing methods in diagnostic laboratory medicine; approved guideline. (CLSI document MM09-A2). 2nd ed. Wayne: Clinical and Laboratory Standards Institute; 2014.
33. Bentley DR, Balasubramanian S, Swerdlow HP, et al. Accurate whole human genome sequencing using reversible terminator chemistry. Nature. 2008;456:53–9.
34. Arvidsson G, Henriksson J, Sander B, Wright AP. Mixed-species RNAseq analysis of human lymphoma cells adhering to mouse stromal cells identifies a core gene set that is also differentially expressed in the lymph node microenvironment of mantle cell lymphoma and chronic lymphocytic leukemia patients. Haematologica. 2018;103:666–78.
35. Hynes SO, Pang B, James JA, et al. Tissue-based next generation sequencing: application in a universal healthcare system. Br J Cancer. 2017;116:553–60.

36. Head SR, Komori HK, LaMere SA, Whisenant T, Van Nieuwerburgh F, Salomon DR, Ordoukhanian P. Library construction for next-generation sequencing: overviews and challenges. Biotechniques. 2014;56:61–4, 66, 68, passim.
37. Etheridge A, Wang K, Baxter D, Galas D. Preparation of small RNA NGS libraries from biofluids. Methods Mol Biol. 2018;1740:163–75.
38. Velizheva NP, Rechsteiner MP, Wong CE, Zhong Q, Rössle M, Bode B, et al. Cytology smears as excellent starting material for next-generation sequencing-based molecular testing of patients with adenocarcinoma of the lung. Cancer Cytopathol. 2017;125:30–40.
39. Guseva NV, Jaber O, Stence AA, Sompallae K, Bashir A, Sompallae R, et al. Simultaneous detection of single-nucleotide variant, deletion/insertion, and fusion in lung and thyroid carcinoma using cytology specimen and an RNA-based next-generation sequencing assay. Cancer Cytopathol. 2018;126:158–69.
40. Troncone G. All-in-one: the dream and reality of molecular cytopathology testing on routine lung cancer smears. Cancer Cytopathol. 2018;126:155–7.
41. Kim MH, Seo HJ, Joung JG, Kim JH. Comprehensive evaluation of matrix factorization methods for the analysis of DNA microarray gene expression data. BMC Bioinformatics. 2011;12 Suppl 13:S8.
42. Lira ME, Choi YL, Lim SM, Deng S, Huang D, Ozeck M, et al. A single-tube multiplexed assay for detecting ALK, ROS1, and RET fusions in lung cancer. J Mol Diagn. 2014;16:229–43.
43. Lira ME, Kim TM, Huang D, Deng S, Koh Y, Jang B, et al. Multiplexed gene expression and fusion transcript analysis to detect ALK fusions in lung cancer. J Mol Diagn. 2013;15:51–61.
44. Sunami K, Furuta K, Tsuta K, Sasada S, Izumo T, Nakaoku T, et al. Multiplex diagnosis of oncogenic fusion and MET exon skipping by molecular counting using formalin-fixed paraffin embedded lung adenocarcinoma tissues. J Thorac Oncol. 2016;11:203–12.
45. Zhao W, Choi YL, Song JY, Zhu Y, Xu Q, Zhang F, et al. ALK, ROS1 and RET rearrangements in lung squamous cell carcinoma are very rare. Lung Cancer. 2016;94:22–7.
46. Fang DD, Zhang B, Gu Q, Lira M, Xu Q, Sun H, et al. HIP1-ALK, a novel ALK fusion variant that responds to crizotinib. J Thorac Oncol. 2014;9:285–94.

Chapter 7
FISH Testing of Cytology Specimens: Pre-analytic, Analytic, and Post-analytic Considerations

Karen D. Tsuchiya, Laura J. Tafe, and Julia A. Bridge

Abbreviations

ABL1	ABL proto-oncogene 1
ALK	Anaplastic lymphoma kinase or ALK receptor tyrosine kinase
BCL2	B-cell CLL/lymphoma 2
BCR	Breakpoint cluster region

K. D. Tsuchiya (✉)
Department of Laboratories, Seattle Children's Hospital, Seattle, WA, USA
e-mail: karen.tsuchiya@seattlechildrens.org

L. J. Tafe
Laboratory for Clinical Genomics and Advanced Technologies, Department of Pathology and Laboratory Medicine, Dartmouth-Hitchcock Medical Center, Lebanon, NH, USA
e-mail: laura.j.tafe@hitchcock.org

J. A. Bridge
Departments of Pathology/Microbiology, Pediatrics and Orthopedic Surgery, University of Nebraska Medical Center/Nebraska Medicine, Omaha, NE, USA
e-mail: jbridge@unmc.edu

S. Roy-Chowdhuri et al. (eds.), *Molecular Diagnostics in Cytopathology*, https://doi.org/10.1007/978-3-319-97397-5_7

bp	Basepair
BRAF	v-Raf murine sarcoma viral oncogene homolog B
CCND1	Cyclin D1
DAPI	4′,6-diamidino-2-phenylindole
EDTA	Ethylenediaminetetraacetic acid
EML4	Echinoderm microtubule-associated protein-like 4
ERBB2	Erb-b2 receptor tyrosine kinase 2 (HER2)
ERG	ERG, ETS transcription factor
ETV6	ETS variant 6
EWSR1	Ewing sarcoma breakpoint region 1
FFPE	Formalin fixed paraffin embedded
FISH	Fluorescence *in situ* hybridization
FNA	Fine-needle aspirate
HER2	Human epidermal growth factor receptor 2 (ERBB2)
IGH	Immunoglobulin heavy chain
ISH	*In situ* hybridization
Kb	Kilobase
KMT2A	Lysine methyltransferase 2A
LBC	Liquid-based cytology
Mb	Megabase
MLL	Mixed-lineage leukemia
MYC	v-myc avian myelocytomatosis viral oncogene homolog
MYCN	v-myc myelocytomatosis viral oncogene homolog, neuroblastoma-derived
Pap	Papanicolaou
PML	Promyelocytic leukemia
RARA	Retinoic acid receptor alpha
ROS1	ROS proto-oncogene 1, receptor tyrosine kinase
RT-PCR	Reverse transcription-polymerase chain reaction
RUNX1	Runt-related transcription factor 1
SS18	Synovial sarcoma translocation chromosome 18

Key Terminology

Aneuploidy	An abnormal number of chromosomes in a cell (e.g., monosomy, trisomy, tetrasomy, etc.)
Bacterial artificial chromosome	A construct or vector used for cloning segments of DNA with a typical size of approximately 150–350 Kb
Chromosomal rearrangements	General term that encompasses chromosomal translocations, inversions, and insertions
Cutoff	The threshold above which a result is considered positive and below which a result is considered negative
Interphase	A phase of the cell cycle in which chromatin is decondensed; contrast to metaphase in which chromatin is condensed and individual chromosomes can be visualized
Locus	The position of a gene or other specific sequences in a chromosome
Polyploidy	The presence of more than two sets of homologous chromosomes

	within a cell (triploidy, tetraploidy, etc.)
Polysomy	The condition in which there may be three or more copies of the chromosome rather than the expected two copies
Signal scoring	The process of enumerating or evaluating probe signals within a nucleus and sometimes determining relative position of probe signals with respect to each other
Touch preparation (touch imprint)	Cytologic preparation where cells are transferred onto a glass slide by touching the histologic tissue directly to the slide

Key Points

- FISH results should be interpreted in the context of clinical presentation, cytopathology, differential diagnosis, and other ancillary tests
- Pre-analytic variables including type of cytologic preparation, fixative, prior staining, and length of and time to fixation can impact FISH results
- Validation of laboratory-developed FISH assays is specific for each probe and specimen type
- Both the FISH slide processing and scoring are amenable to automation, but automated signal scoring

still requires confirmation by an individual experienced in interpretation of FISH results and familiarity with cytomorphology
- Interpretation of FISH results requires knowledge of probe design, tumor biology and morphology, the spectrum of genetic alterations in different types of neoplasia, and limitations of the technique

Fluorescence *in situ* hybridization (FISH) is a technique that is well suited for detecting many types of genomic abnormalities in cytology specimens. FISH involves hybridization of fluorescently labeled nucleic acid sequences (probes) to complementary nucleic acid sequences (targets) which are typically in the form of metaphase chromosomes obtained from cultured, dividing cells or decondensed chromosomes within interphase nuclei of nondividing cells. Although FISH probes and targets can consist of RNA, this chapter will refer specifically to DNA probes and targets. FISH allows visualization of the physical location of the probe(s) to their target(s) and can be used to interrogate specific areas of the genome. Whole-chromosome loss or deletions of chromosomal loci may correlate with loss of function of specific tumor suppressor genes. In contrast, whole-chromosome gains or amplification of regions within chromosomes may correspond to gain of function of given oncogenes. Chromosomal rearrangements that result in fusion of two genes, or juxtapositioning of a gene and a regulatory element, can be responsible for novel gene function or gain of function. The technical approach of FISH can be engaged to detect all of these types of genetic abnormalities.

Knowledge of probe design is necessary for optimal probe choice, analysis, and interpretation of results (Fig. 7.1). *Enumeration probes* are used to detect genomic gains and losses. *Centromere probes*, which are composed of alpha satellite DNA (tandemly repeated, 171 bp noncoding blocks of DNA), or locus–/gene-specific (unique sequence) probes are commonly used for the assessment of corresponding copy number. Centromere probes are typically the preferred choice for enumerating whole-chromosome aneuploidies, while locus–/gene-specific probes can be used to detect loss or gain/amplification of a region of interest. For assessment of the latter, a differentially labeled centromere probe or a distinct locus-specific probe located at a distance or on the

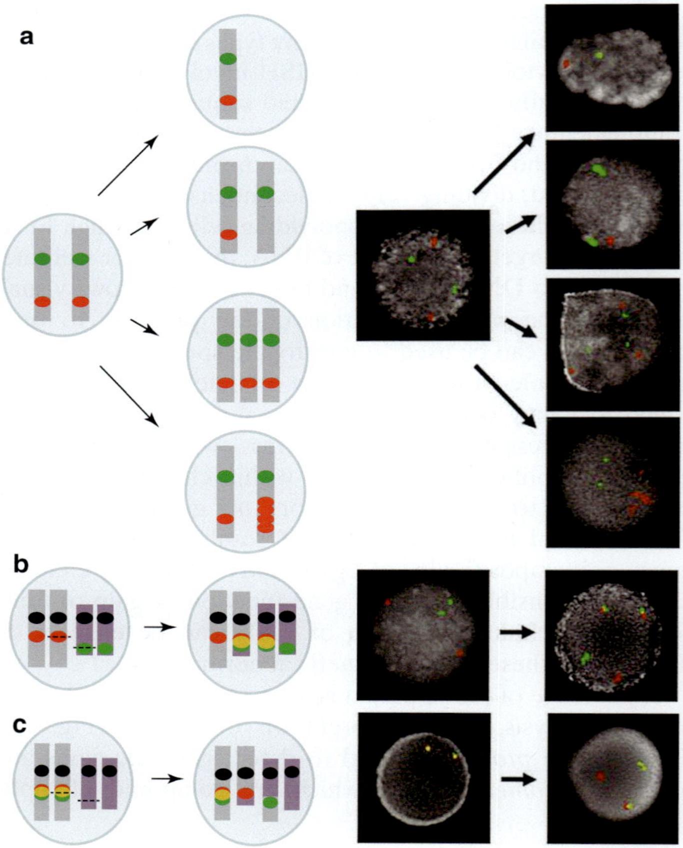

opposite chromosomal arm from the locus of interest is often concurrently employed as a copy number control for ploidy level or ratio calculations. *Dual color, break-apart probes* are locus-specific probes that flank a gene breakpoint region of interest and are designed to detect a rearrangement based on physical separation of the two probes that are labeled with distinct fluorophores. Break-apart probes are optimal for assessing rearrangements of a gene that could have more than one translocation partner, such as *MLL* (*KMT2A*). In contrast, *fusion probes* are composed of two independent fluorophore-labeled DNA probes that span both rearranged gene loci of a specific fusion gene event, allowing for its detection. Fusion probes are most frequently employed when fusions involve consistent gene partners, such as *BCR/ABL1* but may also be of value in identifying or characterizing less common variants as well. The advantage of dual fusion

FIGURE 7.1 Schematic representations (left) and corresponding cytological FISH images (right) illustrating different probe strategies and the abnormalities detected by each. (**a**) Enumeration probe set consisting of a locus-specific probe (red) and a centromere-specific probe (green) on the same chromosome. This probe set can detect aneuploidies, deletions, duplications, and amplifications. The normal diploid state (two green, two red) is on the left, and arrows indicate abnormalities consisting of (from top to bottom) monosomy (one green, one red), deletion (two green, one red), trisomy or triploidy (three green, three red), and amplification (two green, multiple red). (**b**) Dual fusion probe strategy consisting of two differentially labeled, locus-specific probes that span the genes involved in a fusion event. When a balanced rearrangement (translocation or inversion) occurs, there is a break within each probe (dashed lines) and a rearrangement that results in reciprocal juxtaposition of red and green signals to create dual fusion (yellow) signals. (**c**) Break-apart probe strategy consisting of two differentially labeled probes that flank the breakpoint (dashed lines) of one of the gene partners involved in a fusion. In the normal state, there are two juxtaposed red/green (yellow) signals. When a rearrangement (e.g. translocation) occurs, the break-apart probe is split into separate red and green signals

probes is the greater sensitivity and specificity they provide compared to break-apart probes [1]. In addition to dual fusion probes, other less common probe strategies exist for detecting gene fusions (e.g., Vysis *ETV6/RUNX1* ES probe, Abbott Laboratories, Abbott Park, IL).

An appreciation for the limitation of resolution of FISH is also necessary to determine if it is an appropriate technique to use in a given setting or if another technique is warranted. The majority of probes currently used for FISH are in the order of approximately 100–300 Kb in size. Due to probe size and other technical factors, deletions below approximately 50–100 Kb and duplications below approximately 200–300 Kb are difficult to detect in interphase nuclei by FISH. Small inversions cannot be identified using a break-apart probe if the separation is not large enough to visualize two distinct signals.

Although extracted nucleic acid (DNA and RNA)-based assays are also used to detect genetic abnormalities, an advantage of FISH is the ability to visualize results within individual cells, allowing for correlation of results with cellular morphology and distinct cell populations. DNA- and RNA-based assays, in contrast, are performed on nucleic acids that are extracted from a mixture of neoplastic and non-neoplastic cells, resulting in dilution of the target(s) of interest and an inability to correlate results with individual cells. On the other hand, DNA- and RNA-based assays can sometimes identify abnormalities that are below the size resolution of FISH or the analytical sensitivity. For example, the high analytic sensitivity of RT-PCR or quantitative RT-PCR procedures for the detection of fusion mRNA transcripts (one tumor cell in 10^4–10^5 total mononuclear cells) or next-generation sequencing may be preferable depending on the clinical question and available specimen [2, 3]. As with any technique, there are a number of pre-analytic, analytic, and post-analytic considerations that are crucial not only for the success of probe hybridization but also proper interpretation of FISH results. Most of the concepts and principles presented in this chapter are also applicable to bright-field *in situ* hybridization techniques, although there are some differences that are not addressed.

Pre-analytic FISH Considerations

Types of Cytologic Preparations for FISH

A wide range of cytologic preparations have been used for FISH, including touch preparations, unstained cytologic smears, archival stained cytology slides, cytospin preparations, liquid-based cytologic preparations, and formalin or alcohol-fixed, paraffin-embedded cell blocks [4, 5]. Inherent advantages and limitations exist among each preparation type (Table 7.1).For paraffin-embedded cell block material, FISH studies are typically performed on 4–5 μm sections. Sectioning can result in artifactual loss of probe signal due to nuclear truncation. An advantage of touch preparations, smears, cytospins, and liquid-based cytologic preparations over paraffin-embedded cell blocks is that nuclear truncation due to sectioning is not an issue. For paraffin blocks, the problem of nuclear truncation from sectioning can be alleviated by extraction of whole nuclei from thick sections, cores, or microdissected material; however, the trade-off is that tissue architecture is not maintained. Extracted nuclei and other cytologic preparations are not suitable for FISH tests that require intact tissue architecture, such as *HER2* (*ERBB2*) amplification status in primary breast cancer, in which scoring should be limited to invasive tumor [6]. This limitation is not an issue for cytology samples of metastatic tumors including metastatic breast carcinoma. Another drawback of some preparations for FISH is the presence of a significant number of overlapping nuclei. Scoring of overlapping nuclei is not recommended, as their inclusion may cause erroneous signal interpretation. Overlapping nuclei, which can be problematic in paraffin-embedded sections, smears, cytospins, and touch preparations, are much less of an issue in liquid-based cytologic preparations. Touch preparations can only be made from intact tissue, such as a resection or needle biopsy. Given the limitations of each technique, it can be beneficial for laboratories to validate FISH in more than one type of preparation.

TABLE 7.1 Advantages and disadvantages of different cytologic preparations for FISH

Preparation type	Advantages	Disadvantages
Touch preparation	No nuclear truncation artifact Less processing time than FFPE, cytospins, liquid-based cytology	Requires intact tissue Low-cellularity specimens with abundant fibrous stroma may result in sparsely cellular slides Overlapping nuclei can cause difficulty scoring signal Nuclear distortion due to crushing during slide preparation May experience autofluorescent background that obscures signals
FFPE cell block	Allows for correlation with adjacent H&E- or IHC-stained section Preservation of morphology and partial tissue architecture Cell blocks made from aspirates may be enriched for tumor cells	Probe signal loss due to nuclear truncation from sectioning Overlapping nuclei can cause difficulty scoring signals May have autofluorescent background that obscures signals May have inadequate tumor cellularity

TABLE 7.1 (continued)

Preparation type	Advantages	Disadvantages
Cytology smear	No nuclear truncation artifact Previously stained slides can be used Only technique that allows rapid on-site determination of specimen adequacy at time of procedure Smears made from aspirates may be enriched in tumor cells	Overlapping nuclei can cause difficulty scoring signals Nuclear distortion due to crushing during slide preparation May have autofluorescent background that obscures signals
Cytospin	No nuclear truncation artifact Cytospins made from aspirates may be enriched for tumor cells Cells are concentrated in a smaller area	Overlapping nuclei can cause difficulty scoring signals May have inadequate cellularity
Liquid-based cytology	No nuclear truncation artifact Thin, monolayer preparation minimizing nuclear overlap Less background than other preparations Less hands-on time than many other preparations Cells are concentrated in a smaller area	More expensive than other cytologic preparations Special instrumentation needed for slide preparation May have inadequate cellularity

Multiple studies that have assessed the performance of FISH on cytologic preparations have shown variable results. There are dozens of specimen and FISH processing variables between laboratories that could be responsible for differences in FISH success, even on the same type of cytologic preparation. Monaco et al. evaluated FISH on cases of B-cell non-Hodgkin lymphoma using unstained, air-dried smears made from fine-needle aspirates (FNAs) [7]. Out of 106 cases, a positive or negative FISH result was obtained in 93 cases (87.7%), while 13 cases (12%) yielded an indeterminate result, and only 2 cases (1.9%) failed hybridization. Bozzetti et al. performed FISH for *ALK* and *ROS1* rearrangements on either fresh unstained, air-dried smears or stained smears [8]. *ALK* FISH was successful in 49 out of 55 cases (89%), although 5 out of 14 destained smears either lacked hybridization or presented difficulties with signal visualization due to background fluorescence. The background fluorescence was attributed to a "high hematic component" that was not present in the unstained smears which were fixed in Carnoy's solution prior to FISH. *ROS1* FISH was successful in all 12 of their cases that were attempted (eight fresh smears and four destained smears). Bravaccini and coworkers experienced *ALK* FISH failure in 19 out of 72 cases (26%) from prospectively collected cytologic smears of transbronchial aspirates that were fixed using Cytofix and PAP-stained [9]. The majority of their failed cases were attributed to sample inadequacy or overlapping cells and not hybridization failure, which emphasizes the need for proper preparation of smears by trained personnel.

Other studies have evaluated archival smears for FISH suitability. Bentz and coworkers performed FISH for the t(11;14), which results in juxtaposition of *CCND1* with *IGH* and overexpression of *CCND1*, in ten cases of mantle cell lymphoma using archival cytology slides that had been stained with either Papanicolaou (PAP) or Diff-Quik stain [10]. All ten cases were positive for the translocation. Richmond et al. observed a 15% FISH failure rate in archival PAP-stained cytology slides from 60 cases of non-Hodgkin lymphoma or reactive lymphoid tissue using a dual fusion probe that identifies *BCL2/IGH* rearrangements [11]. This decreased success rate may be due to the Pap stain, as others have found that Pap-stained compared to Diff-Quik-stained smears demonstrate DNA degradation as a function of time [12]. Betz et al. compared FISH for *ALK* rearrangements in paraffin-embedded cell blocks vs. archival Diff-Quik-stained smears prepared from the same 32 cases of metastatic lung carcinoma [13]. Results were obtained in all 32 cases and concordance was observed in all but one case. The single discordant case was positive for an *ALK* rearrangement in the destained smear but negative in the cell block. RT-PCR performed on the cell block of this case confirmed the presence of an *EML4/ALK* fusion transcript. Zito-Marino et al. have summarized results from several published studies of FISH for *ALK* rearrangements performed on conventional smears and cell blocks [14].

FISH studies can also be performed on the same slides following immunocytochemical staining provided diaminobenzidine, which results in nuclear autofluorescence, has not been used as a chromogen [5]. An advantage of performing FISH on previously stained cytologic preparations is that the same cells can be sequentially evaluated with the use of an automated platform (see FISH slide analysis and scoring under *Analytic FISH Considerations*).

Cytospin preparations made from a number of different specimen types have been shown to be suitable for FISH. A retrospective review of FISH performed on cytospin preparations from 298 non-Hodgkin lymphoma FNAs at one institution demonstrated a success rate of 95.3% [15]. In another study, FISH analysis for the presence of *BCR/ABL1* or *PML/RARA* fusions was successful on all 24 cytospins prepared from bone marrow or peripheral blood [16]. Moreover, a FISH result was obtained in 12 h for all 24 cytospin preparations, compared to an average of 4 days for interphase FISH on cultured cells. Zellweger et al. successfully used FISH on cytospins from voided urine to assist in predicting recurrence of bladder cancer in large series of patients [17].

Cytospins prepared from brushings of resected or biopsied central nervous system tumors have also been used for 1p/19q FISH [18]. This technique avoided the impediment of signal scoring from truncated, overlapping nuclei in formalin-fixed, paraffin-embedded (FFPE) sections. The authors compared FISH on the cytospins to FISH on FFPE sections from the same tumors. FISH was successful in all but two of the cytospins which failed due to low cellularity. In contrast, FISH failed in four of the FFPE cases because of weak signals. This brush cytology/cytospin technique may be useful as an alternative to touch preparations made from friable tissue that tends to result in unacceptable cell clumping. For tumors that are extremely fibrous or contain bone, another alternative to touch preparations that we have used is to gently scrape the surface of the specimen with a scalpel and then smear the scraped cells onto a slide or resuspend them in fixative for a cytospin preparation.

Liquid-based cytology (LBC) has been widely adopted for the collection and preparation of both gynecologic and non-gynecologic cytology samples. Many studies have demonstrated that LBC provides a reliable and reproducible source material for a number of ancillary tests, including CISH [19]. For example, *SS18* and *EWSR1* chromogenic ISH on LBC samples was sensitive and specific for detection of the appropriate gene rearrangement in ten cases of synovial sarcoma and in nine cases of Ewing sarcoma [20]. In another study, *ALK* FISH was successful in 99.1% (228 out of 230) of non-small cell lung cancer ThinPrep samples obtained from FNA, bronchial brush, pleural fluid, pericardial fluid, or peritoneal fluid [21].

Cytology Fixatives and FISH

While formalin fixation is standard for tissues, alcohol fixatives are often used for cytologic preparations. A number of studies in the previous section demonstrated that alcohol-fixed and various LBC-fixed cytology specimen types are compatible with FISH. One study that directly compared alcohol-fixed cell blocks, formalin-fixed cell blocks, and FFPE tissue specimens for the detection of *ALK* gene rearrangements by FISH showed hybridization success rates of 100% of 34 alcohol-fixed cell blocks, 82% of 22 formalin-fixed cell blocks, and 96.6% of 58 FFPE tissues [22]. The FISH failures in this study were attributed to insufficient tumor cell numbers, and not the type of fixative. Abati et al. obtained probe signals of equivalent quality using cytology specimens fixed by a variety of methods including 95% ethanol, methanol, and Carnoy's solution [23]. They also did not observe any difference in probe signals or specimen adhesion on positively charged vs. non-charged slides, although charged slides are often necessary for adhesion of paraffin-embedded sections or cells. Fixatives containing acidic components (Bouin's, Davidson's AFA) have been shown to yield suboptimal FISH/ISH results, as have decalcification solutions containing strong acidic components [24–28]. Multiple studies have demonstrated that EDTA decalcification is superior to acid decalcification for FISH [24, 26–28]; however, there is some evidence that 5% or even 10% formic acid decalcification can yield successful FISH results in trephine biopsies if incubation periods are short [26, 27]. The advantage of formic acid decalcification is that it is faster than EDTA.

Length of Fixation and Time to Fixation

HER2 FISH/ISH guidelines in breast and gastric cancer stipulate that specimens should ideally be placed in fixative within 1 h of collection and fixed for 6–72 h [6, 29]. Babic et al. demonstrated that underfixation in formalin-based fixatives resulted in weak FISH/ISH signals, while overfixation was not as problematic [25]. Another study also showed that prolonged formalin fixation did not adversely impact FISH results, but a delay of 6 h to fixation did have a negative impact on FISH results [30]. Khoury et al. performed a delay to fixation study on *HER2* ISH in invasive breast cancer and found that while there was no statistically significant effect on

HER2/centromere17 ratio even after an 8-h delay to fixation, there was a statistically significant trend in signal loss after a 1-h delay [31]. In addition, artifacts such as nuclear bubbling and background began to appear after 30-min to 1-h delay in fixation, which could lead to difficulties with signal scoring. Portier et al. also found that delay to fixation of up to 3 h did not have a deleterious effect on *HER2* ISH results [32]. However, in contrast to the study by Khoury et al., they did not see degradation of signal intensity with up to a 3-h delay to fixation. After 3 h, FISH, but not bright-field ISH, showed a degradation of signal intensity.

Analytic FISH Considerations

Cytology specimens are advantageous for FISH because results can be obtained with as few as 50 or even 20 tumor nuclei in some clinical settings, such as *HER2* status in breast or gastroesophageal carcinoma [6, 29]. In contrast to molecular techniques that require extracted DNA, FISH is not necessarily limited by a minimum percentage of tumor cells within a background of non-neoplastic cells, as long as a sufficient number of tumor nuclei can be identified and scored. When a specific cell type needs to be distinguished for analysis, FISH testing performed in a cytogenetics laboratory should engage a pathologist for confirmation of appropriate cell selection, ideally with the pathologist visualizing the findings at the fluorescent microscope or on a fully digitalized scanned slide preparation [29, 33, 34].

Processing Cytology Slides for FISH

The processing steps involved in FISH include slide pretreatment, denaturation of probe and slide to obtain single-stranded DNA, hybridization, post-hybridization washes, nuclear DNA counterstaining, slide examination, and nuclear signal scoring.

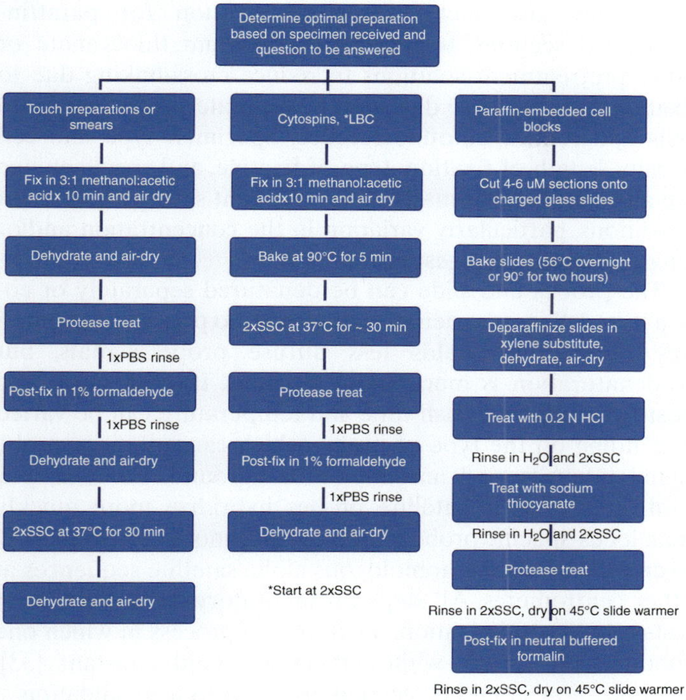

FIGURE 7.2 Flowchart summarizing slide treatment for FISH for different cytologic preparations. LBC liquid-based cytology, HCl hydrochloric acid, N normal, PBS phosphate-buffered saline, SSC saline sodium citrate

Slide pretreatment is necessary for preparing the cells for probe penetration and efficient hybridization (Fig. 7.2). Unfixed preparations such as touch preparations, smears, or cytospins should be fixed prior to hybridization to prevent cells from detaching from the slide and to preserve nuclear morphology. Typical fixation for FISH involves incubation in 3:1 methanol/acetic acid for 10–20 min followed by air-drying. Slide baking prior to processing can improve adherence to the slide and nuclear morphology; however, excessive baking can also decrease hybridization efficiency [35]. Slide pretreatment steps may also include deparaffinization for paraffin-embedded sections, treatment with sodium thiocyanate or other pretreatment solutions to reduce cross-linking due to fixation, and protease digestion to facilitate probe entry into cells and reduce autofluorescence. Specimen type and cell density, length of fixation, type of fixative, and specimen age are all variables that may require different slide pretreatment conditions, particularly variation in the concentration and/or length of protease digestion.

The probes and slide can be denatured separately or co-denatured. Separate denaturation tends to preserve morphology better and yields less diffuse probe signals, but co-denaturation is much more efficient. Hybridization and post-hybridization wash time and temperature can be varied depending on the type of probe, which can influence probe signal intensity and amount of background. For example, centromeric alpha satellite probes hybridize more quickly than locus-specific probes, but they have more of a propensity to cross hybridize to homologous alpha satellite sequences at other centromeres. All steps for laboratory-developed FISH tests require optimization, an empirical process in which one condition is varied, while others are held constant [33]. Optimization should be carried out prior to test validation.

FISH Test Validation

For US laboratories using FDA-approved probes, all steps of the procedure, including signal scoring and interpretation, should be followed according to manufacturer specifications. Any deviation from the manufacturer-approved package insert for an FDA-approved FISH test, as well as any laboratory-developed FISH test, requires validation. Not only does each different probe or probe set require a separate validation, but also the same probes applied to different specimen types (e.g., FFPE vs. direct smears) require their own validation [36].

Validation of laboratory-developed FISH tests entails confirmation of probe localization, determination of probe sensitivity and specificity, and establishment of normal cutoff values. Detailed description of these processes is beyond the scope of this document and can be found elsewhere [33]; however, a few points are worth noting. A limitation of interphase FISH testing is that for most probes, technical artifacts can cause a low percentage of cells to have the abnormal signal pattern in question. As a consequence, cutoffs (i.e., the percentage of nuclei with an abnormal signal pattern that are required to determine when a specimen is a true positive for the abnormality in question) need to be determined for each individual probe. A common method for determining the normal cutoff for a given probe is to score a specified number of known normal controls, determine how often the abnormal signal pattern is observed, and then apply a statistical test to account for variation between scorers, runs, etc. [33].The normal control tissue should be comprised of cells that mimic as closely as possible the size of tumor nuclei that will be evaluated by FISH. For example, tonsil or thymus could be used as normal controls for small blue round cell tumors. As mentioned previously, different specimen preparations and changes in other FISH variables require separate validation. It should also be kept in mind that for FFPE FISH, different cutoffs would need to be determined for different section thicknesses, particularly when enumeration FISH probes are employed. A 4 μm section will lead to increased nuclear truncation artifact compared to a 6 μm section. Therefore, once a cutoff is determined for a given section thickness, either that thickness should be used for all testing, or separate cutoffs need to be determined.

FISH Slide Analysis and Scoring

Analysis of the hybridized slide should occur in a manner in which scoring of signals from tumor nuclei can be confirmed whenever possible. Evaluation of an adjacent stained slide to confirm scoring of tumor nuclei is more easily accomplished with certain types of preparations compared to others.

For example, an adjacent H&E stained section from an FFPE cell block may be more representative of the hybridized slide than an independently stained smear or touch preparation slide. However, an adjacent touch preparation slide can sometimes be stained with a conventional cytology stain to document presence and abundance of tumor cells. In specimens with a low tumor fraction, it may be difficult to differentiate benign from malignant cells on the DAPI-counterstained FISH slide which does not provide good nuclear morphology. Automated platforms are available that allow identification of target cells of interest by conventional staining or immunocytochemistry and then analysis of the same cells after subsequent probe hybridization. Briefly, images of stained cells are captured, subsequently subjected to FISH, and then target cells of interest are relocated by virtue of software that is coupled with an automated stage [5, 22].

Individuals involved in signal scoring should understand the FISH probe design, the precise mapped location of the probe(s), probe behavior, and normal, classic abnormal, and any variant abnormal signal patterns. Only nuclei with internal control signal(s) should be scored. Controls may consist of the same target locus on the homologous chromosome. For example, an *MLL* break-apart probe could be deleted on one chromosome 11. However, nuclei with a deletion should still consistently demonstrate an *MLL* signal from the other chromosome 11 homolog. Controls may also consist of a centromere probe or a probe for another locus on the same chromosome as the target locus. Including more than one control probe, such as a centromeric probe from a chromosome other than the chromosome of interest, might also be useful for a sense of the ploidy status.

For manual scoring, two individuals validated on the specific probes being used should score without knowledge of each other's result. Criteria should be established for a third scorer in the event of a discrepant result. If the FISH test is for disease monitoring, scorers should have knowledge of the abnormal signal pattern established in prior testing. The number of nuclei scored should be the same as the number used to establish cutoffs during validation.

FISH Automation

Many of the steps involved in FISH testing are amenable to automation, depending on the test volume and workflow of a laboratory. Automation for both slide processing (Table 7.2) and slide analysis (Table 7.3) is available. Some of the benefits of automated slide processing systems include increased throughput, standardization of protocols which decreases variability between technologists, and decreased hands-on technologist time [37]. Many of these platforms have an open-access probe step so that a laboratory can process cases for multiple different probe sets simultaneously. A potential drawback includes the need for a backup or redundant system or method in case the instrument breaks down. Moreover, occasional cases may require greater flexibility in the parameters of the pretreatment steps that can be afforded more readily through manual processing.

Automated slide scanners and readers that can aid in the scoring of FISH signals are also available. Manual scoring of FISH slides is labor-intensive, with slides typically being scored by two technologists followed by doctoral-level review and confirmation. Manual scoring introduces inter-reader variability, and there may be challenges in reviewing the specific cells that were scored. Automated systems require strict validation or verification and sometimes integration with preexisting laboratory information systems. After validating the computer algorithms, signal scoring is more standardized. However, hybridized slides still need to be reviewed prior to automated scoring for selection of regions with appropriate morphology and signal quality. Additionally, automated scoring results of each case should be confirmed by inspection of captured FISH images. Thus, automated slide scoring may result in decreased hands-on technical time in high-volume FISH laboratories [41], but the time savings may not be as

Table 7.2 Automated processors for FISH

Instrument	Manufacturer	Specifications	Comments	Reference
ThermoBrite elite	Leica biosystems	Deparaffinization Pretreatment Probe denaturation and hybridization Post-hybridization wash Process up to 12 slides per run	Open access for probing Manual probing, counterstaining, and cover slipping	[37]; http://www.leicabiosystems.com/clinical-microscopy-surgery-radiology/cytogenetics/products/leica-thermobrite-elite/
VP2000/VIP2000	Abbott Laboratories, Abbott Park, Illinois, USA	Deparaffinization Pretreatment Process 8–50 slides per run	Utilizes Vysis ThermoBrite system for denaturation/hybridization	https://www.molecular.abbott/us/en/products/instrumentation/vp-2000-processor-vip2000-processor
Little dipper	SciGene corporation, Sunnyvale, CA	Pre- and post-hybridization processing 1–24 slides per run	Manual probing, counterstaining, and cover slipping	http://www.scigene.com/details.php?pid=1167
Dako Omnis	Dako, Denmark A/S; Agilent Technologies, Santa Clara, CA	No manual user interaction from loading the FFPE slides to unloading the stained slides Up to 15 FISH slides	Continuous loading Different staining protocols simultaneously Also runs IHC	[38]; http://www.agilent.com/en-us/products/dako-omnis-solution-for-ihc-ish/dako-omnis

TABLE 7.3 Slide scanners and reader instruments

Instrument	Manufacturer	Specifications	Comments	Reference
BioView Accord plus (single slide stage) Allegro plus (8-slide stage) Duet-3 (50-slide loader) Encore (100–/200-slide loader)	Rehovot, Israel	Olympus BX41 microscope Slide scanning, scoring, and classification Report generation	Allows for tissue mapping of H&E and FISH slides Separate review and analysis workstations	[39] http://bioview.com/products/
Metafer slide scanning workstation with Isis imaging software and Neon Metafer imaging software platform	MetaSystems, Altlussheim, Germany	Slide scanning, scoring, and classification Report generation	Allows for tissue mapping of H&E and FISH slides	[40] https://metasystems-international.com/us/applications/patho/
Ariol system	Leica biosystems imaging, Inc.	Leica DM6000 B microscope 4-, 8-, or 200-slide capacity		http://www.leicabiosystems.com/digital-pathology/aperio-digital-pathology-slide-scanners/products/ariol/

significant compared to automating the slide processing steps. An advantage of automated slide scanning systems is that they typically have some flexibility and capacity for image analysis beyond FISH to include immunohistochemistry slides and also research applications including tissue microarray and multiplex fluorescence analysis.

Post-analytic FISH Considerations

Knowledge of the spectrum and characteristics of genomic abnormalities in a particular neoplasm, probe design including location with respect to rearrangement breakpoints, tumor biology, cellular morphology, differential diagnosis, and the literature are all essential for proper interpretation of FISH results.

Interpretation of Results in the Context of Specific Neoplasms and Genomic Abnormalities

ALK gene rearrangements in non-small cell lung cancer, which are most commonly the result of an inversion in the short arm of chromosome 2 that results in an *EML4/ALK* fusion, can be detected using a break-apart probe. However, there are intrinsic challenges with assessment of this *ALK* rearrangement because the inversion does not result in as much signal separation as a translocation between different chromosomes, and thus it is vital to become attuned to this subtle alteration. In addition, with the FDA-approved *ALK* break-apart probe, single red signal(s) (3′ or telomeric end) with loss of green signal(s) is considered positive for a rearrangement. In other neoplasms, loss of the 5′ or 3′ end of a break-apart probe could either indicate positivity for a gene rearrangement resulting in a fusion event or a partial deletion of the gene that does not create a fusion [42]. In some scenarios, duplication or amplification of a probe may result in gain of an oncogene, whereas in others it can indicate a gene fusion event. For example, in sporadic pilocytic astrocytoma, a duplication in 7q34 that can be detected by a variety of methods, including FISH, results in a *KIAA1549/BRAF* fusion [43, 44].

Interpretation of Results in the Context of Probe Design

Knowledge of probe mapping with respect to the target gene and the breakpoints of a specific abnormality, including breakpoint variability, is critical for accurate interpretation of FISH results. For example, *MYC* breakpoints in B-cell malignancies are highly variable, sometimes requiring the use of probes both downstream and upstream of the gene itself to detect a rearrangement [45, 46]. Therefore, it is not unusual for one *MYC* probe to fail to demonstrate a rearrangement while another gives a positive result, prompting some laboratories to reflex to a second *MYC* probe if the first is negative.

Interpretation of Results in the Context of Tumor Biology and Cytomorphology

An example of the need to understand tumor biology for proper FISH interpretation can occur in the setting of an abnormal FISH result that is just above normal cutoff. Although a result near cutoff can be seen in hematologic neoplasms when assessing minimal residual disease, one must question the possibility of a false-positive result if FISH is being performed for a driver abnormality in a diagnostic sample with a high tumor fraction.

The t(14;18) is one example of the importance of correlation of FISH results with cytomorphology. This translocation, resulting in rearrangement of *IGH* and *BCL2*, is seen in the majority of follicular lymphomas, although it is also present in about 15% of cases of diffuse large B-cell lymphomas.

Therefore, a positive t(14;18) result cannot be assumed to be diagnostic of follicular lymphoma [11].

Interpretation of Results in the Context of Literature and Guidelines

Proper interpretation of FISH results also requires knowledge of the literature and published recommendations, as in the example of amplification interpretation. There is no single definition of amplification, which varies depending on tumor type and may be based on clinical parameters such as response to treatment or prognosis. Typically, gain of a single copy does not fit a definition of amplification, but the number of copies required for amplification is not consistent across tumor types. For example, the definition of *HER2* amplification in breast cancer takes into account both the ratio of *HER2* to chromosome 17 centromere signals and the absolute number of *HER2* signals. These specific criteria, including integration of HER2 immunoexpression analysis, have evolved over time and are based on response to trastuzumab [6]. *MYCN* amplification in neuroblastoma is defined as greater than four-fold increase in *MYCN* signals compared to reference probe signals and is based on unfavorable clinical behavior [47]. The use of a control probe from the centromere or opposite arm of the chromosome containing the test probe target is often recommended for distinguishing amplification from polysomy, which may not have the same biologic consequence as amplification of a specific gene or region. Similarly, increased copy number of probes from a single chromosome cannot distinguish between polysomy and polyploidy.

Figure 7.3 illustrates the complexities that can be involved when interpreting FISH results. The case is from a 12-year-old who presented with a chest wall mass. A miniscule needle biopsy was obtained by interventional radiology. Touch preparation slides were made for preliminary cytology diagnosis and FISH; the remainder of the biopsy was formalin fixed and paraffin embedded. Morphology and immunostaining (CD99 strong membranous staining, myogenin, and cytokeratin AE1/3 negative) were consistent with a diagnosis of Ewing sarcoma. FISH with a commercially available *EWSR1* break-apart probe (Fig. 7.3a) was first performed on a touch preparation slide and repeated on an FFPE section to confirm the results, which were similar in both preparations. Only approximately 30% of the nuclei showed separation of one red and green signal, and the distance between the separated signals was less than expected for an *EWSR1* rearrangement resulting from a translocation with another chromosome (Fig. 7.3a). Review of the adjacent H&E stained FFPE slide showed that the majority of the biopsy consisted of tumor. Therefore, not only was the signal separation less than expected, but the percentage of nuclei with signal separation was low for the amount of tumor present, given that an *EWSR1* rearrangement would be expected to be present in most, if not nearly all of the tumor cells. In this case, the low percentage of positive nuclei is likely due to the small distance between split signals, which may not allow the signal separation to be resolved in many nuclei. This *EWSR1* break-apart probe result is not conclusive, but it is suggestive of an *EWSR1* rearrangement. Equivocal or even negative FISH results in Ewing sarcoma using the *EWSR1* break-apart probe have been described with variant *EWSR1* fusions involving *ERG* instead of the more common *FLI1* partner [48–50]. These *EWSR1/ERG* fusions may require alternative fusion probe FISH strategies or other molecular methods for detection due to the complex nature of the rearrangement, which involves a 22q inversion and insertion of 5′*EWSR1* into *ERG* on 21q [48–50]. FISH performed on the tumor in Fig. 7.3 using laboratory-developed, differentially labeled probes that span *EWSR1* and *ERG* confirmed an *EWSR1/ERG* fusion (Fig. 7.3b).

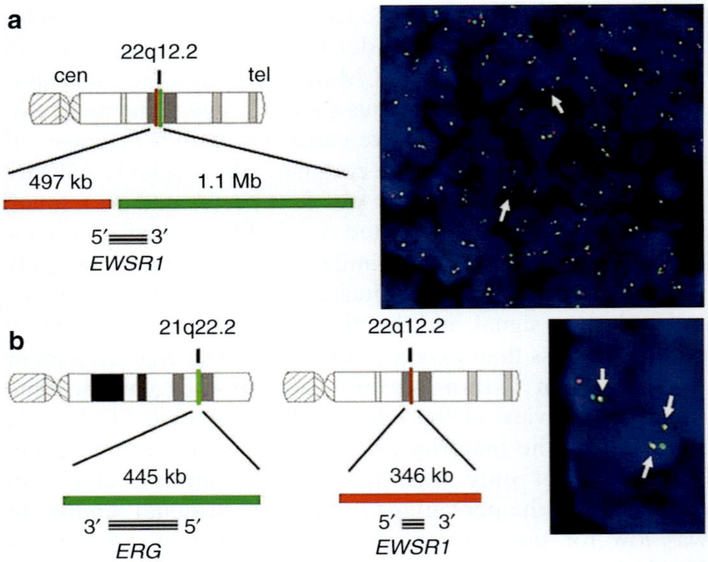

Figure 7.3 FISH performed on a Ewing sarcoma with an *EWSR1/ERG* fusion. (**a**) Map of *EWSR1* break-apart probe (left) and representative image of this probe hybridized to the tumor (right). Red and green bars represent the two halves of the break-apart probe in relation to the *EWSR1* gene. Arrows indicate representative nuclei with signal separation suggestive of an *EWSR1* rearrangement. (**b**) Map of *EWSR1* and *ERG* differentially labeled probes that span the genes (left) and representative image of this probe set hybridized to the tumor (right). Arrows indicate yellow fusion signals resulting from an *EWSR1/ERG* fusion

Limitations of FISH

As with any technology, FISH has its limitations, and there are many examples of cases in which FISH results are negative, but results utilizing an orthogonal method are positive and vice versa. False-negative FISH results can be due to a variety of variables, such as failure to score tumor nuclei or atypical rearrangements. For example, complex rearrangements, or submicroscopic insertions of part of a gene into another gene, have been documented to result in fusions that yield false-negative FISH results [48–50] (Figs. 7.3 and 7.4). The reverse is also true, and there are many examples of cases that are positive by FISH but negative by other methodologies. Break-apart probes may give a positive FISH result when RT-PCR is negative because of a rearrangement with a variant fusion partner that is not detected by the specific PCR primers used in the assay. Aberrant molecular results can also be encountered even if known fusion partners with unusual breakpoints are involved [51]. False-positive and false-negative FISH results can also be caused by misinterpretation of signal patterns. The possibility of a false-negative or false-positive result must always be considered when a FISH result is incongruent with morphology and other ancillary test results (Table 7.4).

Summary

The morphologic assessment of various types of cancer within a cytologic preparation may present challenges that can be further complicated when the quantity or quality of the sample falls short of processing requirements for ancillary studies, including an assessment of relevant molecular markers. Embracing the use of the various molecular methodologies with their differing strengths and weaknesses in the formulation of a diagnosis improves accuracy considerably as well as provides or predicts key features of tumor behavior such as progression and response to therapeutics. FISH is a method that is highly suitable for cytologic preparations, as tissue requirements are minimal and analysis permits direct *in situ* morphologic correlation. Familiarity with the pre-analytic and analytic factors that affect the success of FISH

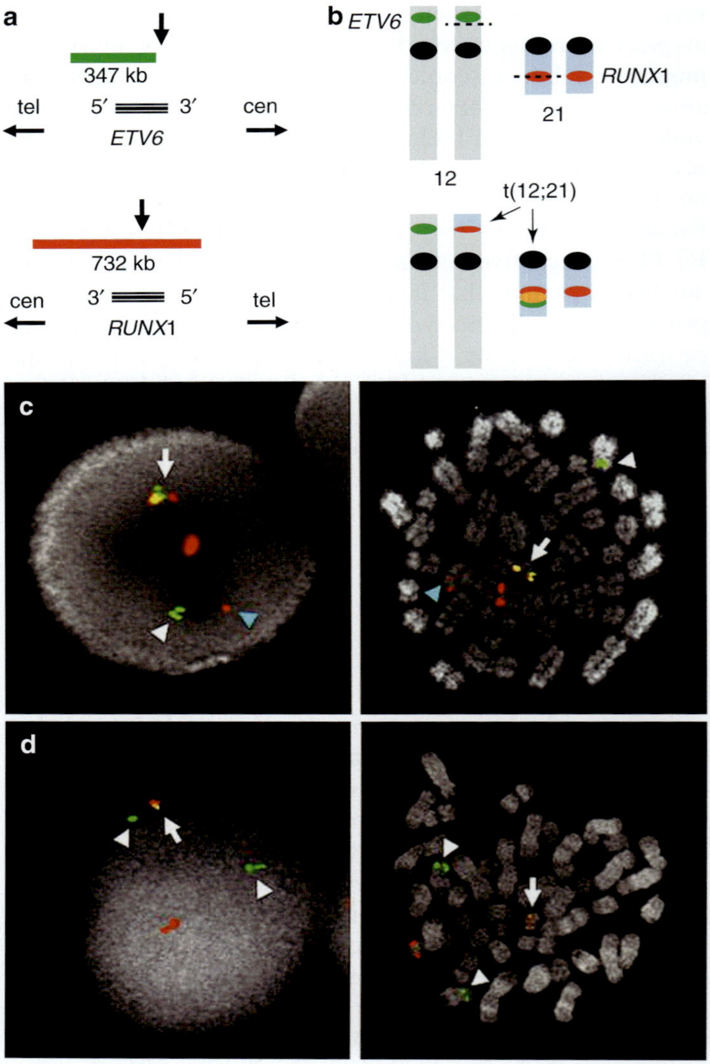
a
347 kb
tel
5′ 3′
cen
ETV6
732 kb
cen
3′ 5′
tel
RUNX1
b
ETV6
RUNX1
21
12
t(12;21)
c
d

FIGURE 7.4 FISH results illustrating a typical *ETV6/RUNX1* fusion resulting from a t(12;21) that occurs in acute lymphoblastic leukemia and a variant fusion due to an insertion of *ETV6* into *RUNX1*. (**a**) Probe map of the Vysis *ETV6/RUNX1* ES (extra signal) probe (Abbott Laboratories, Abbott Park, IL). The *ETV6* probe is labeled in green and the *RUNX1* probe is labeled in red. The location of the most common breakpoints relative to each gene and probe is designated by the vertical arrows. For *ETV6*, breakpoints are typically in the 15 kb intron 5, and for *RUNX1*, most breakpoints occur within the 155 kb intron 1 or the 5.5 kb intron 2. The direction of the centromere (cen) and telomere (tel) relative to the 5′ and 3′ ends of the genes is shown. (**b**) Schematic representation of the *ETV6* probe on 12p, *RUNX1* probe on 21q, location of breakpoints (dashed lines) with respect to the probes (top), and a typical t(12;21) showing relocation of probes and the subsequent signal pattern (bottom). Note that the breakpoint in 21q occurs within the *RUNX1* probe and the breakpoint in 12p occurs centromeric to the *ETV6* probe, resulting in relocation of a small red signal to 12p and an entire green signal to 21q to form a fusion signal. (**c**) Interphase (left) and metaphase (right) images from a typical t(12;21). There is an *ETV6/RUNX1* fusion signal on the derivative chromosome 21 (arrow), a small red *RUNX1* signal translocated from 21q to 12p (aqua arrowhead), a green *ETV6* signal on the normal 12p, and a red *RUNX1* signal on the normal chromosome 21. (**d**) Interphase (left) and metaphase (right) images from an insertion of a portion of the *ETV6* gene into *RUNX1*. In contrast to a typical *ETV6/RUNX1* fusion resulting from a t(12;21), both green signals are still located on the short arms of both chromosomes 12 (white arrowheads), and the two red signals are roughly equivalent in size and still located on the long arms of both chromosomes 21, with one chromosome 21 showing a barely visible fusion signal due to insertion of a portion of the green *ETV6* signal into *RUNX1*. These small fusion signals that result from insertions can be easily missed depending on the size of the inserted material

Table 7.4 Problematic scenarios encountered in interpretation of FISH results

Scenario	Possible explanations	Actions
The FISH result is unexpectedly negative given morphology and results of other ancillary tests	Specimen tested contains insufficient tumor cells	Review adjacent FFPE section or other stained slides for tumor content; repeat FISH with alternative slide if possible; consider possibility of true false-negative result if molecular test reveals low-level positivity
	Variant rearrangement below resolution of FISH or not detected with probe design/location	Consider FISH with alternative probe or orthogonal confirmatory molecular test
The FISH result is unexpectedly positive given morphology and results of other ancillary tests	Incorrect interpretation of FISH result	Consider false positive if result is low-level/close to cutoff or atypical abnormal signal pattern (see below); consider FISH with alternative probe or orthogonal molecular test

The FISH result gives an abnormal signal pattern that is atypical (e.g., break-apart probe with loss of 5′ or 3′ probe signal instead of split signals)	Could represent true-positive result (e.g., 5′ loss of signal positive for *ALK* rearrangement)	Determine if the pattern makes sense in light of whether or not the gene analyzed is contributing to the 5′ or 3′ end of the active fusion of interest; consider alternative testing for abnormality (different FISH probes, molecular test)
	Could represent true-negative result (e.g., some cases with loss of *MLL* are negative for a rearrangement)	Consult literature; if not previously reported, consider alternative testing for abnormality (different FISH probes, molecular test)
FISH results with alternative probes for the same locus give conflicting results	Could represent a true-positive or true-negative result	Review probe mapping in relation to gene/locus and known breakpoints; consider molecular testing

performance on clinical cytopathologic specimens and the measures to overcome them is necessary for optimal test performance. Knowledge of post-analytic factors is critical for proper interpretation of FISH results.

Acknowledgments The authors thank Billy Davis and Xiao-Qiong Liu for their assistance with the figures.

References

1. Brockman SR, Paternoster SF, Ketterling RP, Dewald GW. New highly sensitive fluorescence in situ hybridization method to detect PML/RARA fusion in acute promyelocytic leukemia. Cancer Genet Cytogenet. 2003;145(2):144–51.
2. Roy-Chowdhuri S, Goswami RS, Chen H, Patel KP, Routbort MJ, Singh RR, et al. Factors affecting the success of next-generation sequencing in cytology specimens. Cancer Cytopathol. 2015;123(11):659–68.
3. Bridge JA. Reverse transcription-polymerase chain reaction molecular testing of cytology specimens: pre-analytic and analytic factors. Cancer Cytopathol. 2017;125(1):11–9.
4. Knoepp SM, Roh MH. Ancillary techniques on direct-smear aspirate slides: a significant evolution for cytopathology techniques. Cancer Cytopathol. 2013;121(3):120–8.
5. Savic S, Bubendorf L. Common fluorescence in situ hybridization applications in cytology. Arch Pathol Lab Med. 2016;140(12):1323–30.
6. Wolff AC, Hammond ME, Hicks DG, Dowsett M, McShane LM, Allison KH, et al. Recommendations for human epidermal growth factor receptor 2 testing in breast cancer: American Society of Clinical Oncology/College of American Pathologists clinical practice guideline update. J Clin Oncol. 2013;31(31):3997–4013.
7. Monaco SE, Teot LA, Felgar RE, Surti U, Cai G. Fluorescence in situ hybridization studies on direct smears: an approach to enhance the fine-needle aspiration biopsy diagnosis of B-cell non-Hodgkin lymphomas. Cancer. 2009;117(5):338–48.
8. Bozzetti C, Nizzoli R, Tiseo M, Squadrilli A, Lagrasta C, Buti S, et al. ALK and ROS1 rearrangements tested by fluorescence in

situ hybridization in cytological smears from advanced non-small cell lung cancer patients. Diagn Cytopathol. 2015;43(11):941–6.

9. Bravaccini S, Tumedei MM, Ulivi P, Zoli W, Calistri D, Candoli P, et al. ALK translocation detection in non-small cell lung cancer cytological samples obtained by TBNA or EBUS-TBNA. Cytopathology. 2016;27(2):103–7.
10. Bentz JS, Rowe LR, Anderson SR, Gupta PK, McGrath CM. Rapid detection of the t(11;14) translocation in mantle cell lymphoma by interphase fluorescence in situ hybridization on archival cytopathologic material. Cancer. 2004;102(2):124–31.
11. Richmond J, Bryant R, Trotman W, Beatty B, Lunde J. FISH detection of t(14;18) in follicular lymphoma on Papanicolaou-stained archival cytology slides. Cancer. 2006;108(3):198–204.
12. Killian JK, Walker RL, Suuriniemi M, Jones L, Scurci S, Singh P, et al. Archival fine-needle aspiration cytopathology (FNAC) samples. untapped resource for clinical molecular profiling J Mol Diagn. 2010;12(6):739–45.
13. Betz BL, Dixon CA, Weigelin HC, Knoepp SM, Roh MH. The use of stained cytologic direct smears for ALK gene rearrangement analysis of lung adenocarcinoma. Cancer Cytopathol. 2013;121(9):489–99.
14. Zito Marino F, Rossi G, Brunelli M, Malzone MG, Liguori G, Bogina G, et al. Diagnosis of anaplastic lymphoma kinase rearrangement in cytological samples through a fluorescence in situ hybridization-based assay: cytological smears versus cell blocks. Cancer Cytopathol. 2017 May;125(5):303–12.
15. da Cunha Santos G, Ko HM, Geddie WR, Boerner SL, Lai SW, Have C, et al. Targeted use of fluorescence in situ hybridization (FISH) in cytospin preparations: results of 298 fine needle aspirates of B-cell non-Hodgkin lymphoma. Cancer Cytopathol. 2010;118(5):250–8.
16. Horton Y, Ford A, MacKie MJ, Johnson PR. Rapid detection of BCR/ABL and PML/RARA using fluorescence in situ hybridization in cytospin preparations. Clin Lab Haematol. 2000;22(2):97–102.
17. Zellweger T, Benz G, Cathomas G, Mihatsch MJ, Sulser T, Gasser TC, et al. Multi-target fluorescence in situ hybridization in bladder washings for prediction of recurrent bladder cancer. Int J Cancer. 2006;119(7):1660–5.
18. Srebotnik-Kirbis I, Limback-Stokin C. Application of brush cytology for FISH-based detection of 1p/19q codeletion in oligodendroglial tumors. J Neuro-Oncol. 2016;129(3):415–22.

19. Martini M, Capodimonti S, Cenci T, Bilotta M, Fadda G, Larocca LM, et al. To obtain more with less: Cytologic samples with ancillary molecular techniques-the useful role of liquid-based cytology. Arch Pathol Lab Med. 2018;142(3):299–307.
20. Kumagai A, Motoi T, Tsuji K, Imamura T, Fukusato T. Detection of SYT and EWS gene rearrangements by dual-color break-apart CISH in liquid-based cytology samples of synovial sarcoma and Ewing sarcoma/primitive neuroectodermal tumor. Am J Clin Pathol. 2010;134(2):323–31.
21. Minca EC, Lanigan CP, Reynolds JP, Wang Z, Ma PC, Cicenia J, et al. ALK status testing in non-small-cell lung carcinoma by FISH on ThinPrep slides with cytology material. J Thorac Oncol. 2014;9(4):464–8.
22. Rosenblum F, Hutchinson LM, Garver J, Woda B, Cosar E, Kurian EM. Cytology specimens offer an effective alternative to formalin-fixed tissue as demonstrated by novel automated detection for ALK break-apart FISH testing and immunohistochemistry in lung adenocarcinoma. Cancer Cytopathol. 2014;122(11):810–21.
23. Abati A, Sanford JS, Fetsch P, Marincola FM, Wolman SR. Fluorescence in situ hybridization (FISH): a user's guide to optimal preparation of cytologic specimens. Diagn Cytopathol. 1995;13(5):486–92.
24. Alers JC, Krijtenburg PJ, Vissers KJ, van Dekken H. Effect of bone decalcification procedures on DNA in situ hybridization and comparative genomic hybridization. EDTA is highly preferable to a routinely used acid decalcifier. J Histochem Cytochem. 1999;47(5):703–10.
25. Babic A, Loftin IR, Stanislaw S, Wang M, Miller R, Warren SM, et al. The impact of pre-analytical processing on staining quality for H&E, dual hapten, dual color in situ hybridization and fluorescent in situ hybridization assays. Methods. 2010;52(4):287–300.
26. Brown RS, Edwards J, Bartlett JW, Jones C, Dogan A. Routine acid decalcification of bone marrow samples can preserve DNA for FISH and CGH studies in metastatic prostate cancer. J Histochem Cytochem. 2002;50(1):113–5.
27. Neat MJ, Moonim MT, Dunn RG, Geoghegan H, Foot NJ. Fluorescence in situ hybridisation analysis of bone marrow trephine biopsy specimens; an additional tool in the diagnostic armoury. J Clin Pathol. 2013;66(1):54–7.
28. Schrijver WA, van der Groep P, Hoefnagel LD, Ter Hoeve ND, Peeters T, Moelans CB, et al. Influence of decalcification pro-

cedures on immunohistochemistry and molecular pathology in breast cancer. Mod Pathol. 2016;29(12):1460–70.
29. Bartley AN, Washington MK, Ventura CB, Ismaila N, Colasacco C, Benson AB 3rd, et al. HER2 testing and clinical decision making in Gastroesophageal adenocarcinoma: guideline from the College of American Pathologists, American Society for Clinical Pathology, and American Society of Clinical Oncology. Arch Pathol Lab Med. 2016;140(12):1345–63.
30. Yamashita-Kashima Y, Shu S, Yorozu K, Hashizume K, Moriya Y, Fujimoto-Ouchi K, et al. Importance of formalin fixing conditions for HER2 testing in gastric cancer: immunohistochemical staining and fluorescence in situ hybridization. Gastric Cancer. 2014;17(4):638–47.
31. Khoury T, Liu Q, Liu S. Delay to formalin fixation effect on HER2 test in breast cancer by dual-color silver-enhanced in situ hybridization (dual-ISH). Appl Immunohistochem Mol Morphol. 2014;22(9):688–95.
32. Portier BP, Wang Z, Downs-Kelly E, Rowe JJ, Patil D, Lanigan C, et al. Delay to formalin fixation 'cold ischemia time': effect on ERBB2 detection by in-situ hybridization and immunohistochemistry. Mod Pathol. 2013;26(1):1–9.
33. Mascarello JT, Coley LD, Dowling PK, Garcia MV, Jewell SS, Philip R, et al. Fluorescence in situ hybridization methods for clinical laboratories; approved guideline. 2nd ed. Wayne: Clinical and Laboratory Standards Institute; 2013.
34. Lindeman NI, Cagle PT, Beasley MB, Chitale DA, Dacic S, Giaccone G, et al. Molecular testing guideline for selection of lung cancer patients for EGFR and ALK tyrosine kinase inhibitors: guideline from the College of American Pathologists, International Association for the Study of Lung Cancer, and Association for Molecular Pathology. Arch Pathol Lab Med. 2013;137(6):828–60.
35. Lawce HJ, Sanford JS. Fluorescence in situ hybridization (FISH). In: Arsham MS, Barch MJ, Lawce HJ, editors. The AGT Cytogenetics laboratory manual. 4th ed. Hoboken: John Wiley & Sons, Inc.; 2017. p. 717–824.
36. Mascarello JT, Hirsch B, Kearney HM, Ketterling RP, Olson SB, Quigley DI, et al. Section E9 of the American College of Medical Genetics technical standards and guidelines: fluorescence in situ hybridization. Genet Med. 2011;13(7):667–75.
37. Tafe LJ, Allen SF, Steinmetz HB, Dokus BA, Cook LJ, Marotti JD, et al. Automated processing of fluorescence in-situ hybrid-

ization slides for HER2 testing in breast and gastro-esophageal carcinomas. Exp Mol Pathol. 2014;97(1):116–9.
38. Viale G, Paterson J, Bloch M, Csathy G, Allen D, Dell'Orto P, et al. Assessment of HER2 amplification status in breast cancer using a new automated HER2 IQFISH pharmDx (Dako Omnis) assay. Pathol Res Pract. 2016;212(8):735–42.
39. Zwaenepoel K, Merkle D, Cabillic F, Berg E, Belaud-Rotureau MA, Grazioli V, et al. Automation of ALK gene rearrangement testing with fluorescence in situ hybridization (FISH): a feasibility study. Exp Mol Pathol. 2015;98(1):113–8.
40. Thakral G, Wey A, Rahman M, Fang R, Lum C. Agreement of different methods for tissue based detection of HER2 signal in invasive breast Cancer. Pathol Oncol Res. 2017;23(1):79–84.
41. Stevens R, Almanaseer I, Gonzalez M, Caglar D, Knudson RA, Ketterling RP, et al. Analysis of HER2 gene amplification using an automated fluorescence in situ hybridization signal enumeration system. J Mol Diagn. 2007;9(2):144–50.
42. Barber KE, Ford AM, Harris RL, Harrison CJ, Moorman AV. MLL translocations with concurrent 3′ deletions: interpretation of FISH results. Genes Chromosomes Cancer. 2004;41(3):266–71.
43. Jones DT, Kocialkowski S, Liu L, Pearson DM, Backlund LM, Ichimura K, et al. Tandem duplication producing a novel oncogenic BRAF fusion gene defines the majority of pilocytic astrocytomas. Cancer Res. 2008;68(21):8673–7.
44. Sievert AJ, Jackson EM, Gai X, Hakonarson H, Judkins AR, Resnick AC, et al. Duplication of 7q34 in pediatric low-grade astrocytomas detected by high-density single-nucleotide polymorphism-based genotype arrays results in a novel BRAF fusion gene. Brain Pathol. 2009;19(3):449–58.
45. Einerson RR, Law ME, Blair HE, Kurtin PJ, McClure RF, Ketterling RP, et al. Novel FISH probes designed to detect IGK-MYC and IGL-MYC rearrangements in B-cell lineage malignancy identify a new breakpoint cluster region designated BVR2. Leukemia. 2006;20(10):1790–9.
46. Munoz-Marmol AM, Sanz C, Tapia G, Marginet R, Ariza A, Mate JL. MYC status determination in aggressive B-cell lymphoma: the impact of FISH probe selection. Histopathology. 2013;63(3):418–24.
47. Ambros PF, Ambros IM, Brodeur GM, Haber M, Khan J, Nakagawara A, et al. International consensus for neuroblastoma molecular diagnostics: report from the international

Neuroblastoma risk group (INRG) biology committee. Br J Cancer. 2009;100(9):1471–82.
48. Peled N, Palmer G, Hirsch FR, Wynes MW, Ilouze M, Varella-Garcia M, et al. Next-generation sequencing identifies and immunohistochemistry confirms a novel crizotinib-sensitive ALK rearrangement in a patient with metastatic non-small-cell lung cancer. J Thorac Oncol. 2012;7(9):e14–6.
49. Campbell LJ, Oei P, Brookwell R, Shortt J, Eaddy N, Ng A, et al. FISH detection of PML-RARA fusion in ins(15;17) acute promyelocytic leukaemia depends on probe size. Biomed Res Int. 2013;2013:164501.
50. Chen S, Deniz K, Sung YS, Zhang L, Dry S, Antonescu CR. Ewing sarcoma with ERG gene rearrangements: a molecular study focusing on the prevalence of FUS-ERG and common pitfalls in detecting EWSR1-ERG fusions by FISH. Genes Chromosomes Cancer. 2016;55(4):340–9.
51. Safar A, Wickert R, Nelson M, Neff JR, Bridge JA. Characterization of a variant SYT-SSX1 synovial sarcoma fusion transcript. Diagn Mol Pathol. 1998;7(5):283–7.

Chapter 8
Molecular Cytopathology Correlations: Interpretation of Molecular Diagnostic Results

Sinchita Roy-Chowdhuri

Abbreviations

ASCUS	Atypical squamous cells of undetermined significance
AUC	Atypical urothelial cells
BRAF	v-raf murine sarcoma viral oncogene homolog B
DNA	Deoxyribonucleic acid
EGFR	Epidermal growth factor receptor
FISH	Fluorescence *in situ* hybridization
FNA	Fine-needle aspiration
GNA11	Guanine nucleotide-binding protein subunit alpha-11
GNAQ	Guanine nucleotide-binding protein G(q) subunit alpha
H&E	Hematoxylin and eosin
HPV	Human papilloma virus
IgH	Immunoglobulin heavy chain

S. Roy-Chowdhuri
MD Anderson Cancer Center, The University of Texas,
Houston, TX, USA
e-mail: sroy2@mdanderson.org

S. Roy-Chowdhuri et al. (eds.), *Molecular Diagnostics in Cytopathology*, https://doi.org/10.1007/978-3-319-97397-5_8

PCR	Polymerase chain reaction
QNS	Quantity not sufficient
TCR	T-cell receptor
TKI	Tyrosine kinase inhibitor

Key Terminology

Allele	Variant form of a gene. Each gene has two copies that are inherited from each parent and may differ from each other resulting in a variant form or allele
Analytic sensitivity	Lowest limit of detection of an assay where it reliably and reproducibly detects the target analyte
Germline mutation	Inherited genetic alterations that occur in the reproductive/germ cells (i.e., sperm and eggs) and becomes incorporated into the DNA of every cell in the body. Germline mutations are passed from parents to offspring and are also referred to as hereditary mutations
Heterozygous	Most diploid cells such as tumor cells contain two different alleles at any gene locus
Macrodissection	Tissue extraction from a slide without the need of a microscope (usually large area that can be grossly visualized)
Microdissection	Tissue extraction requiring a dissecting microscope or by laser capture microscopy (usually from small areas demarcated on a slide that cannot be well-visualized without a microscope)
Mutant	Any form of an allele other than the wild type is a variant or mutant allele. While variants can represent polymorphisms common to the popula-

	tion (>1% of the population), mutant usually refers to variation that are detected in <1% of the population
Resistance mutation	Acquired somatic mutation that develops as a mechanism of resistance against a targeted therapy
Sample cellularity	Total number of nucleated cells within a sample that contributes to the total DNA yield
Sensitizing mutation	Somatic mutation that will make the patient sensitive to treatment by a specific targeted therapy
Somatic mutation	Genetic alteration acquired by a tumor cell that can be passed to the progeny of the mutated tumor cell during cell division. Somatic mutations that cause cancer will be present only within the tumor where they occur
Tumor enrichment	The process of demarcating tumor-rich areas on a slide to increase the tumor fraction in a sample during tissue extraction
Tumor fraction	Percentage of tumor cells in a sample. The analytic threshold for T% is defined as the minimum amount of tumor DNA that can be reliably detected in a background of wild-type DNA. Calculated by the total number of tumor cells divided by the total number of all nucleated cells. Also referred to as tumor cellularity and tumor proportion
Wild type	A phenotype/genotype/gene that predominates in a natural population. Wild-type allele is the one that is the most common one in the natural population

Key Points

- Always interpret molecular results in context of the clinical and cytopathologic findings
- Use molecular assays as an ancillary study that complements the cytologic findings and helps guide the final diagnosis
- Understand the basic principles and limitations of the molecular assay being used for appropriate molecular cytopathologic correlation
- Reevaluate the cytology sample anytime there is a negative molecular result to exclude the possibility of a false-negative result
- Review the cytology together with the clinical history when there is an unexpected molecular result or novel finding or when the molecular results are discordant with the tumor type/clinical context

The widespread implementation of molecular testing in cytopathology specimens has highlighted the importance of a basic understanding of the principles of molecular assays [1–4]. While an in-depth knowledge of molecular assay test development and technical detail may not be needed by the cytopathologist, an appreciation of the key elements of assay interpretation and reporting is important for molecular cytopathologic correlation [5]. Understanding the basic principles of molecular diagnostics and how factors related to specimen selection and handling influence molecular assay results will ultimately lead to better selection of cytology tissue for molecular testing [6].

For instance, the analytic sensitivity of an assay directly relates to the proportion of tumor cells within a sample (Fig. 8.1). In other words, the higher the analytic sensitivity of an assay, the better it is at analyzing samples with low tumor fractions [1, 7]. Therefore, to avoid the risk of a false-negative result, a cytopathologist selecting a low tumor fraction tissue sample for molecular testing needs to opt for an assay with a

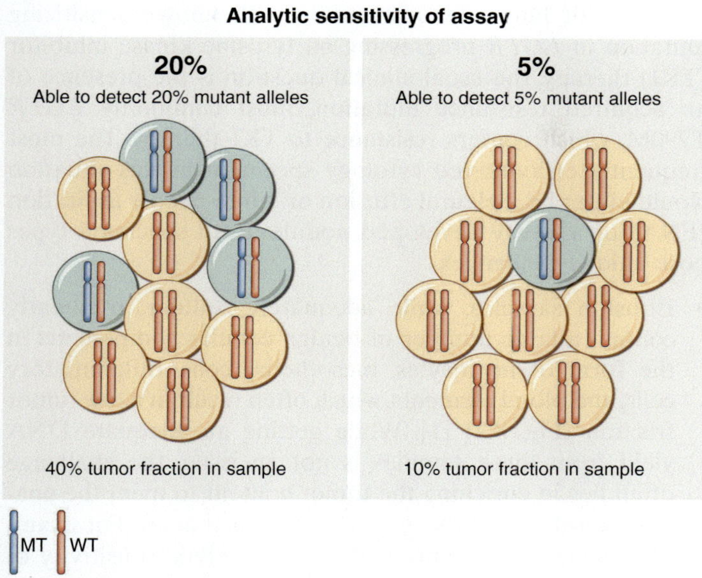

FIGURE 8.1 The analytic sensitivity of a molecular assay is directly related to the proportion of tumor cells within the sample. Assuming most tumor cells are heterozygous, a sample with 40% tumor cells will have only 20% of the alleles that are mutant. Therefore, in this sample, an assay with a minimum analytic sensitivity of 20% is needed to detect the mutant allele present only in the tumor cells. Similarly, a sample with only 10% tumor cells will require an assay with an analytic sensitivity of at least 5% to reliably detect the 5% mutant alleles present within the sample. Abbreviations: MT mutant allele, WT wild-type allele

high analytic sensitivity (see Chap. 4 for more details). This just underscores the need for clear communication between the cytopathologist sending tissue for molecular testing and the molecular laboratory performing the assay with clear guidelines outlining selection/rejection criteria for each of the assays performed [6].

The interpretation of molecular test results also requires a working knowledge of the molecular pathology of the selected tumor and the clinical context. For example, in a patient with lung adenocarcinoma with known sensitizing mutation in *EGFR* progressing on tyrosine kinase inhibitor (TKI) therapy, the usual clinical question is the presence of an acquired resistance mutation, most commonly *EGFR* T790M, which confers resistance to TKI therapy. The most frequently encountered cytology specimen in this situation would either be a pleural effusion or a fine-needle aspiration (FNA) of a newly developed nodule. Both specimen types pose unique challenges.

- Effusion samples, while adequately cellular, frequently contain a large number of benign cellular components in the form of histiocytes, mesothelial cells, inflammatory cells, and blood elements, which often result in a low tumor fraction (Fig. 8.2) [1]. While getting an adequate DNA yield from these samples is not an issue, the challenge often lies in enriching the tumor content to meet the analytic sensitivity of the *EGFR* mutational assay. For example, Sanger sequencing with a low analytic sensitivity of 15–20% would require a tumor sample to be enriched to comprise at least 30–40% tumor fraction to be adequate for analysis. In these situations, selecting a high-sensitivity assay that aligns with the low tumor fraction is critical to avoid risking a false-negative result. It is important to remember that tumor fraction can be enhanced in some situations by circling tumor-rich areas on the slide for macro- or microdissection and eliminating areas that have

Figure 8.2 A Papanicolaou-stained cytospin preparation of a pleural fluid where most areas in the slide show small clusters and scattered malignant cells admixed with numerous non-tumor cells (top panel). The tumor fraction in this sample is, therefore, diluted by the benign cells in the background. However, the areas near the edge of the preparation show higher tumor fraction (bottom panel) and have been circled for microdissection. This tumor mapping increases the tumor fraction in the extracted sample (circled tumor-rich areas), but at the cost of lowering the total number of cells that could be used for extraction (entire slide)

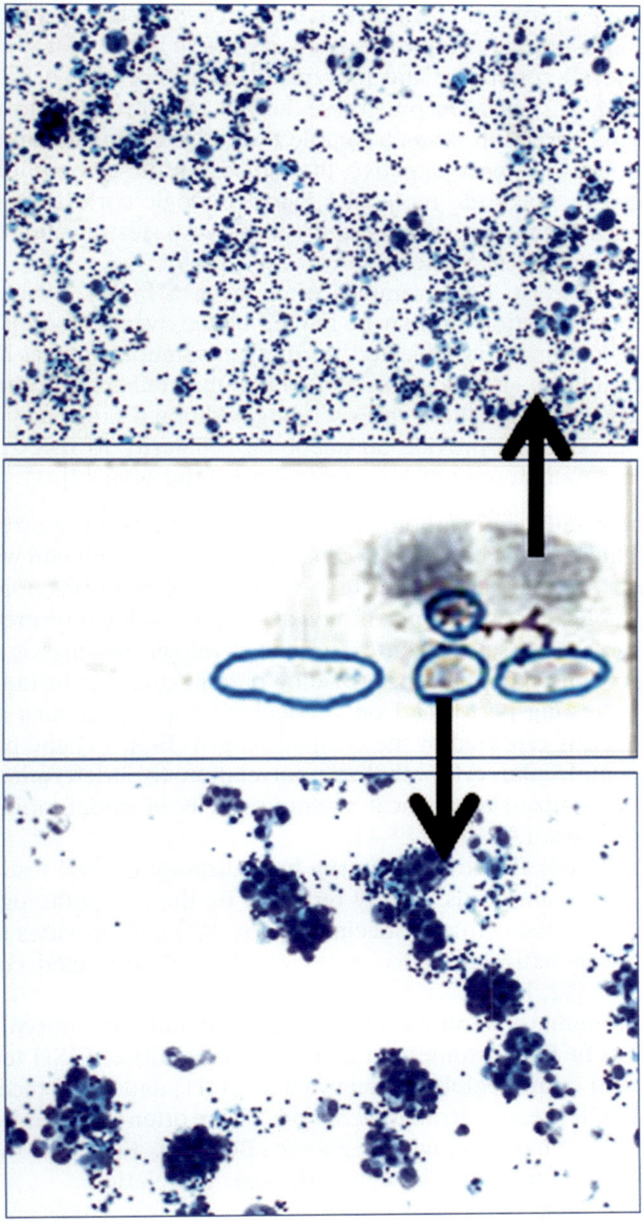

higher proportions of benign cells [1, 6–8]. While this technique improves tumor fraction, it does so at the cost of the overall cellularity and may result in a lower DNA yield (Fig. 8.2) [7]. Despite these heroic measures to ensure tumor fraction, when a sample tested for resistance mutation comes back negative, the onus is on the cytopathologist to make the molecular cytopathologic correlation to ensure that an appropriate sample was tested and the result reflects a true negative.

- In contrast, FNA samples often have a highly enriched tumor fraction but may be limited by the overall amount of cellular material collected, resulting in a sample that has low cellularity and a low DNA yield that may fail amplification. Therefore, for these cases sending additional slides may be necessary to provide an adequate cellularity to meet the minimum input DNA requirements of the assay [7].

Molecular cytopathologic correlations are a two-way street, and the responsibility of the cytopathologist does not end with the triage and selecting of tissue for molecular testing. Once the molecular assay is performed and reported, the interpretation of the assay in context of the cytologic findings is an important component of providing patient care. For instance, HPV testing performed on cervical cytology specimens are frequently reported by the cytopathologist (Box. 8.1) and provide molecular cytopathologic correlation to indeterminate cases finalized as atypical squamous cells of undetermined significance (ASCUS) [9–11].

Similarly, fluorescence *in situ* hybridization (FISH) testing on urine samples is usually reported by the cytopathologist reviewing the cytology specimen (Box. 8.2) and provides the necessary correlation for cases of atypical urothelial cells (AUC) [12, 13].

In hematolymphoid malignancies, immunophenotyping results by flow cytometry and molecular results of FISH testing and immunoglobulin heavy chain (IgH) and T-cell receptor (TCR) gene rearrangements [14, 15] are often incorporated into the final cytologic diagnosis (Box. 8.3, Fig. 8.3), thus providing the molecular cytopathologic correlation.

Box 8.1 A sample cytopathology report showing the cytologic results of the Pap test with the HPV test results in an addendum. The molecular test is interpreted in context of the cytomorphologic assessment.

Specimen source:
Cervix, liquid-based prep

Specimen adequacy:
Satisfactory for evaluation
Endocervical/transformation zone component present

Diagnosis:
Atypical squamous cells of undetermined significance (ASCUS)

Supplemental report:
Cervista(TM) HPV HR assay is POSITIVE for high-risk type(s) of HPV.

The HPV assay was performed using the Cervista(TM) high-risk HPV DNA test (Hologic, Madison, WI). The HPV high-risk panel tests for human papillomavirus (HPV) types 16, 18, 31, 33, 35, 39, 45, 51, 52, 56, 58, 59, 66, and 68. A positive test indicates the presence of one or more HPV types.

Control samples were run with appropriate results.

While the assays are performed and interpreted by qualified molecular pathologists/geneticists, the clinicopathologic correlation remains the responsibility of the cytopathologist reviewing the cytology sample [6]. Therefore, other high complexity molecular testing such as DNA-based assays, gene expression analyses, and proteomic assays that are routinely performed using cytology specimens for diagnostic, predictive, and prognostic information need to be interpreted in

Box 8.2 A sample urine cytology report with the fluorescence *in situ* hybridization (FISH) testing results correlated with the final interpretation. A subsequent follow-up biopsy showed high-grade urothelial carcinoma.

Specimen source:
A. Urine, voided

Gross description:
50 ml. yellow fluid

Diagnosis:
Few atypical urothelial cells, suspicious for high-grade urothelial carcinoma (see comment)

Comments:
Fluorescence *in situ* hybridization studies using the UroVysion kit demonstrated 25 of 25 cells analyzed with an abnormal signal pattern which equates to a positive result (4 or more cells is a positive result defined as cells with polysomy for probed areas on at least two of the following chromosomes, 3, 7, 17, and 9p21, 12 or more cells with no signal for chromosome 9 and/or 10, or more cells with 4 signals for each probe). These findings suggest the presence of high-grade urothelial carcinoma; however slides prepared for cytomorphologic evaluation do not display such worrisome features. Consequently, since there is a disconnect between the UroVysion findings and cytomorphology, a more definitive diagnosis is not rendered. Continued close follow-up and/or cystoscopy with biopsy is therefore recommended.

Box 8.3 A sample cytopathology report of a lymph node fine-needle aspiration (FNA) with morphologic evaluation, flow cytometry, and immunohistochemical results, supporting a diagnosis of high-grade B-cell lymphoma. In addition, fluorescence *in situ* hybridization (FISH) performed using a break-apart probe showed a *MYC* rearrangement (Fig. 8.3) that supports the final cytopathologic interpretation.

Specimen source:
A. Lymph node, left inguinal, FNA

Gross description:
2 cm mass

Diagnosis:
Large B-cell lymphoma, favor high grade (see comment)

Comment:
The neoplastic cells are large and highly atypical with lobation of the nuclei. Concurrent flow cytometry immunophenotyping demonstrates a kappa-restricted B-cell population that is positive for CD5 (partial), CD10, CD19, CD20, CD22, CD38, and CD44 but negative for CD11c, CD23, CD30, CD34, CD43, CD200, and lambda light chains.

Immunoperoxidase stains performed on cytospin preparations confirm the presence of a kappa-restricted population of B cells and positive CD20 stain. CD3 highlights background T cells. The proliferation rate (Ki-67) is approximately 90%. EBER ISH is negative.

c-MYC status by FISH was ordered on a cytospin preparation, and the result will be reported separately.

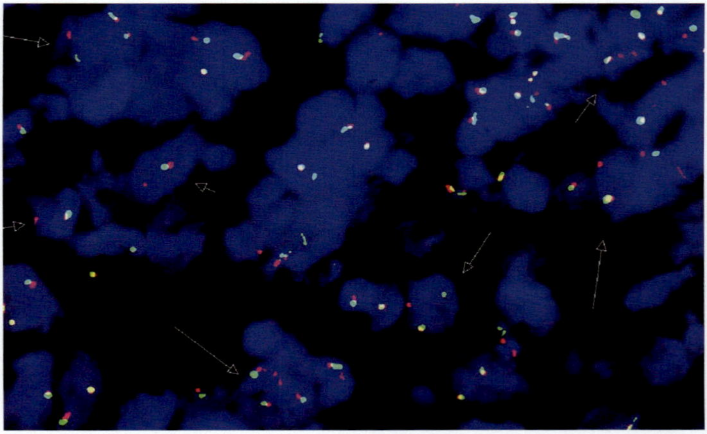

Figure 8.3 Fluorescence *in situ* hybridization (FISH) performed on a cytospin preparation using a break-apart probe shows *MYC* rearrangement (arrows) that supports the final cytopathologic interpretation of a high-grade large cell lymphoma

context of the clinical and cytopathologic findings, making the role of the cytopathologist critical in correlating these results [16]. Some common scenarios outlining the role of the cytopathologist in interpreting and correlating molecular testing results are highlighted in Table 8.1.

TABLE 8.1 Common scenarios for the cytopathologist with molecular cytopathology correlations

Response to the molecular result	Molecular cytopathologic correlation
Molecular result: negative *True negative* vs *false negative*	
"The mutational analysis did not detect any somatic mutations"	Review the sample that was sent for testing, and make sure it had adequate tumor fraction to ensure the result is not a false-negative
	If a small tumor-rich area was circled, check if lab truly employed microdissection, since extracting the entire slide instead of the designated tumor-rich area might dilute the mutant allele and cause false-negative results
	In case of cell blocks, where the unstained deeper sections may not always match the tissue section in the H&E slide (that serves as a guide), extracting from subsequent levels might miss the actual circled tumor-rich area, especially if the circled area is small and focal

(continued)

TABLE 8.1 (continued)

Response to the molecular result	Molecular cytopathologic correlation
"How can the molecular result be negative? The primary tumor tested on the outside showed a mutation"	Compare the morphology. The current tumor tested may be a different primary. Additional ancillary studies, such as immunostaining, may be needed for further evaluation
	The methodology for testing may be different, and analytic sensitivities can be different. Check to make sure the current assay has a high analytic sensitivity to preclude a false-negative result
	Check the outside molecular report for the coverage of the assay. In hotspot-based mutation testing, the assays may not be analyzing the same codons in the gene. It is important to verify that the coverage of the current assay includes the same area where the mutation was detected by the prior assay
Molecular result: quantity not sufficient (QNS)	
"I sent the required 10 unstained slides from the cell block to the molecular lab. How could the assay fail?"	Review the sample that was sent for testing, and make sure it had adequate cellularity. Low cellularity cell blocks will likely need more unstained slides sent, often more than what the usual policy is. Cases with borderline DNA yield can frequently be made "adequate" by sending in additional slides

TABLE 8.1 (continued)

"The smears I sent to the molecular lab had abundant cells. Why did the test fail?"	If smears were sent for testing that had adequate cellularity, check the glass slides post-extraction to ensure the cells were actually scraped/lifted off the slides. Tissue extraction techniques vary, and sometimes slides may retain cells even post-extraction
Molecular result: positive, *but…*	
"Wait…there's a mutation in *never-heard-of-that-before* gene? What does that mean?"	When a novel mutation is detected, it is may be worthwhile checking some of the databases that catalog somatic mutations in different tumor types. Always check validity of "somatic" claims by performing a literature search and reviewing the article
When the mutation detected doesn't make sense to the tumor type	While it is possible to have any mutation, in any tumor type (it's a tumor; it's allowed to do whatever it wants), certain mutations are well characterized in certain tumor types, and detecting them in another tumor would be uncommon. Therefore, (i) confirming for possible sample mix-up and (ii) reviewing the tumor type and doing immunostains to confirm the primary tumor site may be necessary
The mutation detected in the metastasis doesn't match the mutation profile of the primary tumor	While metastatic tumors may have some discordance with the mutation profile of the primary tumor from a divergent subclonal population in the metastasis, it is important to ensure (i) the metastasis does not represent a different primary tumor and (ii) rule out the possibility of a specimen mix-up

(continued)

TABLE 8.1 (continued)

Response to the molecular result	Molecular cytopathologic correlation
When the test result is unexpectedly positive	If a FISH result is unexpectedly positive (morphologically benign specimen) or novel mutations detected are unusual, it may be necessary to exclude the possibility of a false-positive molecular result. Having clear communication with the molecular pathologist is often key to resolving these situations
Molecular result: clues to a puzzle? *Some examples*	
"There's a *GNAQ* mutation in this metastatic melanoma to the liver. But the patient's known primary tumor in the skin had a *BRAF* V600E mutation"	When the mutation profile is unexpected, it is helpful to explore the possibilities. *GNAQ* (and *GNA11*) mutations are mostly seen in uveal melanomas, and these tumors frequently metastasize to the liver. In this situation, it would be necessary to recommend having the patient evaluated for a possible uveal melanoma
"There's an *EGFR* T790M mutation, but this is a new lung adenocarcinoma patient who has not been treated with TKI yet"	*EGFR* T790M is the most commonly acquired resistance mutation to TKI therapy. So in a treatment-naïve patient, explore the possibility of a germline mutation. Testing the peripheral blood or a normal tissue sample may be helpful
"There is an *IDH1* and *KRAS* mutation in this adenocarcinoma of unknown primary liver FNA"	Certain mutations are well characterized in specific tumor types that may serve as diagnostic clues. For instance, *IDH1* and *KRAS* mutations are often seen in cholangiocarcinomas and therefore in this situation would prompt the clinician to evaluate for a potential cholangiocarcinoma

References

1. Aisner DL, Sams SB. The role of cytology specimens in molecular testing of solid tumors: techniques, limitations, and opportunities. Diagn Cytopathol. 2012;40(6):511–24.
2. Salto-Tellez M, Koay ES. Molecular diagnostic cytopathology: definitions, scope and clinical utility. Cytopathology. 2004;15(5):252–5.
3. Schmitt FC. Molecular cytopathology and flow cytometry: pre-analytical procedures matter. Cytopathology. 2011;22(6):355–7.
4. Schmitt FC. Demystifying molecular cytopathology. Int J Surg Pathol. 2010;18(3 Suppl):213S–5S.
5. Goals and objectives for molecular pathology education in residency programs. The Association for Molecular Pathology Training and Education Committee. J Mol Diagn. 1999;1(1):5–15.
6. Roy-Chowdhuri S, Aisner DL, Allen TC, Beasley MB, Borczuk A, Cagle PT, et al. Biomarker testing in lung carcinoma cytology specimens: a perspective from members of the pulmonary pathology society. Arch Pathol Lab Med. 2016;14(11):1267–72.
7. Roy-Chowdhuri S, Stewart J. Preanalytic variables in cytology: lessons learned from next-generation sequencing-the MD Anderson experience. Arch Pathol Lab Med. 2016;140(11):1191–9.
8. Eberhard DA, Giaccone G, BE J, Non-Small-Cell Lung Cancer Working Group. Biomarkers of response to epidermal growth factor receptor inhibitors in Non-Small-Cell Lung Cancer Working Group: standardization for use in the clinical trial setting. J Clin Oncol. 2008;26(6):983–94.
9. Levi AW, Kelly DP, Rosenthal DL, Ronnett BM. Atypical squamous cells of undetermined significance in liquid-based cytologic specimens: results of reflex human papillomavirus testing and histologic follow-up in routine practice with comparison of interpretive and probabilistic reporting methods. Cancer. 2003;99(4):191–7.
10. Steinman S, Smith D, Chandler N, Dhurandhar B, Di Filippo L, Scheiber-Pact M, Mody DR. Morphologic, patient and interpreter profiles of high-risk human papillomavirus-positive vs.-negative cases of atypical squamous cells of undetermined significance. Acta Cytol. 2008;52(3):279–85.
11. Zhao C, Moriarty AT, Ghofrani M, Husain M, Tambouret RH, Laucirica R, et al. Human papillomavirus testing and reporting rates in 2012: results of a College of American Pathologists national survey. Arch Pathol Lab Med. 2015;139(6):757–61.

12. Virk RK, Abro S, Martinez de Ubago JM, Pambuccian SE, Quek ML, Wojcik EM, et al. The value of the UroVysion(R) FISH assay in the risk-stratification of patients with "atypical urothelial cells" in urinary cytology specimens. Diagn Cytopathol. 2017;45(6):481–500.
13. Miki Y, Neat M, Chandra A. Application of The Paris System to atypical urine cytology samples: correlation with histology and UroVysion(R) FISH. Cytopathology. 2017;28(2):88–95.
14. Venkatraman L, Catherwood MA, Patterson A, Lioe TF, McCluggage WG, Anderson NH. Role of polymerase chain reaction and immunocytochemistry in the cytological assessment of lymphoid proliferations. J Clin Pathol. 2006;59(11):1160–5.
15. Zhang S, Abreo F, Lowery-Nordberg M, Veillon DM, Cotelingam JD. The role of fluorescence in situ hybridization and polymerase chain reaction in the diagnosis and classification of lymphoproliferative disorders on fine-needle aspiration. Cancer Cytopathol. 2010;118(2):105–12.
16. Vigliar E, Malapelle U, de Luca C, Bellevicine C, Troncone G. Challenges and opportunities of next-generation sequencing: a cytopathologist's perspective. Cytopathology. 2015;26(5):271–83.

Part III
Clinical Relevance

Chapter 9
Human Papillomavirus (HPV) Testing of Head and Neck Cancers

Eleanor Russell-Goldman and Jeffrey F. Krane

Abbreviations

AJCC	American Joint Committee on Cancer
CAP	College of American Pathologists
DNA	Deoxyribonucleic acid
EBER	EBV-encoded RNA
EBV	Epstein-Barr virus
FFPE	Formalin fixed paraffin embedded
FNA	Fine-needle aspiration
HPV	Human papillomavirus
hrHPV	High-risk HPV
IHC	Immunohistochemistry
ISH	*In situ* hybridization

E. Russell-Goldman · J. F. Krane (✉)
Department of Pathology, Harvard Medical School,
Brigham and Women's Hospital, Boston, MA, USA
e-mail: erussell-goldman@bwh.harvard.edu;
jkrane@bwh.harvard.edu

S. Roy-Chowdhuri et al. (eds.), *Molecular Diagnostics in Cytopathology*, https://doi.org/10.1007/978-3-319-97397-5_9

N	Nodes (extent of lymph node involvement by metastatic disease in TNM staging)
OPSQCC	Oropharyngeal squamous cell carcinoma
PCR	Polymerase chain reaction
Rb	Retinoblastoma
RNA	Ribonucleic acid
SQCC	Squamous cell carcinoma
T	Tumor (primary tumor description in TNM staging)

Key Terminology

IHC A laboratory technique that allows the visualization of specific antigens in tissue by conjugating them to complementary antibodies with a reporter molecule. Common reporters are enzymes such as horseradish peroxidase. Enzymatic activation of the reporter leads to the production of a colored product that can be visualized with light microscopy

ISH A DNA or RNA detection method that uses complementary probes to bind and identify specific DNA or RNA sequences. The probes can be conjugated to fluorescent or chromogenic reporter molecules, which can be detected using fluorescence or light microscopy, respectively

PCR Molecular method that exponentially amplifies DNA sequences targeted by specific primers using a heat-stable DNA polymerase. This allows identification of targeted DNA sequences and their subsequent sequencing or other manipulations, if required

Key Points

- HPV-positive OPSQCC have a better prognosis and outcome than conventional head and neck SQCC
- HPV 16 is the most common HPV type associated with OPSQCC
- p16 IHC is a commonly used surrogate marker for hrHPV detection and is highly sensitive and moderately specific in surgical pathology specimens; however criteria for detecting hrHPV using p16 in cytology specimens is not well defined
- In surgical pathology specimens, p16 IHC is recommended as the first-line test for HPV and may be supplemented with other testing modalities if needed
- hrHPV can be detected using DNA and RNA isolation techniques that are highly specific and have variable sensitivity
- Current CAP guidelines recommend HPV testing in all cytologic material in cases of known or suspected OPSQCC when the HPV status is unknown or in cases of metastatic SQCC of unknown primary
- There is currently no preferred first-line test for cytology specimens
- While a positive p16 IHC result is considered to be at least 70% nuclear and cytoplasmic staining of at least moderate intensity in surgical pathology specimens, in cytologic material, the threshold for a positive p16 result needs to be individually validated in each laboratory
- Equivocal p16 IHC can be followed up by HPV PCR or ISH testing
- hrHPV testing performed on cytology specimens should be rigorously validated and interpreted with caution
- Negative HPV testing results in cytologic material should be repeated if a subsequent surgical pathology specimen becomes available
- In cases of metastatic SQCC of unknown primary, EBER testing should be performed either concurrently with HPV testing or in cases that prove to be HPV negative

Head and neck cancers encompass a variety of tumor types of the upper aerodigestive tract and salivary glands. Work over recent decades has shown significant molecular and clinical differences among head and neck tumor types. One of the most notable advances has been the recognition of human papillomavirus (HPV)-associated oropharyngeal squamous cell carcinoma (OPSQCC) as a distinct epidemiologic, morphologic, and molecular variant from non-HPV-associated head and neck squamous cell carcinoma [1]. High-risk HPV (hrHPV) has been detected in 70% of oropharyngeal carcinomas and is often associated with a nonkeratinizing basaloid morphology and a distinct clinical course with a more favorable outcome [2–5]. In particular, HPV type 16 has been shown to be most commonly associated with OPSQCC, being found in approximately 90% of cases, with HPV 18 being present in the majority of the remainder of cases [1, 6]. Although HPV has been detected in other head and neck carcinomas, the role and significance of HPV in these tumor types is less well defined [7]; therefore, HPV testing is currently only recommended for known or suspected cases of primary OPSQCC [8].

The HPV status of OPSQCC has been shown to be an independent prognostic factor for survival [5], and patients are now considered for deintensified therapy regimes in clinical trials based on tumor HPV status [4]. The recently published American Joint Committee on Cancer (AJCC) 8th Edition Cancer Staging System now considers high-risk HPV-associated (p16-positive) OPSQCC in its own chapter and incorporates different staging based on whether an OPSQCC is p16 positive or p16 negative [9]. These important insights have been gained from studies evaluating p16/HPV status on surgical pathology specimens.

There are two main scenarios in which the role of fine-needle aspiration (FNA) is increasingly important in the diagnosis and management of these HPV-associated OPSQCC patients. Firstly, many patients have metastatic nodal disease at initial presentation, as HPV-associated OPSQCC commonly presents with low tumor (T) but high nodal (N) stage disease. FNA of involved lymph nodes, rather than a biopsy of the known primary site, is often the diagnostic method of choice. The second scenario is in patients presenting with metastatic disease of unknown primary site. This is the mode of presentation in 34% of patients with HPV-associated OPSQCC [10], making cytologic material often the only substrate available for both diagnosis and molecular work-up. In patients with metastatic SQCC of unknown primary site, Epstein-Barr virus (EBV)-associated nasopharyngeal carcinoma is also an important consideration. *In situ* hybridization for EBV-encoded RNAs (EBER) should be performed in HPV-negative specimens or tested concurrently with HPV.

The use of FNA material for HPV detection poses its own unique advantages and challenges. Metastatic OPSQCC can often present as necrotic and cystic nodal deposits with scant viable material for testing and a necrotic background that may interfere with testing [11]. Nevertheless, FNA remains an effective, low-cost, and minimally invasive method to rapidly evaluate a patient presenting with lymphadenopathy of unknown primary. Molecular testing of FNA material is also of particular value in patients presenting with SQCC following a history of a prior HPV-positive OPSQCC. In the lung, p16 testing can be used on FNA specimens to distinguish between metastases from an OPSQCC and a primary lung basaloid SQCC, which may be difficult to distinguish on morphological or clinical grounds alone. In this scenario, a positive p16 result is not entirely specific for HPV but suggests a metastasis in patients with a known history of HPV OPSQCC [12]. The recently published College of American Pathologists (CAP) guidelines for HPV testing in head and neck carcinoma now recommend hrHPV testing in all FNA specimens of SQCC in patients with known but previously untested OPSQCC, in patients with a suspected OPSQCC, or in a patient with metastatic SQCC of unknown primary [8]. Currently there is no specific recommendation for a preferred testing methodology in cytology specimens, but regardless of which testing method is used, internal laboratory validation must be performed. If a hrHPV test is negative in a cytology specimen, follow-up hrHPV testing should be performed on subsequent surgical pathology specimens, if and when they become available. The discussion below addresses the main types of testing methodologies available and how they relate to HPV testing in cytologic material, predominantly referring to cell block preparations with additional discussion of newer liquid-based testing modalities (summarized in Table 9.1).

p16 Immunohistochemistry

The most frequently used HPV testing modality in surgical pathology material is p16 immunohistochemistry (IHC). This method detects the presence of the p16INK4a protein, a cell cycle regulator, which is upregulated during HPV infection and has been shown to be a reliable surrogate marker for hrHPV infection [13]. p16 IHC is the preferred first-line surrogate marker for the detection of hrHPV in surgical pathology specimens as it is highly sensitive, widely available, and relatively inexpensive to perform. The most commonly used p16 antibody is the E6H4 clone (Ventana Medical Systems, Inc., Oro Valley, AZ), which has recently been found to be the most specific and reliable p16 antibody in OPSQCC specimens, even at dilute concentrations [14, 15]; however, CAP guidelines do not specifically endorse any specific antibody or technique for p16 IHC [8]. In histologic tissue specimens, p16 is a highly sensitive marker (up to 100%) for the detection of HPV but has a specificity of approximately 80% [16–18]. CAP guidelines recommend at least 70% moderate to strong nuclear and cytoplasmic p16 positivity in tumor cells in order to report a positive result [8]. Currently, these guidelines refer mainly to surgical pathology specimens, with all testing carried out on formalin-fixed, paraffin-embedded (FFPE) tissue; there is no clear consensus on the interpretation of p16 IHC on cytologic material. Recent studies have attempted to answer this question and found p16 testing on

TABLE 9.1 HPV testing methods in cytology

Method	Substrate	Widely available	HPV types tested	Correlates with in vivo viral activity	Sensitivity	Specificity	Positivity threshold in cytologic material
p16 IHC	Cell block	Yes	hrHPV	Yes	High	Moderate (varies with clinical context)	Not established
PCR	Cell block or smear material	Yes	LR and HR	No	High	Low	Not established
RNA ISH	Cell block	No	LR and HR[a]	Yes	High	High	Not established
DNA ISH	Cell block	No	LR and HR[a]	No	Low	High	Not established
Liquid-phase detection	Liquid-based cytology or smear material	Yes	HR	No	Likely high	Likely high	Not established

Abbreviations: *HR* high risk, *LR* low risk

[a]Although both LR and hrHPV probes are commercially available, LR testing is not routinely recommended

cytologic material resulted in variable sensitivities and specificities with suggested cutoffs for positivity ranging from 10% to 90% [11, 19, 20]. It is, therefore, prudent to interpret limited p16 IHC staining on cytologic material with caution, as specimen processing, low cellularity, and the presence of necrosis may all affect staining. CAP guidelines indicate that the threshold for determining a p16-positive result in cytologic material needs to be individually validated in each laboratory. We favor reporting p16 positivity on a cytology specimen when there is strong nuclear and cytoplasmic staining in the majority of cells in an at least moderately cellular specimen (Fig. 9.1). In cases with an equivocal result, subsequent HPV detection methods can be performed, as discussed below. A potential pitfall in the interpretation of p16 immunostaining is that p16 positivity has been reported in a number of non-HPV-related SQCC, in addition to other tumor types, including oropharyngeal small cell carcinoma, sinonasal undifferentiated carcinoma, clear cell carcinoma of the salivary glands, and HPV-related multiphenotypic sinonasal carcinoma [21–24]. Indeed, p16 positivity has also been reported in benign lymphoepithelial cysts [25]. Therefore, as p16 is a surrogate marker for HPV infection, a positive p16 result should always be interpreted in the context of the cytomorphology and the given clinical and radiological information. Despite these potential confounders, CAP guidelines consider p16 positivity alone adequate evidence of an HPV-associated OPSQCC when there is a known oropharyngeal primary or when there is a metastatic SQCC of unknown primary in upper or middle jugular lymph nodes with typical nonkeratinizing morphology [8].

→

Figure 9.1 FNA of HPV-associated OPSQCC. (**a**) The cell block demonstrates characteristic basaloid cells with mitotic activity and apoptotic debris (×1000). (**b**) Positive p16 immunocytochemistry on cell block material demonstrates strong and diffuse nuclear and cytoplasmic staining in the majority of cells (×1000). (**c**) Concurrent positive HR DNA ISH is seen as punctate dot-like hybridization signals in tumor nuclei (×1000)

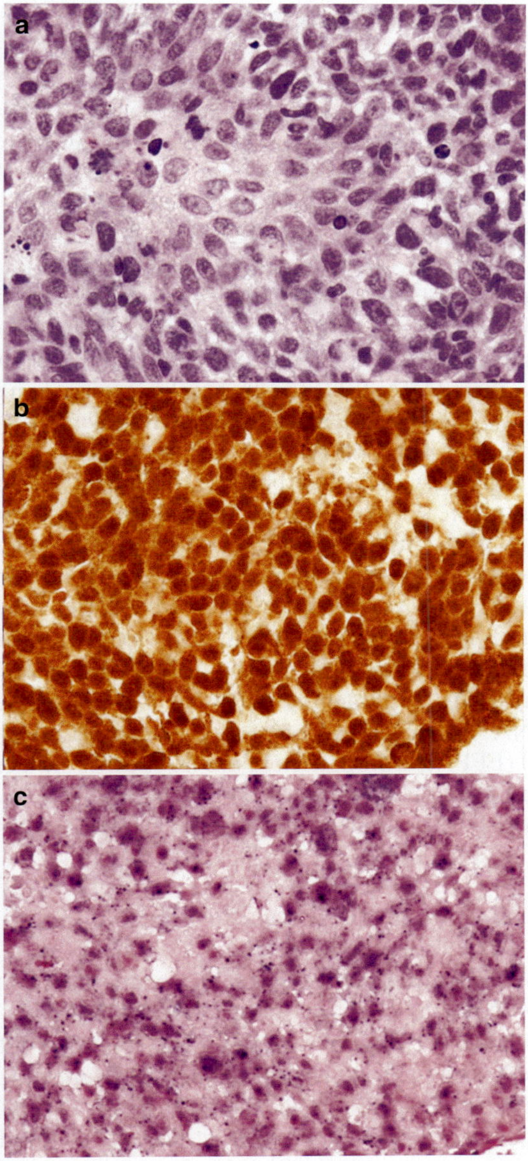

RNA *In Situ* Hybridization (ISH)

The demonstration of transcriptionally active hrHPV is considered a gold standard for the diagnosis of a HPV-related malignancy. Viral oncoproteins E6 and E7 play an essential role in pathogenesis as they bind and disrupt cell cycle regulators TP53 and retinoblastoma (Rb) proteins, respectively [26]. The detection of E6/E7 mRNA by *in situ* hybridization (ISH) allows the direct visualization of hrHPV transcripts in FFPE tissue using chromogenic probes and light field microscopy. RNA ISH has been shown to be a sensitive marker for the presence of hrHPV and may be more sensitive than DNA ISH due to amplification of mRNA in the sample. RNA ISH has been shown to have strong agreement with p16 immunostaining, with a concordance rate of 96.4% [27]. RNA ISH may be able to detect cases of HPV infection when low copy numbers result in a negative DNA ISH result [28]. Until recently, RNA ISH has not been widely available as the hybridization and staining process were not automated. Recent work has demonstrated the utility of an automated hrHPV E6/E7 RNA ISH method which can detect the 18 most common types of HPV in a single assay, with sensitivity approaching 100% in OPSQCC specimens [29]. RNA ISH can be performed on cytology cell block material (FFPE), although there are no specific studies examining any potential differences between HPV RNA ISH in cytology cell blocks and surgically obtained FFPE tissue.

DNA *In Situ* Hybridization (ISH)

DNA ISH uses DNA probes, which are complementary to HPV viral DNA sequences, to detect HPV DNA in FFPE. Chromogenic probes allow direct visualization of HPV DNA in tumor cells using light microscopy, whereas fluorescent probes can also be used with fluorescence microscopy. DNA ISH is a highly specific method for HPV identification, with only a 1% false-positive rate reported [30]. It has been recommended that a combination of sensitive p16 IHC and specific DNA ISH testing be employed for HPV detection [17]. A recent study evaluated the interpretation of DNA ISH on cytology cell blocks and found that approximately 30% of the cases were scored as difficult or moderately difficult to interpret [31]. The authors cited weak or non-specific staining as a barrier to interpretation and noted that there is often background debris or necrosis which may hinder interpretation. In cases where the result of DNA ISH appears negative or equivocal in a p16-positive cytology case, further hrHPV polymerase chain reaction (PCR)-based testing could be performed as a confirmatory test.

HPV Polymerase Chain Reaction (PCR)

HPV PCR can be performed on FFPE or non-formalin-fixed cytology specimens (smears, liquid-based cytology) and is one of the most commonly used methods for HPV detection. Studies have shown that PCR for HPV DNA is highly sensitive when performed on OPSQCC biopsies [32]. Commonly used primers, GP5+ and GP6+, detect both low- and high-risk HPV DNA [33]. A drawback of the PCR method is that it cannot distinguish between episomal and integrated DNA and therefore may detect the presence of HPV that is not transcriptionally active and therefore not clinically relevant. Specificity can be improved by utilizing multiplex assays such as PCR mass array and targeting the L1 gene of HPV [34]. One study examined PCR testing of scraped FNA smear material and demonstrated that this method had approximately 95% sensitivity and 100% specificity when compared to p16 testing of paired surgical specimens [35].

Liquid-Phase Assays

In addition to immunohistochemical and molecular testing on FFPE tissue, evaluation of HPV status can be performed using liquid-based assays. There are currently five FDA-approved assays that are widely used for the detection of hrHPV in cervical cytology brushings and could be readily applied to head and neck OPSQCC FNA material. One such method is the Hybrid Capture 2 assay (Digene Corporation, Gaithersburg, MD), which is a liquid-phase hybridization assay using RNA probes to detect up to 13 hrHPV types. Pilot studies have demonstrated that the Hybrid Capture 2 assay is comparable to p16 immunohistochemistry and ISH for hrHPV detection in FNA material [36]. Another FDA-approved liquid-phase test for hrHPV types 16 and 18 is the Cervista assay (Hologic Inc., Bedford, MA), which uses a proprietary signal amplification method for the detection of specific DNA sequences. The Cervista assay has been found to have >90% agreement with concurrent p16 or ISH testing for hrHPV in FNA specimens of head and neck OPSQCC [37]. The Cobas 4800 test (Roche Molecular Systems, Pleasanton, CA) is an automated platform that performs real-time PCR on extracted DNA to detect hrHPV 16/18 and 12 additional high-risk strains. It has been demonstrated that the Cobas 4800 test has >90% agreement with concurrent p16 or DNA ISH testing for hrHPV in FNA specimens of head and neck OPSQCC and has a sensitivity of 100% and specificity of 86% [38]. The overall benefits of liquid-phase testing include the fact that special specimen processing requirements are minimal and the process is automated, resulting in greater reproducibility and short turnaround times. The high sensitivity and quick turnaround make liquid-based testing especially attractive as a screening test for patients with suspected hrHPV-associated OPSQCC.

Summary

The implementation of HPV testing in head and neck carcinomas, namely, OPSQCC, has revolutionized the management and prognosis for patients with hrHPV-positive OPSQCC. These patients may be spared extensive chemotherapy and radiotherapy regimes and overall have better outcomes than patients with conventional OPSQCC. There are a number of testing modalities available for the detection of hrHPV including evaluation of the surrogate marker p16 by IHC and direct detection of the virus by RNA and DNA isolation methods. Both the AJCC and CAP now recommend hrHPV testing as part of the work-up of OPSQCC. A positive p16 is reported for surgical specimens when at least 70% moderate to strong nuclear and cytoplasmic staining is present in tumor cells. The clinical relevance of HPV testing of head and neck carcinomas outside the oropharynx has not been established, and therefore routine HPV testing of these tumors is not currently recommended. The reporting of the HPV status of an OPSQCC should be included in the top-line diagnosis. Tumor grade or differentiation status is not reported as this does not impact prognosis in HPV-positive tumors. Preferred terminology is HPV-positive or p16-positive SQCC with a description of the testing method used and result included in the report.

For cytology specimens, CAP guidelines recommend hrHPV testing on all FNA specimens of known or suspected OPSQCC when hrHPV status has not previously been established and for metastatic SQCC of unknown primary. However, the choice of method of hrHPV testing in cytology specimens is left up to the pathologist or laboratory performing the test.

There is no single perfect test for HPV detection, and as discussed above, each test type has its own limitations and advantages (Table 9.1). Rigorous laboratory validation is essential for all HPV testing methods. The adequacy of the cytology specimen is paramount to reliable HPV testing, and evaluation of adequacy at the time of FNA is recommended to ensure optimal sampling. Until widely validated criteria for HPV testing in cytologic material are established, it is incumbent upon practicing pathologists to judiciously report HPV status and ensure that testing performed at the individual institution is thoroughly validated in order to provide optimal patient care.

References

1. Kreimer AR, Clifford GM, Boyle P, Kreimer AR, Clifford GM, Boyle P, et al. Human papillomavirus types in head and neck squamous cell carcinomas worldwide: a systematic review. Cancer Epidemiol Biomark Prev. 2005;14(2):467–75.

2. Fakhry C, Westra WH, Li S, Cmelak A, Ridge JA, Pinto H, et al. Improved survival of patients with human papillomavirus-positive head and neck squamous cell carcinoma in a prospective clinical trial. J Natl Cancer Inst. 2008;100(4):261–9.
3. Chaturvedi AK, Anderson WF, Lortet-Tieulent J, Paula Curado M, Ferlay J, Franceschi S, et al. Worldwide trends in incidence rates for oral cavity and oropharyngeal cancers. J Clin Oncol. 2013;31(36):4550–9.
4. Krane JF. Role of cytology in the diagnosis and management of HPV-associated head and neck carcinoma. Acta Cytol. 2013;57(2):117–26.
5. Ang KK, Harris J, Wheeler R, Weber R, Rosenthal DI, Nguyen-Tân DF, et al. Human papillomavirus and survival of patients with oropharyngeal Cancer. N Engl J Med. 2010;363(1):24–35.
6. Gillison ML, Koch WM, Capone RB, Spafford M, Westra WH, Wu L, et al. Evidence for a causal association between human papillomavirus and a subset of head and neck cancers. J Natl Cancer Inst. 2000;92(9):709–20.
7. Isayeva T, Li Y, Maswahu D, Brandwein-Gensler M. Human papillomavirus in non-oropharyngeal head and neck cancers: a systematic literature review. Head Neck Pathol. 2012;6(Suppl 1):104–20.
8. Lewis JS Jr, Beadle B, Bishop JA, Chernock RD, Colasacco C, Lacchetti C, et al. Human papillomavirus testing in head and neck carcinomas. Arch Pathol Lab Med. 2018;142(5):559–97.
9. O'Sullivan B, Lydiatt WM, Haughey BH, Brandwein-Gensler M, Glastonbury CM, Shah J. HPV-mediated (p16+) oropharyngeal cancer. In: Amin MB, Edge S, Greene F, Byrd DR, Brookland RK, Washington MK, et al., editors. AJCC cancer staging manual. 8th ed. New York: Springer International Publishing; 2017. p. 113–22.
10. Chernock RD, Lewis JS. Approach to metastatic carcinoma of unknown primary in the head and neck: squamous cell carcinoma and beyond. Head Neck Pathol. 2015;9(1):6–15.
11. Xu B, Ghossein R, Lane J, Lin O, Katabi N. The utility of p16 immunostaining in fine needle aspiration in p16-positive head and neck squamous cell carcinoma. Hum Pathol. 2016;54:193–200.
12. Bishop JA, Ogawa T, Chang X, Illei PB, Gabrielson E, Pai SI, et al. HPV analysis in distinguishing second primary tumors from lung metastases in patients with head and neck squamous cell carcinoma. Am J Surg Pathol. 2012;36(1):142–8.

13. Weinberger PM, Yu Z, Haffty BG, Kowalski D, Harigopal M, Brandsma J, et al. Molecular classification identifies a subset of human papillomavirus- associated oropharyngeal cancers with favorable prognosis. J Clin Oncol. 2006;24(5):736–47.
14. Shelton J, Purgina BM, Cipriani NA, Dupont WD, Plummer D, Lewis JS. P16 immunohistochemistry in oropharyngeal squamous cell carcinoma: a comparison of antibody clones using patient outcomes and high-risk human papillomavirus RNA status. Mod Pathol. 2017;30(9):1194–203.
15. Lewis JS, Shelton J, Kuhs KL, Smith D K. p16 immunohistochemistry in oropharyngeal squamous cell carcinoma using the E6H4 antibody clone: a technical method study for optimal dilution. Head Neck Pathol. 2017;0(0):1–8.
16. Smeets SJ, Hesselink AT, Speel E-JM, Haesevoets A, Snijders PJF, Pawlita M, et al. A novel algorithm for reliable detection of human papillomavirus in paraffin embedded head and neck cancer specimen. Int J Cancer. 2007;121(11):2465–72.
17. Singhi AD, Westra WH. Comparison of human papillomavirus in situ hybridization and p16 immunohistochemistry in the detection of human papillomavirus-associated head and neck cancer based on a prospective clinical experience. Cancer. 2010;116(9):2166–73.
18. Schache AG, Liloglou T, Risk JM, Filia A, Jones M, Sheard J, et al. Evaluation of human papillomavirus diagnostic testing in oropharyngeal squamous cell carcinoma: sensitivity, specificity and prognostic discrimination. Clin Cancer Res. 2012;17(19):6262–71.
19. Jalaly JB, Lewis JS, Collins BT, Wu X, Ma XJ, Luo Y, et al. Correlation of p16 immunohistochemistry in FNA biopsies with corresponding tissue specimens in HPV-related squamous cell carcinomas of the oropharynx. Cancer Cytopathol. 2015;123(12):723–31.
20. Grimes R, Garcia-Buitrago MT, Jorda M, Ganjei-Azar P, Ferrell A, Gomez-Fernandez C. P16INKa immunocytochemistry in fine-needle aspiration cytology smears of metastatic head and neck squamous cell carcinoma. Acta Cytol. 2013;57(1):33–7.
21. Bishop JA, Westra WH. Human papillomavirus-related small cell carcinoma of the oropharynx. Am J Surg Pathol. 2011;35(11):1679–84.
22. Wadsworth B, Bumpous JM, Martin AW, Nowacki MR, Jenson AB, Farghaly H. Expression of p16 in sinonasal undifferentiated carcinoma (SNUC) without associated human papillomavirus (HPV). Head Neck Pathol. 2011;5(4):349–54.

23. Bishop JA, Rooper LM, Chiosea SI, Westra WH. Clear cell carcinoma of salivary glands is frequently p16 positive: a pitfall in the interpretation of oropharyngeal biopsies. Am J Surg Pathol. 2018;42(3):367–71.
24. Bishop JA, Andreasen S, Hang JF, Bullock MJ, Chen TY, Franchi A, et al. HPV-related multiphenotypic sinonasal carcinoma: an expanded series of 49 cases of the tumor formerly known as HPV-related carcinoma with adenoid cystic carcinoma-like features. Am J Surg Pathol. 2017;41(12):1690–701.
25. Cao D, Begum S, Ali SZ, Westra WH. Expression of p16 in benign and malignant cystic squamous lesions of the neck. Hum Pathol. 2010;41(4):535–9.
26. Asiaf A, Ahmad ST, Mohammad SO, Zargar MA. Review of the current knowledge on the epidemiology, pathogenesis, and prevention of human papillomavirus infection. Eur J Cancer Prev. 2014;23(3):206–24.
27. Ukpo OC, Flanagan JJ, Ma XJ, Luo Y, Thorstad WL, Lewis JS. High-risk human papillomavirus E6/E7 mRNA detection by a novel in situ hybridization assay strongly correlates with p16 expression and patient outcomes in oropharyngeal squamous cell carcinoma. Am J Surg Pathol. 2011;35(9):1343–50.
28. Bishop J, Ma X-J, Wang H, Luo Y, Illei PB, Begum S, et al. Detection of transcriptionally active high risk HPV in patients with head and neck squamous cell carcinoma as visualized by a novel E6/E7 mRNA in situ hybridization method. Am J Surg Pathol. 2012;36(12):1874–82.
29. Mills AM, Dirks DC, Poulter MD, Mills SE, Stoler MH. HR-HPV E6/E7 mRNA in situ hybridization. Am J Surg Pathol. 2017;41(5):607–15.
30. Thavaraj S, Stokes A, Guerra E, Bible J, Halligan E, Long A, et al. Evaluation of human papillomavirus testing for squamous cell carcinoma of the tonsil in clinical practice. J Clin Pathol. 2011;64(4):308–12.
31. Miller JA, Allison DB, Maleki Z. Interpretation of HPV DNA in situ hybridization in HPV-related head and neck squamous cell carcinoma: an achievable task in cell block and small biopsy material. J Am Soc Cytopathol. 2017;6(3):89–95.
32. Agoston ES, Robinson SJ, Mehra KK, Birch C, Semmel D, Mirkovic J, et al. Polymerase chain reaction detection of HPV in squamous carcinoma of the oropharynx. Am J Clin Pathol. 2010;134(1):36–41.

33. De Roda Husman AM, Walboomers JMM, Van den Brule AJC, Meijer CJLM, Snijders PJF. The use of general primers GP5 and GP6 elongated at their 3′ ends with adjacent highly conserved sequences improves human papillomavirus detection by PCR. J Gen Virol. 1995;76(4):1057–62.
34. Walline HM, Komarck C, JB MH, Byrd SA, Spector ME, Hauff SJ, et al. High-risk human papillomavirus detection in oropharyngeal, nasopharyngeal, and oral cavity cancers comparison of multiple methods. JAMA Otolaryngol Head Neck Surg. 2013;139(12):1320–7.
35. Channir HI, Grønhøj Larsen C, Ahlborn LB, van Overeem Hansen T, Gerds TA, Charabi BW, et al. Validation study of HPV DNA detection from stained FNA smears by polymerase chain reaction: improving the diagnostic workup of patients with a tumor on the neck. Cancer Cytopathol. 2016;124(11):820–7.
36. Bishop JA, Maleki Z, Valsamakis A, Ogawa T, Chang X, WestraPai SI, et al. Application of the hybrid capture 2 assay to squamous cell carcinomas of the head and neck: a convenient liquid-phase approach for the reliable determination of human papillomavirus status. Cancer Cytopathol. 2012;120(1):18–25.
37. Guo M, Khanna A, Dhillon J, Patel SJ, Feng J, Williams MD, et al. Cervista HPV assays for fine-needle aspiration specimens are a valid option for human papillomavirus testing in patients with oropharyngeal carcinoma. Cancer Cytopathol. 2014;122(2):96–103.
38. Kerr DA, Pitman MB, Sweeney B, Arpin RN, Wilbur DC, Faquin WC. Performance of the roche cobas 4800 high-risk human papillomavirus test in cytologic preparations of squamous cell carcinoma of the head and neck. Cancer Cytopathol. 2014;122(3):167–74.

Chapter 10
Human Papillomavirus (HPV) Testing on Cervical Cytology Specimens

Ming Guo

Abbreviations

ACOG	American College of Obstetricians and Gynecologists
ACS	American Cancer Society
AGC	Atypical glandular cell
ASCCP	American Society of Colposcopy and Cervical Pathology
ASC-H	Atypical squamous cells, cannot exclude high-grade squamous intraepithelial lesion
ASCP	American Society of Clinical Pathology
ASCUS	Atypical squamous cells of undetermined significance

M. Guo
Department of Pathology, The University of Texas MD Anderson Cancer Center, Houston, TX, USA
e-mail: mguo@mdanderson.org

S. Roy-Chowdhuri et al. (eds.), *Molecular Diagnostics in Cytopathology*, https://doi.org/10.1007/978-3-319-97397-5_10

CIN	Cervical intraepithelial neoplasm
CIN2	Cervical intraepithelial neoplasia, grade 2
CIN3	Cervical intraepithelial neoplasia, grade 3
DNA	Deoxyribonucleic acid
HC2	Hybrid capture 2
HPV	Human papilloma virus
hr	High risk
HSIL	High-grade squamous intraepithelial lesion
LEEP	Loop electrosurgical excision procedure
LSIL	Low-grade squamous intraepithelial lesion
Pap test	Papanicolaou test
PCR	Polymerase chain reaction
RNA	Ribonucleic acid
SGO	Society of Gynecologic Oncology
USPSTF	United States Preventive Services Task Force
VAIN	Vaginal intraepithelial neoplasia

Key Terminology

Clinical sensitivity	To correctly predict high-grade cervical intraepithelial lesion, CIN2+ by a HPV testing assay
High-risk HPV (hrHPV)	HPV16, 18, 31, 33, 35, 39, 45, 51, 52, 56, 58, 59, 66, and 68 genotypes etiologically associated with cervical cancer and precancerous lesions

Key Points

- Integration of HPV testing in cervical cancer screening is one of the most significant advances for cervical cancer prevention in the USA in the past decades
- HPV testing, alone or in conjunction with Pap cytology, shows convincing clinical evidence of improved cervical cancer screening efficacy compared to Pap cytology only screening
- HPV testing was recommended in conjunction with Pap cytology or as a primary screening tool by the American Cancer Society (ACS), American Society of Colposcopy and Cervical Pathology (ASCCP), and American Society for Clinical Pathology (ASCP) guidelines for cervical cancer prevention with specific recommendations on age for screening, for screening intervals, and for women with specific Pap testing results
- HPV testing for cervical cancer screening can increase the efficacy of cervical cancer screening to identify cervical precancerous lesions
- The limitations of HPV testing in cervical cancer prevention include complexity of screening algorithms, women's age, screening intervals, Pap cytology stratification, and multiple FDA-approved, commercially available HPV testing assays
- HPV testing assay and testing strategy should be selected to best fit patient care in a given clinical setting

Cervical cancer is one of the major malignancies in women globally, ranking the fourth most common carcinomas following breast, colorectal, and lung cancer, with 528,000 new cases diagnosed worldwide each year [1]. In the USA, the incidence of cervical cancer has significantly declined over the past 50 years primarily due to systemic cervical cancer screening with the Papanicolaou (Pap) cytology and subsequently incorporated with human papillomavirus (HPV) tests [2, 3]. In 2016, the newly diagnosed cervical cancer cases were estimated to be 12,900 with 4120 deaths [4], representing more than 50% decline of cervical cancer incidence in the past 30 years [3].

In the past two decades, significant advances have been made in cervical cancer prevention following the milestone discovery that oncogenic or high-risk HPV (hrHPV) is the major etiological factor for carcinogenesis of cervical cancer and precancers [5]. More than 90% of cervical cancer and cervical precancerous lesions (i.e., high-grade cervical intraepithelial neoplasia grade 2 or 3 (CIN2+)) are associated with 13–14 hrHPV genotypes [6–10]. These discoveries have led to a significant evolving of cervical cancer screening with incorporation of hrHPV testing [11–13] as well as HPV vaccination for cervical cancer prevention in the USA.

The hrHPV DNA or RNA tests have been recommended in the USA in conjunction with the Pap cytology test or as a primary screening for cervical cancer prevention [12, 14–17]. Before hrHPV testing was incorporated, Pap cytology testing had been used for cervical cancer screening in the USA for decades and became the most successful cancer screening tool that helped to significantly reduce the incidence of cervical cancer in the screened population [18].

HPV is a family of non-enveloped double-stranded DNA viruses and the most common sexually transmitted pathogen. Currently, hrHPV or oncogenic HPV includes HPV16, 18, 31, 33, 35, 39, 45, 51, 52, 56, 58, 59, 66, and 68 genotypes. Of these, HPV16 and HPV18 are the most clinically relevant hrHPV genotypes that are associated with more than 70% of cervical carcinoma and the most predictive marker for the risk of

CIN3 [7, 9, 19–26]. Because of this, HPV16/18 genotyping was separately recommended in the American Cancer Society (ACS), American Society of Colposcopy and Cervical Pathology (ASCCP), and American Society for Clinical Pathology (ASCP) guidelines for cervical cancer screening for both HPV/Pap cytology co-testing and HPV primary screening [12, 16]. Some HPV genotypes were classified as low-risk HPV because they were identified as etiologic factors for genital warts rather than cervical cancer. The low-risk HPV includes HPV6, 11, 40, 42, 43, 44, 53, 54, 61, 72, 73, and 81. Although HPV6 and HPV11, which account for 90% of genital warts, were included in HPV vaccines, the low-risk HPVs are not recommended in cervical cancer screening because there is no convincing evidence to link low-risk HPVs to cervical cancer or precancers [27, 28]. HPV infections occur commonly in the basal/stem cells in the transformation zone of the cervix to form either episomal or integrated forms in host cells. The integrated form of hrHPV is critical for HPV-mediated cell transformation that has a significantly higher clinical implication than the episomal form of hrHR HPVs. Integration of hrHPV into the host DNA results in the deletion of the HPV E2 reading frame, releasing E2 suppressing effects on the expression of the E6 and E7 oncogenes [29, 30]. The E6 and E7 oncoproteins interact with p53 and pRB that consequently results in the degradation of these tumor suppressor proteins, leading to uncontrolled cell proliferation and chromosomal instability and eventually development of precancer lesions and carcinoma [31, 32]. Because E6 and E7 expression is a hallmark of HPV DNA integration [32, 33], detecting mRNA of E6 and E7 is highly specific for predicting CIN2+ during cervical cancer screening [34].

HPV infection is very common in young women with predominantly transient HPV infection with little or no clinical implications [35]. Epidemiologically, HPV infection in women in the USA reaches a maximal level in the mid-20s and declines with age [35]. Most of the infections are cleared by the host immune system within 9–12 months [36]. However, the immunity is usually short-lived or ineffective in preventing future infections by the same or different HPV genotypes [37, 38]. Only a small fraction of women who cannot effectively eliminate the hrHPV and have persistent infection with one or multiple hrHPVs (most frequently by HPV16) are at risk of developing CIN3+ [39]. The aim of introducing HPV test for cervical cancer screening, either primary HPV screening or in conjunction with Pap cytology test, is to identify the small fraction of women who have persistent hrHPV infection and are at a high risk of CIN2+. Once a CIN2+ is confirmed by a diagnostic colposcopy/biopsy, the loop electrosurgical excision procedure (LEEP) or a cone excision is recommended to eliminate the CIN2+ lesions to prevent the cervical dysplastic lesion progression [40].

It has been well recognized that a single positive HPV test result may not be clinically relevant because most HPV infection is transient and most CINs regress with no clinical implications [41]. The incidence of cervical cancer in women gradually increases with age, and the peak of incidence occurs a decade after the peak of HPV prevalence [42]. Due to the very high HPV prevalence and the low incidence of cervical precancerous lesions in young women, HPV testing is not cost-effective and has a limited predictive value for CIN3+ in women aged 30 years and younger. Consequently, HPV test as a co-testing with Pap cytology was not recommended in women aged 29 and younger or as a primary HPV testing for women aged 24 and younger in the USA [12, 15, 16]. In addition to the age factor, HPV testing has been recommended in conjunction with Pap cytology test with a triage algorithm in order to achieve an optimal efficacy of cervical cancer screening. However, the combination of HPV and Pap cytology testing results, the women's age, and the re-screening intervals resulted in a highly complicated screening system for patient's triage and follow-up steps [16]. For these reasons, HPV primary screening was recommended as an alternative to the current Pap cytology test for cervical cancer screening in the USA in 2015 [12].

The Current Recommendations of HPV Testing for Cervical Cancer Prevention

In the USA, the current guidelines for cervical cancer prevention were updated in 2012 by the American Cancer Society (ACS), American Society of Colposcopy and Cervical Pathology (ASCCP), and American Society for Clinical Pathology (ASCP) [16] and separately by the United States Preventive Services Task Force (USPSTF) [43]. In 2015, HPV primary screening was recommended by the ASCCP and the Society of Gynecologic Oncology (SGO) [12]. These guidelines were reiterated by the American College of Obstetricians and Gynecologists (ACOG) in 2016 [44]. Age recommendation for cervical cancer screening is as follows:

1. No screening for women who are 20 years and younger or 66 years and older who have no history of dysplasia.
2. Pap cytology testing with a 3-year screening interval for women who are 21–29 years old.
3. HPV/Pap cytology co-testing with a 5-year screening interval for women who are 30–65 years old.
4. For HPV primary screening, women who are 25–65 years old are recommended for cervical cancer screening.

For both HPV primary screening and HPV/Pap cytology co-testing, HPV test was recommended in conjunction at certain levels with Pap cytology test in these guidelines for cervical cancer prevention (Table 10.1).

Table 10.1 Recommendations for using HPV testing for cervical cancer prevention[a]

Age-based recommendation
<20 or >65 years of age: no screening
21–29 years of age: cytology alone every 3 years with an option of reflex HPV testing for women with ASCUS
30–65 years of age: HPV co-screening along with Pap test every 5 years

(continued)

Table 10.1 (continued)

In conjunction with Pap cytology
ASCUS (21 years and older)
Pap/HPV+ co-testing results: HPV16/18 genotyping
LSIL in postmenopausal women
Post-colposcopy management of women with AGC or ASC-H
Post-colposcopy management of women 21 years or older with ASCUS or LSIL
Posttreatment surveillance
Primary HPV screening
25–65 years of age: primary HPV screening every 5 years, if tested negative
HPV16/18 genotyping test, colposcopy referral if positive
Non-HPV16/18 positive (12 hrHPV genotypes), Pap cytology triage

[a]The guidelines by the American Cancer Society, American Society for Colposcopy and Cervical Pathology, and American Society for Clinical Pathology

HPV and Pap Cytology Co-testing

Indications In 2004, ACS and the ASCCP recommended HPV and Pap cytology co-testing for cervical cancer prevention [45]. The consensus guidelines issued in 2006 by ASCCP for cervical cancer prevention recommended HPV and Pap cytology co-testing for women aged 30 years and older with a 3-year screening interval [15], and the screening interval was extended to 5 years in the 2012 consensus guidelines [16].

Advantages Based on the published data of clinical trial studies, women with HPV and Pap cytology co-testing had increased detection rates of CIN3+ and decreased the incidence of CIN3+ during the follow-up periods compared to the Pap cytology test-only screening [46, 47]. The extended screening interval for HPV and Pap cytology co-testing was recommended to reduce unnecessary follow-up testing and the associated morbidity as well as the costs while maintaining the testing efficacy similar to that of Pap cytology screening test at 3-year screening interval.

Concerns The efficacy of the 5-year HPV/Pap co-screening interval was established by comparing its efficacy with the efficacy of the 3-year Pap test screening interval [48, 49]. Controversial opinions were raised on whether a 5-year screening interval is safe for women with negative HPV/Pap co-testing results [50, 51]. Increased cumulative CIN3+ or carcinoma incidence for 5-year follow-up has been reported compared to those of 3-year follow-up periods [48, 49, 52, 53]. Whether the 5-year screening interval of HPV/Pap cytology co-testing implies a potentially suboptimal screening efficacy needs to be evaluated by more observatory clinical studies or clinical trials [54]. Nevertheless, it is rational to conclude that the screening efficacy of HPV/Pap co-testing is higher than that of Pap cytology test only which has been widely used in the USA for a long time.

HPV Primary Screening

Indications In 2015, the first US guideline of HPV primary screening for cervical cancer prevention was issued [12]. Shortly before the recommendation, the US FDA approved the Cobas HPV assay (Roche Diagnostics, Indianapolis, IN), one of the commercially available HPV testing assays, as a primary cervical cancer screening method. For cervical cancer screening, this is a milestone that may transform cervical cancer prevention from the primarily Pap cytology-based screening, widely used in the USA for more than half a century, to HPV-based molecular screening.

Advantages The randomized clinical trials in Europe and observational studies in the USA provided evidences supporting HPV primary screening for cervical cancer prevention [52, 53, 55–57]. It is rational to replace Pap cytology test-only screening by HPV primary screening because HPV/Pap cytology co-testing presently has not completely replaced Pap cytology test-only screening in the USA and there is no recommendation for HPV/Pap cytology co-testing in Canada and the European countries [58]. The obvious advantages of HPV primary screening include its significantly improved simplicity and reduced costs compared to Pap/HPV co-testing with only a small percentage of HPV-positive women needing the additional Pap test triage and follow-up. As a result, an increased reproducibility of cervical cancer screening is expected. HPV16/18 genotyping integrated in the HPV primary screening algorithm has a clear advantage in predicting more clinically relevant cases of CIN3+ associated with HPV16/18.

Concerns The FDA approval and the ASCCP guideline for HPV primary screening in the USA raised controversy [59]. The major concern is the possible false-negative HPV test results in cervical cancer [60, 61]. The relatively lower HPV sensitivity for detecting cervical cancer can be attributed to the low HPV copy numbers in carcinoma that may fall below the detection cutoff of the commercially available HPV assays [62, 63]. The clinical implications of the negative HPV results in patients with cervical carcinoma are not clear. There are few published data showing the rate of CIN3+ detected by Pap cytology test but missed by HPV testing. Consequently, to evaluate the efficacy and the safety of HPV primary screening, it is necessary to document the incidence of CIN3+ cases detected by Pap test but missed by HPV test. More clinical studies/trials are required to conclude whether HPV primary screening is more efficient than or equivalent to HPV/Pap cytology co-testing for cervical cancer screening.

Special Issues of HPV Testing in Conjunction with Pap Cytology Test

Women with a Pap Cytology Test Result of Abnormal Squamous Cells of Undetermined Significance (ASCUS)

Indications In conjunction with Pap cytology, reflex HPV testing is recommended for a small percentage of women with mildly abnormal Pap test results, i.e., ASCUS (Table 10.1). In 2002, ASCCP issued the first guidelines to incorporate HPV testing for cervical cancer screening [64]. The guidelines recommended the use of HPV testing as a preferred strategy for the triage of women with ASCUS Pap results.

Advantages The ASCUS/LSIL Triage Study (ALTS) and a recently published observational study, the Kaiser Permanente Northern California (KPNC) study, showed that the risk of CIN3+ in women with ASCUS/HPV+ testing was significantly higher [65, 66].

Concerns The HPV-positive rate in women with ASCUS is age-dependent with the HPV-positive rate declining from younger women (21–29 years) to older women (30–65 years) in different clinical settings [66–70]. The sensitivity for predicting CIN2+ decreased in older compared to younger women [67, 71]. It is possible that the decreased clinical sensitivity for CIN3+ in women with ASCUS in older age groups is associated with cervical atrophy that can cause suboptimal Pap sampling and/or reduced HPV copy numbers in older women [62, 72].

Women with Pap-Negative/HPV-Positive Co-testing Result

Indications When HPV/Pap cytology co-testing or HPV primary screening with reflex Pap cytology testing is used for cervical cancer screening, there is a small percentage of women with HPV-positive/Pap-negative test results [73]. Current recommendation is genotyping test for HPV16 or both HPV16 and HPV18 or repeating HPV/Pap co-testing in 12 months to determine if further evaluation by colposcopy is required [16].

Advantages Women with HPV16-positive testing results have a significantly higher risk for CIN3+ than women with non-HPV16 hrHPV results [7, 20–25]. In the long-term follow-up studies, the risk of CIN3+ was also significantly higher in women with a positive HPV16/18 genotype than in those with non-16/18 hrHPV genotypes [7, 19, 24]. Clinically, reflex HPV16/18 genotyping for women with HPV-positive/Pap-negative co-testing results may improve the efficacy of cervical cancer screening [21, 74–76]. These findings support the clinical utility of reflex HPV16/18 genotyping in women with HPV-positive/Pap-negative co-testing results.

Concerns Because HPV16-associated CIN3+ accounted for 74–77% of these cases in North America [8], there is a certain risk for CIN3+ in women with a negative reflex HPV16/18 genotyping results. To detect non-16/18 hrHPV-associated CIN3+/VAIN3+, an annual follow-up HPV/Pap co-testing is still necessary.

HPV Testing Assays and Validation

To date, a total of seven commercially available HPV testing assays under five commercial brand names were approved by US FDA for cervical cancer screening (Table 10.2). For hrHPV testing, the assays are designed to collectively test 13–14 hrHPVs.

1. Hybrid Capture 2 (HC2, Qiagen, Valencia, CA): HC2 is the first FDA-approved HPV testing assay that has been widely used in the USA in ThinPrep Pap cytology specimens with extensive published technical and clinical studies including several large clinical trials [55, 78, 79]. HC2 is a non-PCR-based HPV assay with a unique design of RNA-DNA hybridization for 13 high-risk HPV types. Even though HC2

HPV assay lacks both internal control for specimen adequacy determination and the capability of HPV16/18 genotyping, it is still the benchmark being used for HPV assay validation and to compare for the HPV testing efficacy.

2. Cervista HPV HR and Cervista HPV16/18 assays (Hologic, Marlborough, MA): These two HPV assays are also non-PCR-based HPV testing assays in ThinPrep Pap cytology specimens with unique design to detect hrHPVs and approved by the FDA. These assays have the advantage of internal control and the capability of HPV16/18 genotyping (Table 10.2). The disadvantage of the Cervista HPV assays is that HPV16/18 genotyping and hrHPV testing are not in a single testing platform and need to be tested separately.

Table 10.2 The US FDA-approved HPV testing assays

	HC2[a]	**Cervista HPV**	**Aptima HPV**	**Cobas HPV**	**BD Onclarity HPV**
PCR-based	No	No	Yes	Yes	Yes
Amplification	Signal	Signal	E6, E7 RNA	E6, E7 DNA	E6, E7 DNA
HPV detection[b]	13 types	14 types	14 types	14 types	14 types
HPV genotyping	No	HPV16, 18	HPV16, 18, 45	HPV16, 18,	HPV16, 18, 45
Internal controls	No	Yes	Yes	Yes	Yes
Equivocal zone	Yes	No	No	No	No
Company	Qiagen	Hologic	Hologic	Roche	Becton, Dickinson and Company

Reprinted and updated by permission from Springer Nature, Ge and Guo [77], © 2017

[a]Hybrid Capture 2

[b]HPV types:

13 high-risk HPV types: HPV16, 18, 31, 33, 35, 39, 45, 51, 52, 56, 58, 59, 68

14 high-risk HPV types: HPV16, 18, 31, 33, 35, 39, 45, 51, 52, 56, 58, 59, 66, 68

3. Cobas HPV assay (Roche Diagnostics, Indianapolis, IN): Cobas HPV assay is an FDA-approved HPV assay for HPV/Pap cytology co-testing and HPV primary screening (Table 10.3) in both ThinPrep and SurePath Pap specimens. The advantage of Cobas HPV assay is a highly automated and a robust test to provide HPV16/18 genotyping results and hrHPV results in the same platform that allows a specific triage for women with positive HPV16 or 18 during HPV primary screening. Cobas is a PCR-based HPV testing assay. The Cobas HPV was designed to have a completely sealed testing system and special chemical reaction design to eliminate potential cross contamination. An arbitrary cutoff was set for a positive result in order to exclude the less clinically relevant cases. Cobas HPV assay is the first FDA-approved HPV assay in SurePath Pap cytology specimens.
4. Aptima HPV and Aptima HPV16 18/45 assays (Hologic, Marlborough, MA): The two HPV assays are the only HPV

TABLE 10.3 Timeline of major clinical applications of HPV testing assays approved by the US FDA

Clinical applications[a]	2003	2009	2011	2015	2016	2018
Reflex for ASCUS	HC2[b]	Cervista HR	Cobas, Aptima HPV 16/18/45		Cobas (Sure Path)	BD Onclarity (SurePath)
HPV/Pap Co-testing	HC2[b]	Cervista HR	Cobas, Aptima HPV		Cobas (Sure Path)	BD Onclarity (SurePath)
Reflex HPV16/18		Cervista HPV16/18	Cobas, Aptima HPV16/18/45			
Primary screening				Cobas	Cobas (Sure Path)	BD Onclarity (SurePath)

Reprinted and updated by permission from Springer Nature, Ge and Guo [77], © 2017
[a]HPV testing assays unspecified for Pap cytology specimens were approved by FDA for ThinPrep Pap cytology specimen only
[b]Hybrid Capture 2

testing assays designed to target HPV mRNA. Since mRNAs are reliable indicators of active E6/E7 transcription, the HPV E6 or E7 mRNA detected by Aptima HPV assays is considered more clinically relevant than HPV DNA in predicting CIN3+. Aptima HPV assays are highly automated with the ability to detect HPV16, HPV18, and HPV45 genotypes. However, a separate test is required for HPV16/18/45 genotyping.

5. BD Onclarity HPV assay (Becton, Dickinson and Company, Sparks, MD): This HPV detecting assay was recently approved by the US FDA for cervical cancer screening in SurePath Pap cytology specimen, including HPV/Pap cytology co-testing and HPV primary screening. Similar to Cobas, Onclarity has an arbitrary cutoff set for a positive result in order to exclude the less clinically relevant cases. Onclarity HPV assay is highly automated, robust assay providing results of 11 hrHPV and HPV16, 18, and 45 genotypes on the same test run. For cervical specimen collected in SurePath medium, Onclarity HPV assay is an alternative choice to Cobas HPV assay for HPV testing.

To date, the FDA approved most of HPV testing assays specifically in ThinPrep Pap cytology, which is one of the liquid-based Pap cytology tests used in the USA. In 2016 and 2018, FDA approved Cobas HPV assay and BD Onclarity HPV assay for SurePath Pap specimen, respectively (Table 10.3). Although both ThinPrep and SurePath Pap tests are FDA-approved Pap cytology assays for cervical cancer screening, SurePath Pap cytology showed a significantly lower unsatisfactory rate than ThinPrep for Pap cytology testing [80]. Validation studies involving a comparative analysis with a clinically validated HPV testing assay in the same screening population are necessary for "off-label" use of HPV testing in SurePath specimens. HC2 HPV assay was considered as a reference standard [81]. To date, published validation studies for SurePath were limited. The only published clinical trial study using the dual Pap cytology sampling method with ThinPrep and SurePath Pap demonstrated comparable HC2 clinical sensitivities between SurePath and

ThinPrep for CIN2/3 [82]. In this study, SurePath Pap showed a lower failure rate of DNA extraction for HPV testing as compared to ThinPrep. The failure rates of DNA extraction in either ThinPrep or SurePath Pap specimens for HPV testing and its impact on HPV testing have not been adequately reported and need to be studied. With the advance of HPV detection technology and FDA-approved HPV testing assays for SurePath Pap cytology specimens on the market, more options of HPV testing assays are available for cervical cancer screening. It becomes critical to choose the HPV testing assay that fits specific clinical demands in practice.

References

1. WHO. Latest world cancer statistics. 2013. Available from: http://www.iarc.fr/en/media-centre/pr/2013/pdfs/pr223_E.pdf
2. Howlader N, Noone A, Krapcho M, editors. SEER cancer statistics review, 1975–2010. Bethesda: National Cancer Institute; 2015.
3. Sheets SSF. Cervix uteri cancer. National Cancer Institute Surveillance, Epidemiology and End Results Program. 2015. Available online: http://www.seer.cancer.gov/statistics/html/cervix.html
4. Siegel RL, Miller KD, Jemal A. Cancer statistics, 2016. CA Cancer J Clin. 2016;66(1):7–30.
5. Crosbie EJ, Einstein MH, Franceschi S, Kitchener HC. Human papillomavirus and cervical cancer. Lancet. 2013;382(9895):889–99.
6. Walboomers JM, Jacobs MV, Manos MM, Bosch FX, Kummer JA, Shah KV, et al. Human papillomavirus is a necessary cause of invasive cervical cancer worldwide. J Pathol. 1999;189(1):12–9.
7. Monsonego J, Cox JT, Behrens C, Sandri M, Franco EL, Yap PS, et al. Prevalence of high-risk human papilloma virus genotypes and associated risk of cervical precancerous lesions in a large U.S. screening population: data from the ATHENA trial. Gynecol Oncol. 2015;137(1):47–54.
8. Smith JS, Lindsay L, Hoots B, Keys J, Franceschi S, Winer R, et al. Human papillomavirus type distribution in invasive cervical cancer and high-grade cervical lesions: a meta-analysis update. Int J Cancer. 2007;121(3):621–32.
9. de Sanjose S, Quint WG, Alemany L, Geraets DT, Klaustermeier JE, Lloveras B, et al. Human papillomavirus genotype attribu-

tion in invasive cervical cancer: a retrospective cross-sectional worldwide study. Lancet Oncol. 2010;11(11):1048–56.
10. Bosch FX, Lorincz A, Munoz N, Meijer CJ, Shah KV. The causal relation between human papillomavirus and cervical cancer. J Clin Pathol. 2002;55(4):244–65.
11. Saslow D, Solomon D, Lawson HW, Killackey M, Kulasingam SL, Cain J, et al. American Cancer Society, American Society for Colposcopy and Cervical Pathology, and American Society for Clinical Pathology screening guidelines for the prevention and early detection of cervical cancer. CA Cancer J Clin. 2012;62(3):147–72.
12. Huh WK, Ault KA, Chelmow D, Davey DD, Goulart RA, Garcia FA, et al. Use of primary high-risk human papillomavirus testing for cervical cancer screening: interim clinical guidance. J Low Genit Tract Dis. 2015;136(2):178–82.
13. Practice Bulletin No. 156: obesity in pregnancy: correction. Obstet Gynecol. 2016;128(6):1450.
14. Wright TC Jr, Schiffman M, Solomon D, Cox JT, Garcia F, Goldie S, et al. Interim guidance for the use of human papillomavirus DNA testing as an adjunct to cervical cytology for screening. Obstet Gynecol. 2004;103(2):304–9.
15. Wright TC Jr, Massad LS, Dunton CJ, Spitzer M, Wilkinson EJ, Solomon D, et al. 2006 consensus guidelines for the management of women with abnormal cervical screening tests. J Low Genit Tract Dis. 2007;11(4):201–22.
16. Saslow D, Solomon D, Lawson HW, Killackey M, Kulasingam SL, Cain JM, et al. American Cancer Society, American Society for Colposcopy and Cervical Pathology, and American Society for Clinical Pathology screening guidelines for the prevention and early detection of cervical cancer. J Low Genit Tract Dis. 2012;16(3):175–204.
17. Massad LS, Einstein MH, Huh WK, Katki HA, Kinney WK, Schiffman M, et al. 2012 updated consensus guidelines for the management of abnormal cervical cancer screening tests and cancer precursors. J Low Genit Tract Dis. 2013;17(5 Suppl 1):S1–S27.
18. Vesco KK, Whitlock EP, Eder M, Lin J, Burda BU, Senger CA, et al. Screening for cervical cancer: a systematic evidence review for the US Preventive Services Task Force. Rockville: US Preventive Services Task Force Evidence Syntheses, Formerly Systematic Evidence Reviews; 2011.
19. Khan MJ, Castle PE, Lorincz AT, Wacholder S, Sherman M, Scott DR, et al. The elevated 10-year risk of cervical precancer and

cancer in women with human papillomavirus (HPV) type 16 or 18 and the possible utility of type-specific HPV testing in clinical practice. J Natl Cancer Inst. 2005;97(14):1072–9.
20. Schiffman M, Wentzensen N. Human papillomavirus infection and the multistage carcinogenesis of cervical cancer. Cancer Epidemiol Biomark Prev. 2013;22(4):553–60.
21. Wright TC Jr, Stoler MH, Sharma A, Zhang G, Behrens C, Wright TL, et al. Evaluation of HPV-16 and HPV-18 genotyping for the triage of women with high-risk HPV+ cytology-negative results. Am J Clin Pathol. 2011;136(4):578–86.
22. Castle PE, Stoler MH, Wright TC Jr, Sharma A, Wright TL, Behrens CM. Performance of carcinogenic human papillomavirus (HPV) testing and HPV16 or HPV18 genotyping for cervical cancer screening of women aged 25 years and older: a subanalysis of the ATHENA study. Lancet Oncol. 2011;12(9):880–90.
23. Katki HA, Wacholder S, Solomon D, Castle PE, Schiffman M. Risk estimation for the next generation of prevention programmes for cervical cancer. Lancet Oncol. 2009;10(11):1022–3.
24. Kjaer SK, Frederiksen K, Munk C, Iftner T. Long-term absolute risk of cervical intraepithelial neoplasia grade 3 or worse following human papillomavirus infection: role of persistence. J Natl Cancer Inst. 2010;102(19):1478–88.
25. Kitchener HC, Gilham C, Sargent A, Bailey A, Albrow R, Roberts C, et al. A comparison of HPV DNA testing and liquid based cytology over three rounds of primary cervical screening: extended follow up in the ARTISTIC trial. Eur J Cancer. 2011;47(6):864–71.
26. Li N, Franceschi S, Howell-Jones R, Snijders PJ, Clifford GM. Human papillomavirus type distribution in 30,848 invasive cervical cancers worldwide: variation by geographical region, histological type and year of publication. Int J Cancer. 2011;128(4):927–35.
27. Castle PE, Maza M. Prophylactic HPV vaccination: past, present, and future. Epidemiol Infect. 2016;144(3):449–68.
28. Thomsen LT, Frederiksen K, Munk C, Junge J, Castle PE, Iftner T, et al. High-risk and low-risk human papillomavirus and the absolute risk of cervical intraepithelial neoplasia or cancer. Obstet Gynecol. 2014;123(1):57–64.
29. Thierry F, Yaniv M. The BPV1-E2 trans-acting protein can be either an activator or a repressor of the HPV18 regulatory region. EMBO J. 1987;6(11):3391–7.

30. Vinokurova S, Wentzensen N, Kraus I, Klaes R, Driesch C, Melsheimer P, et al. Type-dependent integration frequency of human papillomavirus genomes in cervical lesions. Cancer Res. 2008;68(1):307–13.
31. Klingelhutz AJ, Roman A. Cellular transformation by human papillomaviruses: lessons learned by comparing high- and low-risk viruses. Virology. 2012;424(2):77–98.
32. Moody CA, Laimins LA. Human papillomavirus oncoproteins: pathways to transformation. Nat Rev Cancer. 2010;10(8):550–60.
33. Duensing S, Munger K. The human papillomavirus type 16 E6 and E7 oncoproteins independently induce numerical and structural chromosome instability. Cancer Res. 2002;62(23):7075–82.
34. Haedicke J, Iftner T. A review of the clinical performance of the Aptima HPV assay. J Clin Virol. 2016;76(Suppl 1):S40–S8.
35. Dunne EF, Unger ER, Sternberg M, McQuillan G, Swan DC, Patel SS, et al. Prevalence of HPV infection among females in the United States. JAMA. 2007;297(8):813–9.
36. Ho GY, Bierman R, Beardsley L, Chang CJ, Burk RD. Natural history of cervicovaginal papillomavirus infection in young women. N Engl J Med. 1998;338(7):423–8.
37. Garcia-Chacon R, Velasco-Ramirez SF, Flores-Romo L, Daneri-Navarro A. Immunobiology of HPV infection. Arch Med Res. 2009;40(6):443–8.
38. Bosch FX, Burchell AN, Schiffman M, Giuliano AR, de Sanjose S, Bruni L, et al. Epidemiology and natural history of human papillomavirus infections and type-specific implications in cervical neoplasia. Vaccine. 2008;26(Suppl 10):K1–16.
39. Chen HC, Schiffman M, Lin CY, Pan MH, You SL, Chuang LC, et al. Persistence of type-specific human papillomavirus infection and increased long-term risk of cervical cancer. J Natl Cancer Inst. 2011;103(18):1387–96.
40. Wright TC Jr, Massad LS, Dunton CJ, Spitzer M, Wilkinson EJ, Solomon D, et al. 2006 consensus guidelines for the management of women with cervical intraepithelial neoplasia or adenocarcinoma in situ. J Low Genit Tract Dis. 2007;11(4):223–39.
41. Holowaty P, Miller AB, Rohan T, To T. Natural history of dysplasia of the uterine cervix. J Natl Cancer Inst. 1999;91(3):252–8.
42. Rositch AF, Nowak RG, Gravitt PE. Increased age and race-specific incidence of cervical cancer after correction for hysterectomy prevalence in the United States from 2000 to 2009. Cancer. 2014;120(13):2032–8.

43. Moyer VA. Screening for cervical cancer: US Preventive Services Task Force recommendation statement. Ann Intern Med. 2012;156(12):880–91.
44. Practice Bulletin No. 168 summary: cervical cancer screening and prevention. Obstet Gynecol. 2016;128(4):923–5.
45. Bulletins ACoP. ACOG practice bulletin: clinical management guidelines for obstetrician-gynecologists. Number 45, August 2003. Cervical cytology screening (replaces committee opinion 152, March 1995). Obstet Gynecol. 2003;102(2):417–27.
46. Bulkmans NW, Berkhof J, Rozendaal L, van Kemenade FJ, Boeke AJ, Bulk S, et al. Human papillomavirus DNA testing for the detection of cervical intraepithelial neoplasia grade 3 and cancer: 5-year follow-up of a randomised controlled implementation trial. Lancet. 2007;370(9601):1764–72.
47. Naucler P, Ryd W, Tornberg S, Strand A, Wadell G, Elfgren K, et al. Human papillomavirus and Papanicolaou tests to screen for cervical cancer. N Engl J Med. 2007;357(16):1589–97.
48. Dillner J, Rebolj M, Birembaut P, Petry KU, Szarewski A, Munk C, et al. Long term predictive values of cytology and human papillomavirus testing in cervical cancer screening: joint European cohort study. BMJ. 2008;337:a1754.
49. Katki HA, Kinney WK, Fetterman B, Lorey T, Poitras NE, Cheung L, et al. Cervical cancer risk for women undergoing concurrent testing for human papillomavirus and cervical cytology: a population-based study in routine clinical practice. Lancet Oncol. 2011;12(7):663–72.
50. Kinney W, Wright TC, Dinkelspiel HE, DeFrancesco M, Thomas Cox J, Huh W. Increased cervical cancer risk associated with screening at longer intervals. Obstet Gynecol. 2015;125(2):311–5.
51. Dinkelspiel H, Kinney W. State of the science: cervical cancer screening in transition. Gynecol Oncol. 2014;133(3):389–93.
52. Ronco G, Dillner J, Elfstrom KM, Tunesi S, Snijders PJ, Arbyn M, et al. Efficacy of HPV-based screening for prevention of invasive cervical cancer: follow-up of four European randomised controlled trials. Lancet. 2014;383(9916):524–32.
53. Gage JC, Schiffman M, Katki HA, Castle PE, Fetterman B, Wentzensen N, et al. Reassurance against future risk of precancer and cancer conferred by a negative human papillomavirus test. J Natl Cancer Inst. 2014;106(8):1–4.
54. Dinkelspiel H, Fetterman B, Poitras N, Kinney W, Cox JT, Lorey T, et al. Cervical cancer rates after the transition from annual Pap to 3-year HPV and Pap. J Low Genit Tract Dis. 2014;18(1):57–60.

55. Ronco G, Giorgi-Rossi P, Carozzi F, Confortini M, Dalla Palma P, Del Mistro A, et al. Efficacy of human papillomavirus testing for the detection of invasive cervical cancers and cervical intraepithelial neoplasia: a randomised controlled trial. Lancet Oncol. 2010;11(3):249–57.
56. Ronco G, Giorgi-Rossi P, Carozzi F, Confortini M, Dalla Palma P, Del Mistro A, et al. Results at recruitment from a randomized controlled trial comparing human papillomavirus testing alone with conventional cytology as the primary cervical cancer screening test. J Natl Cancer Inst. 2008;100(7):492–501.
57. Wright TC, Stoler MH, Behrens CM, Sharma A, Zhang G, Wright TL. Primary cervical cancer screening with human papillomavirus: end of study results from the ATHENA study using HPV as the first-line screening test. Gynecol Oncol. 2015 Feb;136(2):189–97.
58. Castle PE, de Sanjose S, Qiao YL, Belinson JL, Lazcano-Ponce E, Kinney W. Introduction of human papillomavirus DNA screening in the world: 15 years of experience. Vaccine. 2012;30(Suppl 5):F117–22.
59. Stoler MH, Austin RM, Zhao C. Point-counterpoint: cervical cancer screening should be done by primary human papillomavirus testing with genotyping and reflex cytology for women over the age of 25 years. J Clin Microbiol. 2015;53(9):2798–804.
60. Blatt AJ, Kennedy R, Luff RD, Austin RM, Rabin DS. Comparison of cervical cancer screening results among 256,648 women in multiple clinical practices. Cancer Cytopathol. 2015;123(5):282–8.
61. Zhao C, Li Z, Nayar R, Levi AW, Winkler BA, Moriarty AT, et al. Prior high-risk human papillomavirus testing and Papanicolaou test results of 70 invasive cervical carcinomas diagnosed in 2012: results of a retrospective multicenter study. Arch Pathol Lab Med. 2015;139(2):184–8.
62. Yoshida T, Sano T, Kanuma T, Owada N, Sakurai S, Fukuda T, et al. Quantitative real-time polymerase chain reaction analysis of the type distribution, viral load, and physical status of human papillomavirus in liquid-based cytology samples from cervical lesions. Int J Gynecol Cancer. 2008;18(1):121–7.
63. Cricca M, Morselli-Labate AM, Venturoli S, Ambretti S, Gentilomi GA, Gallinella G, et al. Viral DNA load, physical status and E2/E6 ratio as markers to grade HPV16 positive women for high-grade cervical lesions. Gynecol Oncol. 2007;106(3):549–57.

64. Wright TC Jr, Cox JT, Massad LS, Twiggs LB, Wilkinson EJ, Conference AS-SC. 2001 consensus guidelines for the management of women with cervical cytological abnormalities. JAMA. 2002;287(16):2120–9.
65. Solomon D, Schiffman M, Tarone R, Group AS. Comparison of three management strategies for patients with atypical squamous cells of undetermined significance: baseline results from a randomized trial. J Natl Cancer Inst. 2001;93(4):293–9.
66. Katki HA, Schiffman M, Castle PE, Fetterman B, Poitras NE, Lorey T, et al. Five-year risks of CIN 3+ and cervical cancer among women with HPV testing of ASC-US Pap results. J Low Genit Tract Dis. 2013;17(5 Suppl 1):S36–42.
67. Einstein MH, Martens MG, Garcia FA, Ferris DG, Mitchell AL, Day SP, et al. Clinical validation of the Cervista HPV HR and 16/18 genotyping tests for use in women with ASC-US cytology. Gynecol Oncol. 2010;118(2):116–22.
68. Stoler MH, Wright TC Jr, Sharma A, Apple R, Gutekunst K, Wright TL, et al. High-risk human papillomavirus testing in women with ASC-US cytology results from the ATHENA HPV study. Am J Clin Pathol. 2011;135(3):468–75.
69. Arbyn M, Martin-Hirsch P, Buntinx F, Van Ranst M, Paraskevaidis E, Dillner J. Triage of women with equivocal or low-grade cervical cytology results: a meta-analysis of the HPV test positivity rate. J Cell Mol Med. 2009;13(4):648–59.
70. Cuzick J, Myers O, Hunt WC, Saslow D, Castle PE, Kinney W, et al. Human papillomavirus testing 2007–2012: co-testing and triage utilization and impact on subsequent clinical management. Int J Cancer. 2015;136(12):2854–63.
71. Stoler MH, Wright TC Jr, Sharma A, Zhang G, Apple R, Wright TL, et al. The interplay of age stratification and HPV testing on the predictive value of ASC-US cytology. Results from the ATHENA HPV study. Am J Clin Pathol. 2012;137(2):295–303.
72. Morris BJ. Cervical human papillomavirus screening by PCR: advantages of targeting the E6/E7 region. Clin Chem Lab Med. 2005;43(11):1171–7.
73. Katki HA, Schiffman M, Castle PE, Fetterman B, Poitras NE, Lorey T, et al. Five-year risks of CIN 3+ and cervical cancer among women who test Pap-negative but are HPV-positive. J Low Genit Tract Dis. 2013;17(5 Suppl 1):S56–63.
74. Schiffman M, Burk RD, Boyle S, Raine-Bennett T, Katki HA, Gage JC, et al. A study of genotyping for management of human

papillomavirus-positive, cytology-negative cervical screening results. J Clin Microbiol. 2015;53(1):52–9.
75. Woodard A, Austin RM, Li Z, Beere J. Prevalence of HPV 16/18 genotypes and histopathologic follow-up outcomes in women with negative cytology and positive high-risk HPV test results. J Am Soc Cytopathol. 2015;4:261–6.
76. Guo M, Khanna A, Dawlett M, Patel S, Gong Y, Staerkel G. Efficacy of reflex HPV16/18 genotyping in predicting CIN3/VAIN3 in women with HPVD/Pape results. J Am Soc Cytopathol. 2016;5:31–6.
77. Ge Y, Guo M. Molecular pathology of cervical dysplasia and carcinoma. In: Deavers MT, Coffey DM, editors. Precision molecular pathology of uterine cancer: Springer Nature; New York, NY, USA. 2017;253–78.
78. Ogilvie GS, Krajden M, van Niekerk D, Smith LW, Cook D, Ceballos K, et al. HPV for cervical cancer screening (HPV FOCAL): complete round 1 results of a randomized trial comparing HPV-based primary screening to liquid-based cytology for cervical cancer. Int J Cancer. 2017;140(2):440–8.
79. Zorzi M, Frayle H, Rizzi M, Fedato C, Rugge M, Penon MG, et al. A 3-year interval is too short for re-screening women testing negative for human papillomavirus: a population-based cohort study. BJOG. 2017;124(10):1585–93.
80. Fontaine D, Narine N, Naugler C. Unsatisfactory rates vary between cervical cytology samples prepared using ThinPrep and SurePath platforms: a review and meta-analysis. BMJ Open. 2012;2(2):e000847.
81. Arbyn M, Snijders PJ, Meijer CJ, Berkhof J, Cuschieri K, Kocjan BJ, et al. Which high-risk HPV assays fulfil criteria for use in primary cervical cancer screening? Clin Microbiol Infect. 2015;21(9):817–26.
82. Zhao FH, Hu SY, Bian JJ, Liu B, Peck RB, Bao YP, et al. Comparison of ThinPrep and SurePath liquid-based cytology and subsequent human papillomavirus DNA testing in China. Cancer Cytopathol. 2011;119(6):387–94.

Chapter 11
Molecular Diagnostics in Lung Cytology

Paul A. VanderLaan

Abbreviations

AKT-1	AKT serine/threonine kinase 1
ALK	anaplastic lymphoma kinase or ALK receptor tyrosine kinase
ASCO	American Society of Clinical Oncology
ATS	American Thoracic Society
BRAF	v-raf murine sarcoma viral oncogene homolog B
CAP/IASLC/AMP	College of American Pathologists/International Association for the Study of Lung Cancer/Association for Molecular Pathology
DDR2	discoidin domain receptor tyrosine kinase 2
EBUS-TBNA	endobronchial ultrasound-guided transbronchial needle aspiration

P. A. VanderLaan
Beth Israel Deaconess Medical Center, Harvard Medical School, Boston, MA, USA
e-mail: pvanderl@bidmc.harvard.edu

S. Roy-Chowdhuri et al. (eds.), *Molecular Diagnostics in Cytopathology*, https://doi.org/10.1007/978-3-319-97397-5_11

EGFR	epidermal growth factor receptor
ENB	electromagnetic navigational bronchoscopy
ERBB2	erb-b2 receptor tyrosine kinase 2 (HER2)
FFPE	formalin-fixed paraffin-embedded
FGFR1–4	Fibroblast growth factor receptor 1–4
FISH	fluorescence *in situ* hybridization
FNA	fine-needle aspiration
IASLC/ATS/ERS	International Association for the Study of Lung Cancer/American Thoracic Society/European Respiratory Society
IHC	immunohistochemistry
KIT	KIT proto-oncogene receptor tyrosine kinase
KRAS	Kirsten rat sarcoma viral oncogene homolog
MEK1	mitogen-activated protein kinase kinase 1
MET	MET proto-oncogene, receptor tyrosine kinase
MTOR	mechanistic target of rapamycin
NCCN	National Comprehensive Cancer Network
NF1	Neurofibromin 1
NGS	next-generation sequencing
NRAS	neuroblastoma RAS viral oncogene
NRG1	Neuregulin 1
NSCLC	non-small cell lung cancer
NTRK1–3	neurotrophic tyrosine kinase receptor, type 1–3
PCR	polymerase chain reaction
PD-1	programmed cell death protein 1 (CD279)
PD-L1	programmed death-ligand 1 (CD274)

PDGFRA	platelet-derived growth factor receptor alpha
PIK3CA	phosphatidylinositol-4,5-bisphosphate 3-kinase catalytic subunit alpha
RET	proto-oncogene tyrosine-protein kinase receptor Ret
RIT1	Ras-like without CAAX 1
ROS1	ROS proto-oncogene 1, receptor tyrosine kinase
TKI	tyrosine kinase inhibitor
TPS	tumor proportion score
TSC1/2	tuberous sclerosis 1/2 (TSC1)

Key Terminology

Biomarker	According to the NIH Biomarkers Definitions Working Group, a biomarker is any objectively measurable characteristic that can be used as an indicator of normal biological processes, pathogenic processes, or a pharmacological response to a therapeutic intervention
Driver mutation	Driver mutation refers to somatic alterations in genes (including point mutations, insertions/deletions, and gene fusions) that are responsible for the development and progression of cancer
Immunotherapy	According to the NCI dictionary of cancer terms, immunotherapy is a type of therapy that uses substances to stimulate or suppress the immune system to help the body fight cancer

Key Points

- Molecular and ancillary biomarker testing in lung cancer is a rapidly evolving field, with new testing targets emerging on a regular basis
- Molecular and ancillary biomarker testing has become standard of care in the work-up of advanced-stage NSCLC to direct appropriate choice of therapy
- Guideline recommendations issued by various groups have broadly outlined the requirements for molecular testing, including which targets to test, how to test them, and how the results should be reported
- Immune checkpoint inhibitor therapy has emerged as an important therapeutic modality in NSCLC, and as such routine PD-L1 biomarker testing has also become standard of care
- Cytology specimens by and large have been shown to be adequate testing substrates in the setting of NSCLC

Introduction

Despite the significant advances witnessed over the past few decades in lung cancer screening, diagnosis, and treatment, lung cancer remains the leading cause of cancer death in both men and women, with 2018 estimates accounting for over a quarter of all cancer-related deaths in the United States [1]. Over this time, the medical community has seen an increasing reliance on minimally invasive tissue sampling techniques for the diagnostic work-up of lung cancer, including both transthoracic CT-guided needle biopsies as well as various bronchoscopic-based modalities including EBUS-TBNA and ENB. As such, cytology and small biopsy specimens have become the primary modality for establishing a pathologic diagnosis of lung cancer. On these specimens, traditional cytomorphologic assessment in conjunction with lineage-specific immunohistochemical stains can lead to a precise diagnosis in the majority of cases, differentiating lung adenocarcinomas from squamous cell carcinomas and neuroendocrine tumors, among others. This is reflected in the increased emphasis placed on these cytology and small biopsy specimens in the 2011 IASLC/ATS/ERS classification system for lung adenocarcinomas as well as the most recent 2015 edition of the WHO classification system for tumors of the lung [2, 3].

Over the past decade, it has been increasingly appreciated that ancillary molecular testing performed on these cytology and small biopsy specimens is necessary in order to identify potentially targetable oncogenic driver mutations and assess for biomarkers that can help direct therapeutic decisions by the treating oncologist. Indeed, in patients with advanced-stage non-small cell lung cancer that have an actionable driver mutation identified, treatment with the appropriate targeted therapy leads to improved overall survival compared to standard cytotoxic chemotherapy [4]. Therefore, the cytologist and the cytopathology laboratory now play a critical role for streamlining the pre-analytic factors that can impact ancillary biomarker testing of NSCLC tumor samples [5].

Given the clinical implications that molecular testing has on directing subsequent oncologic care for patients with NSCLC, guidelines have been put forth in recent years by varying professional societies on the subject. The most comprehensive and widely adopted guidelines for the molecular testing of lung cancer specimens was issued in 2013 by the CAP/IASLC/AMP [6] and recently updated in 2018 [7]. These updated guidelines have been endorsed by ASCO with minor modification (discussed later) [8]. Additionally, the NCCN clinical practice guidelines in oncology outline recommendations for molecular and biomarker analysis in NSCLC [9], and more specialized societies such as the Papanicolaou Society of Cytopathology have also published guidelines on the topic [10]. In general, there is overall consensus on the clinically necessary targets that should be tested and how they should be tested, with differences between guidelines largely attributed to the timing of guideline publication given the rapid biomedical advances in the ever-evolving field thoracic oncology. This chapter will provide a broad summary of these molecular testing guideline recommendations with particular attention paid to the implications for cytology specimens and the cytopathology laboratory. In general, the focused summary below will largely stem from the CAP/IASLC/AMP guidelines [6, 7] with notation for when other guideline recommendations may significantly differ.

Molecular Testing in NSCLC

Although the oncologic management of patients with lung cancer is increasingly reliant on characterizing the genomic alterations and biomarker phenotype, it is important to recognize that the pathologic tumor categorization based on cytomorphology and immunohistochemical staining profile remains the cornerstone for treatment decisions. In most cases, before proceeding to ancillary testing, a firm diagnosis of lung adenocarcinoma, squamous cell carcinoma, or neuroendocrine carcinoma (carcinoid, atypical carcinoid, large cell neuroendocrine carcinoma, or small cell carcinoma) should be established. Classic cytomorphologic features, in conjunction with immunostains such as TTF-1 and napsin A (adenocarcinoma), p40 and CK5/6 (squamous cell carcinoma), or TTF-1 and synaptophysin/chromogranin/CD56 (neuroendocrine tumors), can very accurately classify tumors on cytology specimens, as extensively covered elsewhere [2, 3, 11]. This initial characterization is important, as testing algorithms are largely designed around tumor classification.

What Specimens Should Be Tested?

In general, it has become standard of care to test all advanced-stage NSCLCs (i.e., patients who are not surgical candidates) and not limit testing to only patients with suggestive clinical features (such as never smokers, younger patients, and females). Because the overwhelming majority of targetable driver mutations have been identified in lung adenocarcinomas, the recommendation is to test all advanced-stage non-squamous, NSCLC specimens. However, because of the possibility of tumor heterogeneity especially given limited sampling from cytology or small biopsy specimens, the updated CAP/IASLC/AMP guidelines acknowledge that "physicians may use molecular biomarker testing in tumors with histologies other than adenocarcinoma when clinical features indicate a higher probability of an oncogenic driver," such as never smoker or young age. Essentially, minimizing the tumor types that should not be tested helps ensure the maximum number of targetable mutations is identified in the most efficient manner possible.

Although traditionally molecular testing has been primarily run and validated on FFPE tissue (i.e., surgical pathology biopsies or cytology cell block specimens), the updated CAP/IASLC/AMP guidelines now acknowledge that *any* cytology sample with adequate cellularity and preservation can be tested. More specifically, both the NCCN guidelines and the adapted ASCO guidelines specify that cytologic smears (such as those generated during FNA or rapid on-site specimen evaluation) can be used for molecular testing. The caveat to which is that few commercial laboratories accept direct smears for testing at the moment, and specific validation of the specimen type should be performed by the testing laboratory (be it in-house or send-out).

How Quickly Should the Testing Results Be Available?

From the clinician's perspective, the sooner the better! Treatment plans are often kept on hold until the treating oncologist has knowledge of the tumor genotype. Indeed, a recent study demonstrated that less than 20% of lung cancer patients had their tumor molecular testing results available to the medical oncologist at the time of first oncologic consultation; those patients who did have molecular testing results available had significantly shorter time intervals to treatment choice and treatment start than those patients who were still waiting for the testing results [12]. The CAP/IASLC/AMP guidelines recommend the following testing turnaround time benchmarks:

- Testing results should be available within 2 weeks (10 working days) of receiving the specimen in the testing laboratory.
- Laboratory departments should establish processes to ensure that specimens that have a final histopathologic diagnosis are sent to outside molecular pathology laboratories within 3 working days of receiving requests and to intramural molecular pathology laboratories within 24 h.

These testing intervals can pose a logistical challenge, especially in the send-out testing setting, when considering all the steps that can contribute to delays in the process above and beyond the primary testing/analytic phase (such as block retrieval, specimen packaging and transport, accessioning, and report generation). There is some evidence to indicate that these benchmarks can be met when a streamlined process is in place, and ongoing monitoring of individual components can prove to be a valuable quality assurance measure that cytopathology laboratories employ [13, 14].

How Should the Molecular Targets Be Tested?

Traditionally, molecular testing has relied on a one gene-one assay model, with separate reactions/tests run for each target. However, for small biopsy or cytology specimens with a limited amount of tumor material, this approach may not be sustainable as new testing targets emerge. As such, although single-gene assays for the Tier 1 targets (described below) are still recommended as a viable first step, the field is rapidly moving toward multiplexed genetic sequencing panels as the preferred testing modality over multiple single-gene tests in order to provide the breadth of genomic information required for treatment with approved therapy, emerging therapies, or enrollment in clinical trials. For some genomic targets, IHC or FISH remains a viable testing alternative to molecular techniques, such as for *ALK* and *ROS1* [7].

Which Targets Should Be Tested?

The most recent iteration of the guidelines stratifies molecular targets in a tiered system, summarized in Table 11.1. The top tier represents the "must test" group of genes, as these have proven and FDA-approved therapies. This tier includes *EGFR*, *ALK*, and *ROS1* (with ASCO and the NCCN guidelines also including *BRAF* in this mandatory test group). The second tier or category of molecular targets are those that should be tested as part of an extended panel, either initially along with the Tier 1 targets or if the initial Tier 1 target testing reveals no actionable mutations. These "should test" targets include *MET* (specifically the *MET* exon 14 splicing mutation), *RET*, *ERBB2 (HER2)*, and *KRAS*. The former three show promising results from late-stage clinical trials with respect to response to targeted therapies, and *KRAS* mutations if present predict resistance to TKI therapy. Finally, the third tier includes all other emerging genomic alterations that have potential for treatment with targeted therapies, largely in the clinical trial setting. This growing list of "may test" targets include but are not limited to *MEK1/MAP2K1*,

Table 11.1 Current tiered framework for molecular testing targets in NSCLC

Tier 1 **"Must test"**	**Tier 2** **"Should test"**	**Tier 3** **"May test"**
EGFR	*ERBB2/HER2*	*MEK1/MAP2K1*
ALK	*MET*	*FGFR 1–4*
ROS1	*RET*	*NTRK1–3*
BRAF	*KRAS*	*NRG1*
		RIT1
		NF1
		PIK3CA
		AKT1
		NRAS
		MTOR
		TSC1–2
		KIT
		PDGFRA
		DDR2

FGFR 1–4, *NTRK1–3*, *NRG1*, *RIT1*, *NF1*, *PIK3CA*, *AKT1*, *NRAS*, *MTOR*, *TSC1–2*, *KIT*, *PDGFRA*, and *DDR2*, among others. Over time, as FDA drug approvals follow successful clinical trial results that highlight effective therapeutic options for these emerging molecular targets, there should be an escalator effect in these tier classifications, with "may test" targets becoming "should test" and the "should test" targets being elevated to "must test" status.

What Is the Expected Frequency of Genomic Alterations in NSCLC?

The prevalence of these driver mutations in NSCLC varies depending on clinical variables such as age, gender, ethnicity, and smoking status [15, 16]. However, based on data compiled from 6 large studies with a cumulative total of over 25,000 NSCLCs sequenced, the average percentages for each of the 8 major genomic alterations included in the Tier 1 and Tier 2 groups is presented in Fig. 11.1 [17–22]. A brief discussion of each of these targets follows.

EGFR

EGFR is a member of the ErbB family of transmembrane receptor tyrosine kinases that regulate proliferation and apoptosis. Oncogenic driver mutations localize to the tyrosine kinase domain, most clustering in exons 19 and 21. Approximately 85% of *EGFR* activating mutations are the L858R exon 21 mutation and exon 19 small in-frame deletions [23]. A number of approved tyrosine kinase inhibitors (TKIs) including erlotinib, afatinib, and gefitinib have shown efficacy in treating patients with sensitizing *EGFR* mutations; however, disease progression is usually seen after 9–12 months of treatment, most often secondary to the acquisition of a secondary T790M missense mutation in exon 20 that can be treated with osimertinib, a third-generation, irreversible, *EGFR* TKI [24]. *EGFR* mutational testing should be done

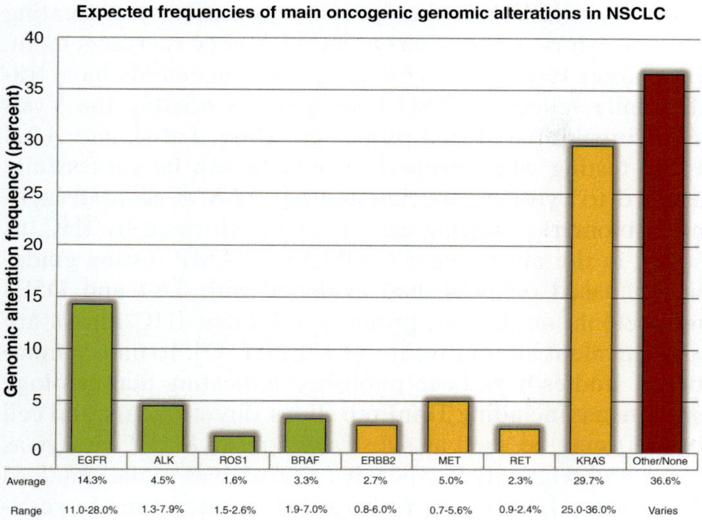

FIGURE 11.1 Frequency of main oncogenic genomic alterations in NSCLC. Values (average and range) are based on reported mutation or gene rearrangement frequencies compiled from six large scale studies [17–22]. The Tier 1 genomic alterations are denoted in green, the Tier 2 targets in gold, and the remaining Tier 3 targets (or no genomic alterations identified) in red

using sequencing or PCR-based techniques, and the updated CAP/IASLC/AMP guideline recommendations state "it is not appropriate to use IHC for *EGFR* mutation testing" [7].

ALK

ALK is a member of the insulin-receptor tyrosine kinase family. In lung cancer *ALK* on chromosome 2 can undergo gene fusion (most frequently with echinoderm microtubule-associated protein-like 4, *EML4*), leading to a constitutively active EML4-ALK fusion protein driving cell division and growth pathways. A growing number of approved oral small-molecule inhibitor TKIs including crizotinib, alectinib, ceritinib, lorlatinib, and brigatinib show efficacy in treating patients whose tumors harbor an *ALK* gene rearrangement. Biomarker testing for *ALK* gene rearrangements have traditionally relied on FISH testing (most notably the Vysis *ALK* break apart FISH probe set, Abbot Labs), and *ALK* FISH testing when properly validated can be successfully applied to cytology specimens [25]. *ALK* gene rearrangement biomarker testing can also be performed by IHC, as stated in the most recent CAP/IASLC/AMP testing guidelines: "based on published evidence with 5A4 and D5F3 monoclonal antibodies, properly validated IHC assays are an equivalent alternative to *ALK* FISH" [7]. To date, a number of studies have been published indicating that cytology specimens (including ThinPrep slides, direct smears, and cell blocks) may be used as substrates for *ALK* IHC assays as quick and relatively inexpensive alternatives to the standard FISH assay [26–28]. As with *EGFR*-mutated tumors, resistance mechanisms eventually develop in *ALK*-rearranged tumors, due to either *ALK*-dependent mechanisms (such as *ALK* kinase secondary mutations) or *ALK*-independent mechanisms. Tumor re-biopsy with reverse transcription polymerase chain reaction (RT-PCR) or sequencing can identify secondary point mutations that can help direct choice of appropriate second- or third-generation *ALK* TKIs [29].

ROS1

Like *ALK*, *ROS1* on chromosome 6 encodes a receptor tyrosine kinase from the insulin-receptor family and can undergo gene rearrangements with a large number of gene targets including *SLC34A2*, *CD74*, *TPM3*, *SDC4*, *EZR*, *LRIG3*, *KDELR2*, *CCDC6*, *CLTC*, *LIMA1*, *MSN*, and *TMEM106B* [30]. The resulting constitutively active kinase signaling of the ROS1-fusion protein drives pathways in cell proliferation, cell survival, and cell migration. Tumors with *ROS1* gene rearrangements show response to the multi-target TKI crizotinib, currently approved by the FDA as first-line treatment in advanced-stage *ROS1*-rearranged NSCLCs. Currently testing for *ROS1* fusions can be achieved through RT-PCR/sequencing techniques for known fusion partners, FISH break-apart probe testing for *ROS1* rearrangements, or *ROS1* IHC. According to the most recent CAP/IASLC/AMP guidelines, any of these methods can be used as screening tests in lung adenocarcinoma patients, though a positive *ROS1* IHC result should be confirmed by molecular or cytogenetic methods [7]. Cytology specimens can serve as adequate substrates for *ROS1* FISH testing if properly validated [25], and a recent study on *ROS1* IHC suggests that cytology cytospins and direct smears can be used when screening for *ROS1* gene rearrangements by IHC [31]. As with *ALK*, resistance to crizotinib eventually develops in virtually all patients with *ROS1*-rearranged tumors, and subsequent RT-PCR/sequencing testing may be useful in identifying secondary point mutations that can be treated with other and emerging TKIs, such as lorlatinib or cabozantinib [29, 32].

BRAF

Unlike the cell surface tyrosine kinases *EGFR*, *ALK*, and *ROS1*, *BRAF* is an intracellular protein kinase involved in the MAP kinase signal transduction pathway. In addition to NSCLC, *BRAF* mutations are encountered in a number of malignancies including melanoma, colorectal carcinoma, papillary thyroid carcinoma, and others. The most commonly encountered activating driver mutation is the V600E (valine to glutamate substitution at amino acid position 600 resulting from a 1799 T > A point mutation). NSCLCs that harbor a *BRAF* V600E mutation respond to the FDA-approved dual small-molecule inhibitory therapy of dabrafenib (*BRAF* inhibitor) and trametinib (*MEK* inhibitor). *BRAF* testing can be performed using PCR/sequencing based methods as well as using IHC with the VE1 clone, though there are no published studies to date on the use of BRAF VE1 IHC on lung cancer cytology specimens. As an expert consensus opinion from the most recent CAP/IASLC/AMP testing guidelines, "BRAF molecular testing is currently not indicated as a routine stand-alone assay outside the context of a clinical trial. It is appropriate to include *BRAF* as part of larger testing panels performed either initially or when routine *EGFR*, *ALK*, and *ROS1* testing is negative [7]." However, both the ASCO endorsement statement on the recent CAP/IASLC/AMP guidelines as well as the NCCN recommendations both elevate *BRAF* to the same "must test" status of *EGFR*, *ALK*, and *ROS1*.

MET

The *MET* proto-oncogene is a cell surface receptor tyrosine kinase for hepatocyte growth factor (ligand) that activates cell signaling pathways for cell survival, migration, proliferation, and epithelial-mesenchymal transition. Genomic alterations in NSCLC for *MET* include gene amplification, activating point mutations in the tyrosine kinase domain, or splice mutations such as the *exon 14 skipping mutation* which interrupts the ubiquitin-mediated degradation of this protein [7]. Although no FDA-approved therapy currently exists for *MET* amplification or exon 14 skipping mutations, the multi-target TKI crizotinib does show efficacy in these tumors [33]. *MET* exon 14 testing can be done by single-gene sequencing or as part of an expanded NGS panel, the latter preferred given the large number and complexity of exon 14 splice sites. *MET* amplification can be tested via FISH or IHC. *MET* is currently classified as a Tier 2 genomic target, with the expert consensus opinion from the most recent CAP/IASLC/AMP testing guidelines stating that "*MET* molecular testing is not indicated as a routine stand-alone assay outside the context of a clinical trial. It is appropriate to include *MET* as part of larger testing panels performed either initially or when routine *EGFR, ALK*, and *ROS1* testing is negative" [7].

RET

RET is a proto-oncogene that encodes for a cell surface receptor tyrosine kinase that is involved in signaling pathways for cellular proliferation, cellular migration, and differentiation. In NSCLC, *RET* gene fusions involve multiple gene targets (most frequently *KIF5B*), which result in constitutive activation of the *RET* signaling pathways [34]. Although no *RET*-specific inhibitor has been developed, trials are ongoing to determine the efficacy of current multi-target TKIs in treating *RET*-rearranged NSCLCs. Testing for *RET* rearrangements is best achieved via FISH- or RT-PCR-based methods, since, unlike *ALK* and *ROS1*, current IHC methods appear to be not sufficiently reliable to detect *RET* rearrangements [7, 34].

ERBB2

The human epidermal growth factor receptor 2 (*ERBB2; HER2*) has long been associated with oncogenesis in breast and gastric cancer but has more recently emerged as an oncogenic driver in NSCLC as well. Oncogenic alterations of the plasma membrane-bound receptor tyrosine kinase include gene amplification as well as exon 20 insertions, the latter likely playing a larger role in NSCLC [30]. These alterations can be either primary genomic alterations in NSCLC or can arise as secondary events as resistance mechanisms in patients with *EGFR* mutations following targeted therapy [7]. Clinical trials are ongoing for treating NSCLC with *ERBB2* alterations with targeted agents including trastuzumab and afatinib [9]. Currently classified as Tier 2 status, *ERBB2* testing in NSCLC is largely PCR/sequencing based and is focused on sequence alterations, specifically insertions and duplications in exon 20. *ERBB2* amplification can also be assayed by FISH, though screening via IHC is not recommended at this time.

KRAS

In contrast to the previously discussed genomic alterations in NSCLC that tend to occur in never-smokers, mutations in the *KRAS* gene are much more common in patients with NSCLC with a smoking history. *KRAS* is a GTPase that is involved in the MAP-kinase (*BRAF/MEK/ERK*) and phosphoinositide-3-kinase (*PI3K*) signaling pathways, with point mutations most commonly in codon 12 leading to continuous proliferative signaling due to impaired feedback regulation [30]. There are currently no specific targetable therapies for *KRAS*-mutated NSCLCs, and at this time, testing for *KRAS* is only useful insomuch that most of these oncogenic driver mutations are mutually exclusive (i.e., a tumor harboring a *KRAS* mutation is unlikely to also have a targetable driver mutation) [7]. Testing for *KRAS* mutations is generally done via PCR-based methods or as part of a larger NGS type panel.

Other Targets in NSCLC

With the use of CGP utilizing panels with hundreds or thousands of assayed genes, the list of rare (generally about 1% or less of all NSCLC) gene mutations continues to grow. The list includes *AKT1*, *NF1*, *PIK3CA*, *NRAS/HRAS*, *MAP2K1(MEK1)*, *STK11*, *MYC*, *RICTOR*, *CDK4/CCND1*, *BRCA1/2*, *NTRK1/NTRK3*, *TSC1/2*, *FGFR1/2*, *CDKN2A*, *PTEN*, and *RIT1*, among others [7]. At this point, the clinical significance of mutations identified in these gene targets is not entirely clear, though preclinical and clinical trials are ongoing to identify potential targetable therapeutics for lung cancers harboring these mutations.

Immune Checkpoint Inhibitor Testing

The past decade has witnessed significant developments in the field of immunotherapy for NSCLC, which has emerged as a major therapeutic choice for tumors that do not harbor a targetable driver mutation. To date, the FDA-approved immune checkpoint inhibitor drugs for NSCLC primarily target the programmed death ligand-receptor axis (PD-L1/PD-1) and in optimally selected patient populations demonstrate superior response rates, survival, and toxicity profiles as compared to conventional chemotherapy [35]. The biomarker selection relies on the assessment of PD-L1 expression via IHC on tumor cells (or in some instances on tumor infiltrating immune cells as well). Different cutoff values for the tumor proportion score (TPS), or the percentage of tumor cells showing partial or complete membranous staining of any intensity for PD-L1, for a given lung cancer biopsy/specimen is used to determine which patients are most likely to respond to immune checkpoint inhibitor therapy. Currently, there are five different drugs that are either FDA-approved or are in late-stage clinical trials for treatment of NSCLC, and each drug has a paired assay consisting of a different antibody clone, run on different staining platforms, and different clinical cutoff definitions of positivity (Table 11.2) [36–38]. This testing complexity is problematic for clinicians and pathology

Table 11.2 PD-L1 immune checkpoint inhibitor drugs, paired IHC assays, and scoring data for NSCLC (as of 2018)

	Biomarker assay		
Drug	**Antibody information**	**IHC platform**	**Scoring criteria**
Nivolumab (Anti-PD-1)	**28–8** Rabbit anti-PD-L1 Epitope: extracellular domain	DAKO pharmDx/ Link 48 Autostainer	**1st line ≥ 50% TPS** (no testing if with platinum doublet chemo) **Second line ≥ 1% TPS**
Pembrolizumab (Anti-PD-1)	**22C3** Mouse anti-PD-L1 Epitope: extracellular domain	DAKO pharmDx/ Link 48 Autostainer	**1st line ≥ 50% TPS** **Second line ≥ 1% TPS**

(continued)

Table 11.2 (continued)

Drug	Biomarker assay Antibody information	IHC platform	Scoring criteria
Atezolizumab (Anti-PD-L1)	**SP142** Rabbit anti-PD-L1 Epitope: intracellular domain	Ventana BenchMark Ultra	**2nd line (no testing needed)** *TCs (TC0–3)* 1%, 5%, 50% cutoffs *TIICs (IC0–3)* In tumor PD-L1+ areas, TICCs at 1%, 5%, 10% cutoffs
Durvalumab (Anti-PD-L1)	**SP263** Rabbit anti-PD-L1 Epitope: extracellular domain	Ventana BenchMark Ultra	**Maintenance therapy for stage III following chemo/XRT** (no testing needed) PACIFIC phase III clinical trials *≥ 25% TPS (high expression)*
Avelumab[a] (Anti-PD-L1)	**73-10** Rabbit anti-PD-L1 Epitope: intracellular domain	DAKO platform	**JAVELIN** phase III clinical trials Second *line ≥ 1% TPS*

[a]Not currently FDA approved for NSCLC. *TC* tumor cells, *TIIC* tumor-infiltrating immune cells, *TPS* tumor proportion score

laboratories alike, which has led to many ongoing studies to compare staining characteristics across the different platforms in the hopes to develop some levels of cross-test comparability [39, 40].

PD-L1 testing recommendations were not included in the 2018 CAP/IASLC/AMP NSCLC molecular testing guidelines (though a separate guideline on the topic is being developed); however, the NCCN NSCLC guidelines recommend testing advanced-stage lung adenocarcinomas as well as lung squamous cell carcinomas for PD-L1 TPS [7, 9]. At this point PD-L1 testing has been only validated on FFPE tissue. There is some uncertainty whether cytology cell block specimens, and more so direct smears or other cytologic preparations, may serve as comparable testing substrates, though few studies have been recently published indicating that FFPE cytology cell blocks may indeed be a comparable testing substrate for PD-L1 IHC just like other molecular tests currently done on these specimens [41–47]. Looking forward, it remains to be seen whether tumor mutation burden as estimated by NGS panel testing may actually emerge as a more reliable biomarker for selecting patients most likely to respond to immune checkpoint inhibitory therapy [48].

Other Emerging Lung Cancer Tests

To date, the vast majority of molecular testing in NSCLC has focused on identifying specific genomic alterations in individual genes to guide selection of targeted therapies for patients who are not surgical candidates. This testing is predicated on having first established a pathologic diagnosis of lung cancer. However, not every pulmonary nodule identified radiologically is malignant, and there is oftentimes ambiguity over which patients should be followed with radiographic surveillance versus those who should progress to an invasive diagnostic procedure (with the associated morbidity and mortality risks they carry). Along these lines, a recently developed bronchial genomic classifier test has been developed [49], much akin to the Afirma genomic classifier test used for indeterminate thyroid nodules (see Chap. 12). Early clinical trials have shown this test to improve the diagnostic accuracy of bronchoscopy for suspected lung cancer, which may be helpful in identifying which lung nodules have a low likelihood of malignancy, and therefore can be followed in a more conservative fashion [49]. As the development of new molecular biomarker tests has the potential for early detection of lung cancer and risk stratification of suspicious pulmonary nodules, the ATS recently issued a consensus statement for guidance on when to determining whether a molecular biomarker for the early detection of lung cancer is ready for clinical use [50].

Conclusions

In summary, cytology specimens represent an increasingly important modality for diagnosis and ancillary testing in lung cancer and as such offer both special opportunities but also challenges with respect to how these specimens are utilized [51, 52]. The identification of oncogenic driver genomic alterations that can be targeted with specific therapeutic agents has ushered in the era of personalized medicine in lung cancer patients. The clinical success of these targeted therapies in appropriately selected patients has elevated the role of ancillary molecular testing to standard of care in patients with advanced-stage lung cancer. As such, the cytopathologist and molecular pathologist have assumed a central role in guiding the care of patients with lung cancer.

References

1. National Cancer Institute (NCI) Surveillance, Epidemiology, and End Results (SEER) program. Cancer Stat Facts: Lung and Bronchus Cancer. https://seer.cancer.gov/statfacts/html/lungb.html. Accessed April 10, 2018.
2. Travis WD, Brambilla E, Noguchi M, et al. Diagnosis of lung cancer in small biopsies and cytology: implications of the 2011 International Association for the Study of Lung Cancer/American Thoracic Society/European Respiratory Society classification. Arch Pathol Lab Med. 2013;137:668–84.
3. Travis WD, Brambilla E, Burke AP, et al., editors. WHO classification of tumours of the lung, pleura, thymus and heart. 4th ed. Lyon: World Health Organization; 2015.

4. Kris MG, Johnson BE, Berry LD, et al. Using multiplexed assays of oncogenic drivers in lung cancers to select targeted drugs. JAMA. 2014;311:1998–2006.
5. Roy-Chowdhuri S, Stewart J. Preanalytic variables in cytology: lessons learned from next-generation sequencing-the MD Anderson experience. Arch Pathol Lab Med. 2016;140:1191–9.
6. Lindeman NI, Cagle PT, Beasley MB, et al. Molecular testing guideline for selection of lung cancer patients for EGFR and ALK tyrosine kinase inhibitors: guideline from the College of American Pathologists, International Association for the Study of Lung Cancer, and Association for Molecular Pathology. Arch Pathol Lab Med. 2013;137:828–60.
7. Lindeman NI, Cagle PT, Aisner DL, et al. Updated molecular testing guideline for the selection of lung cancer patients for treatment with targeted tyrosine kinase inhibitors: guideline from the College of American Pathologists, the International Association for the Study of Lung Cancer, and the Association for Molecular Pathology. Arch Pathol Lab Med. 2018;142:321–46.
8. Kalemkerian GP, Narula N, Kennedy EB, et al. Molecular testing guideline for the selection of patients with lung cancer for treatment with targeted tyrosine kinase inhibitors: American Society of Clinical Oncology Endorsement of the College of American Pathologists/International Association for the Study of Lung Cancer/Association for Molecular Pathology Clinical Practice Guideline Update. J Clin Oncol. 2018;36:911–9.
9. National Comprehensive Cancer Network Clinical Practice Guidelines in Oncology (NCCN Guidelines). Non-Small Cell Lung Cancer (Version 3.2018). https://www.nccn.org/professionals/physician_gls/pdf/nscl.pdf. Accessed April 10, 2018.
10. Layfield LJ, Roy-Chowdhuri S, Baloch Z, et al. Utilization of ancillary studies in the cytologic diagnosis of respiratory lesions: the papanicolaou society of cytopathology consensus recommendations for respiratory cytology. Diagn Cytopathol. 2016;44:1000–9.
11. Zakowski MF. Analytic inquiry: molecular testing in lung cancer. Cancer Cytopathol. 2017;125:470–6.
12. Lim C, Tsao MS, Le LW, et al. Biomarker testing and time to treatment decision in patients with advanced nonsmall-cell lung cancer. Ann Oncol. 2015;26:1415–21.
13. DiStasio M, Chen Y, Rangachari D, Costa DB, Heher YK, VanderLaan PA. Molecular testing turnaround time for non-small cell lung cancer in routine clinical practice confirms

feasibility of CAP/IASLC/AMP guideline recommendations: a single-center analysis. Clin Lung Cancer. 2017;18:e349–56.
14. VanderLaan PA, Chen Y, DiStasio M, Rangachari D, Costa DB, Heher YK. Molecular testing turnaround time in non-small-cell lung cancer: monitoring a moving target. Clin Lung Cancer. 2018;19:e589–90.
15. Yamaguchi N, Vanderlaan PA, Folch E, et al. Smoking status and self-reported race affect the frequency of clinically relevant oncogenic alterations in non-small-cell lung cancers at a United States-based academic medical practice. Lung Cancer. 2013;82:31–7.
16. VanderLaan PA, Rangachari D, Majid A, et al. Tumor biomarker testing in non-small-cell lung cancer: a decade of change. Lung Cancer. 2018;116:90–5.
17. Suh JH, Johnson A, Albacker L, et al. Comprehensive genomic profiling facilitates implementation of the National Comprehensive Cancer Network Guidelines for lung cancer biomarker testing and identifies patients who may benefit from enrollment in mechanism-driven clinical trials. Oncologist. 2016;21:684–91.
18. Jordan EJ, Kim HR, Arcila ME, et al. Prospective comprehensive molecular characterization of lung adenocarcinomas for efficient patient matching to approved and emerging therapies. Cancer Discov. 2017;7:596–609.
19. Collisson EA, Campbell JD, Brooks AN, et al. Cancer genome atlas research network. Comprehensive molecular profiling of lung adenocarcinoma. Nature. 2014;511:543–50.
20. Sholl LM, Aisner DL, Varella-Garcia M, et al. Multi-institutional oncogenic driver mutation analysis in lung adenocarcinoma: the lung cancer mutation consortium experience. J Thorac Oncol. 2015;10:768–77.
21. Illei PB, Belchis D, Tseng LH, et al. Clinical mutational profiling of 1006 lung cancers by next generation sequencing. Oncotarget. 2017;8:96684–96.
22. Barlesi F, Mazieres J, Merlio JP, et al. Routine molecular profiling of patients with advanced non-small-cell lung cancer: results of a 1-year nationwide programme of the French Cooperative Thoracic Intergroup (IFCT). Lancet. 2016;387:1415–26.
23. Sheikine Y, Rangachari D, McDonald DC, et al. EGFR testing in advanced non-small-cell lung cancer, a mini-review. Clin Lung Cancer. 2016;17:483–92.
24. Reck M, Rabe KF. Precision diagnosis and treatment for advanced non-small-cell lung cancer. N Engl J Med. 2017;377:849–61.

25. Tsao M, Hirsch FR, Yatabe Y. IASLC Atlas of ALK and ROS1 Testing in Lung Cancer. 2nd ed. North Fort Meyers, FL: Editorial Rx Press; 2016.
26. Minca EC, Lanigan CP, Reynolds JP, et al. ALK status testing in non-small-cell lung carcinoma by FISH on ThinPrep slides with cytology material. J Thorac Oncol. 2014;9:464–8.
27. Savic S, Bode B, Diebold J, et al. Detection of ALK-positive non-small-cell lung cancers on cytological specimens: high accuracy of immunocytochemistry with the 5A4 clone. J Thorac Oncol. 2013;8:1004–11.
28. Le Quesne J, Maurya M, Yancheva SG, et al. A comparison of immunohistochemical assays and FISH in detecting the ALK translocation in diagnostic histological and cytological lung tumor material. J Thorac Oncol. 2014;9:769–74.
29. Soo RA, Stone ECA, Cummings KM, et al. Scientific advances in thoracic oncology 2016. J Thorac Oncol. 2017;12:1183–209.
30. Calvayrac O, Pradines A, Pons E, Mazières J, Guibert N. Molecular biomarkers for lung adenocarcinoma. Eur Respir J. 2017;49:1601734.
31. Vlajnic T, Savic S, Barascud A, et al. Detection of ROS1-positive non-small cell lung cancer on cytological specimens using immunocytochemistry. Cancer Cytopathol. 2018;126:421–9.
32. Lin JJ, Shaw AT. Recent advances in targeting ROS1 in lung cancer. J Thorac Oncol. 2017;12:1611–25.
33. Drilon A, Cappuzzo F, Ou SI, Camidge DR. Targeting MET in lung cancer: will expectations finally be MET? J Thorac Oncol. 2017;12:15–26.
34. Ferrara R, Auger N, Auclin E, Besse B. Clinical and translational implications of RET rearrangements in non-small cell lung cancer. J Thorac Oncol. 2018;13:27–45.
35. Ferrara R, Mezquita L, Besse B. Progress in the management of advanced thoracic malignancies in 2017. J Thorac Oncol. 2018;13:301–22.
36. Kerr KM. The PD-L1 immunohistochemistry biomarker: two steps forward, one step back? J Thorac Oncol. 2018;13:291–4.
37. Mino-Kenudson M. Immunohistochemistry for predictive biomarkers in non-small cell lung cancer. Transl Lung Cancer Res. 2017;6:570–87.
38. Tsao MS, Kerr KM, Dacic S, Yatabe Y, Hirsch FR. IASLC Atlas of PD-L1 immunohistochemistry testing in lung cancer. 1st ed. North Fort Meyers, FL: Editorial Rx Press; 2017.
39. Hirsch FR, McElhinny A, Stanforth D, et al. PD-L1 immunohistochemistry assays for lung cancer: results from phase 1 of the

blueprint PD-L1 IHC assay comparison project. J Thorac Oncol. 2017;12:208–22.
40. Hendry S, Byrne DJ, Wright GM, et al. Comparison of four PD-L1 immunohistochemical assays in lung cancer. J Thorac Oncol. 2018;13:367–76.
41. Torous VF, Rangachari D, Gallant B, et al. PD-L1 testing using the clone 22C3 pharmDx kit for selection of patients with non-small cell lung cancer to receive immune checkpoint inhibitor therapy: are cytology cell blocks a viable option? J Am Soc Cytopathol. 2018;7:133–41.
42. Noll B, Wang WL, Gong Y, et al. Programmed death ligand 1 testing in non-small cell lung carcinoma cytology cell block and aspirate smear preparations. Cancer Cytopathol. 2018;126:342–52.
43. Russell-Goldman E, Kravets S, Dahlberg SE, Sholl LM, Vivero M. Cytologic-histologic correlation of programmed death-ligand 1 immunohistochemistry in lung carcinomas. Cancer Cytopathol. 2018;126:253–63.
44. Wang H, Agulnik J, Kasymjanova G, et al. Cytology cell blocks are suitable for immunohistochemical testing for PD-L1 in lung cancer. Ann Oncol. 2018;29:1417–22.
45. Ilie M, Juco J, Huang L, Hofman V, Khambata-Ford S, Hofman P. Use of the 22C3 anti-programmed death-ligand 1 antibody to determine programmed death-ligand 1 expression in cytology samples obtained from non-small cell lung cancer patients. Cancer Cytopathol. 2018;126:264–74.
46. Skov BG, Skov T. Paired comparison of PD-L1 expression on cytologic and histologic specimens from malignancies in the lung assessed with PD-L1 IHC 28-8pharmDx and PD-L1 IHC 22C3pharmDx. Appl Immunohistochem Mol Morphol. 2017;25:453–9.
47. Heymann JJ, Bulman WA, Swinarski D, et al. PD-L1 expression in non-small cell lung carcinoma: comparison among cytology, small biopsy, and surgical resection specimens. Cancer Cytopathol. 2017;125:896–907.
48. Carbone DP, Reck M, Paz-Ares L, et al. First-line Nivolumab in stage IV or recurrent non-small-cell lung cancer. N Engl J Med. 2017;376:2415–26.
49. Silvestri GA, Vachani A, Whitney D, et al. A bronchial genomic classifier for the diagnostic evaluation of lung cancer. N Engl J Med. 2015;373:243–51.
50. Mazzone PJ, Sears CR, Arenberg DA, et al. Evaluating molecular biomarkers for the early detection of lung cancer: when

is a biomarker ready for clinical use? An Official American Thoracic Society Policy Statement. Am J Respir Crit Care Med. 2017;196:e15–29.

51. Roy-Chowdhuri S, Aisner DL, Allen TC, et al. Biomarker testing in lung carcinoma cytology specimens: a perspective from members of the pulmonary pathology society. Arch Pathol Lab Med. 2016;140:1267–72.
52. Jain D, Roy-Chowdhuri S. Molecular pathology of lung cancer cytology specimens: a concise review. Arch Pathol Lab Med. 2018;142:1127–33.

Chapter 12
Molecular Diagnostics in Thyroid Cytology

Michiya Nishino

Abbreviations

ATA	American Thyroid Association
AUS/FLUS	Atypia of undetermined significance/follicular lesion of undetermined significance
BRAF	v-raf murine sarcoma viral oncogene homolog B
CALCA	Calcitonin-related polypeptide alpha
CEACAM5	Carcinoembryonic antigen-related cell adhesion molecule 5
cPTC	Classical papillary thyroid carcinoma
DNA	Deoxyribonucleic acid
FN/SFN	Follicular neoplasm/suspicious for follicular neoplasm
FNA	Fine-needle aspiration
FTC	Follicular thyroid carcinoma

M. Nishino
Department of Pathology, Beth Israel Deaconess Medical Center, Harvard Medical School, Boston, MA, USA
e-mail: mnishin1@bidmc.harvard.edu

S. Roy-Chowdhuri et al. (eds.), *Molecular Diagnostics in Cytopathology*, https://doi.org/10.1007/978-3-319-97397-5_12

FV-PTC	Follicular variant of papillary thyroid carcinoma
GC	Genomic Classifier (for ThyroSeq v3)
GEC	Gene Expression Classifier (for Afirma)
GSC	Gene Sequencing Classifier (for Afirma)
HRAS	HRas proto-oncogene, GTPase
KRAS	Kirsten rat sarcoma viral oncogene homolog
KRT7	Cytokeratin 7
MAPK	Mitogen-activated protein kinase
mRNA	Messenger ribonucleic acid
MTC	Medullary thyroid carcinoma
NIFTP	Noninvasive follicular thyroid neoplasm with papillary-like nuclear features
NPV	Negative predictive value
NRAS	Neuroblastoma RAS viral oncogene
PI3K	Phosphoinositide 3-kinase
PIK3CA	Phosphatidylinositol-4,5-bisphosphate 3-kinase catalytic subunit alpha
PPV	Positive predictive value
PTC	Papillary thyroid carcinoma
PTH	Parathyroid hormone
RET-PTC1/3	Gene fusion between tyrosine kinase domain of *RET* (ret proto-oncogene) and *CCD6* gene (PTC1) or *ELE1/RFG/NCOA4* gene (PTC3)
RNA	Ribonucleic acid
ROC	Receiver operating curve
SCG3	Secretogranin III
SCN9A	Sodium voltage-gated channel alpha subunit 9
SLC5A5	Solute carrier family 5 member 5 (also known as *NIS* [sodium/iodide symporter])
SYT4	Synaptotagmin 4
TBSRTC	The Bethesda System for Reporting Thyroid Cytopathology
TCGA	The Cancer Genome Atlas
TERT	Telomerase reverse transcriptase
TG	Thyroglobulin

TP53	Tumor protein p53
TTF-1	Thyroid transcription factor 1 (gene name: *NKX2–1*)

Key Terminology

The Bethesda System for Reporting Thyroid Cytopathology (TBSRTC)	Standardized reporting system for thyroid fine-needle aspiration specimens, consisting of six cytomorphology-based diagnostic categories. Each category is associated with an approximate risk of cancer, which may be used to guide subsequent management decisions
Driver mutation	Refers to somatic alterations in genes (including point mutations, insertions/deletions, and gene fusions) that are responsible for the development and progression of cancer
Gene expression profiling	Analysis of the expression levels of a large panel of genes (mRNA) from cells/tissues, as a measure of the cells' biologic activity
Indeterminate cytology	Refers to the diagnostic categories within TBSRTC that are neither clearly benign nor overtly

	malignant based on cytologic features. Three categories of TBSRTC are considered indeterminate: atypia of undetermined significance/follicular lesion of undetermined significance (AUS/FLUS), follicular neoplasm/suspicious for follicular neoplasm (FN/SFN), and suspicious for malignancy. Most of the ancillary molecular tests described in this chapter are geared toward improving risk stratification among the lower-risk cytologically indeterminate categories (AUS/FLUS and FN/SFN)
microRNA	Short (~22 nucleotide) noncoding RNA that influences gene expression at the posttranscriptional level
microRNA expression profiling	Analysis of the expression levels of a panel of microRNAs from cells/tissues, as a measure of the cells' biologic activity
Negative predictive value (NPV)	For a medical test with a binary classification system, NPV refers to the proportion of patients with a negative test result who do not have the

	disease; i.e., percentage of "true-negative" results among all (true- and false-)negative test results. Corresponds to posttest probability of benignity if the population being tested has similar prevalence of cancer as the cohort in which a test was validated
Noninvasive follicular thyroid neoplasm with papillary-like nuclear features (NIFTP)	Indolent follicular cell-derived thyroid neoplasm characterized by good demarcation, absence of invasive growth, follicular architecture, and nuclear atypia of papillary carcinoma; these tumors were formerly classified as the noninvasive subset of the encapsulated follicular variant of papillary thyroid carcinoma
Positive predictive value (PPV)	For a medical test with a binary classification system, PPV refers to the proportion of patients with a positive test result who have the disease; i.e., percentage of "true-positive" results among all (true- and false-)positive test results. Corresponds to posttest

	risk of disease if the population being tested has similar prevalence of cancer as the cohort in which a test was validated
Sensitivity	For a medical test with a binary classification system, sensitivity refers to the proportion of sick patients who are correctly identified with a positive test result. Tests with high sensitivity have low false-negative rates; consequently, a negative test result is helpful for excluding disease
Specificity	For a medical test with a binary classification system, specificity refers to the proportion of healthy patients who are correctly identified with a negative test result. Tests with high specificity have low false-positive rates; a positive test result is thus helpful for "ruling in" disease

Key Points

- Molecular diagnostics for thyroid cytology specimens is aimed at improving the risk stratification of cytologically indeterminate thyroid nodules
- Test performance can be inferred from positive and negative predictive values (PPV and NPV, respectively) reported by clinical validation studies. However, predictive values are not fixed properties of a diagnostic test. PPV and NPV vary with the prevalence of disease in the tested population
- The four commercially available molecular tests for thyroid FNAs described in this chapter all aim for a high negative predictive value to help identify cytologically indeterminate nodules that can be monitored nonsurgically
- Tests such as ThyGenX/ThyraMIR and ThyroSeq report granular estimates of cancer risk based on genotype. Therefore, the positive predictive value (where the detection of any genetic alteration in the test panel is considered a "positive" result for the purposes of statistical analysis) calculated for these tests does not necessarily reflect the full spectrum of risk stratification these tests offer in clinical practice
- Noninvasive follicular thyroid neoplasm with papillary-like nuclear features (NIFTP) is an indolent tumor for which lobectomy is diagnostically necessary and therapeutically sufficient

What Is the Role of Molecular Testing in Thyroid Cytology?

FNA cytology plays an important role in the evaluation of patients with thyroid nodules. For nodules meeting clinical and ultrasonographic criteria for FNA biopsy, cytomorphologic criteria can be used to place nodules into one of the six interpretive categories outlined by the Bethesda System for Reporting Thyroid Cytopathology (TBSRTC) [1]. Each of these categories is associated with an approximate cancer risk, which in turn helps guide subsequent management decisions (Table 12.1).

TABLE 12.1 The Bethesda System for Reporting Thyroid Cytopathology (TBSRTC)

Category	Risk of malignancy (%) (If NIFTP considered nonmalignant)	Risk of malignancy (%) (If NIFTP considered malignant)	Usual management
Nondiagnostic	5–10%	5–10%	Repeat FNA with ultrasound
Benign	0–3%	0–3%	Clinical and sonographic follow-up
Atypia/follicular lesion of undetermined significance (AUS/FLUS)	6–18%	10–30%	Repeat FNA, molecular testing, or lobectomy
Follicular neoplasm/suspicious for follicular neoplasm (FN/SFN)	10–40%	25–40%	Molecular testing, lobectomy
Suspicious for malignancy	45–60%	50–75%	Near-total thyroidectomy or lobectomy
Malignant	94–96%	97–99%	Near-total thyroidectomy or lobectomy

Adapted by permission from Springer Nature, Overview of Diagnostic Terminology and Reporting, Baloch et al. [1]

At the extreme ends of TBSRTC, management options are fairly straightforward (Fig. 12.1). Nodules classified as cytologically "benign" (Bethesda-II) have a low cancer risk

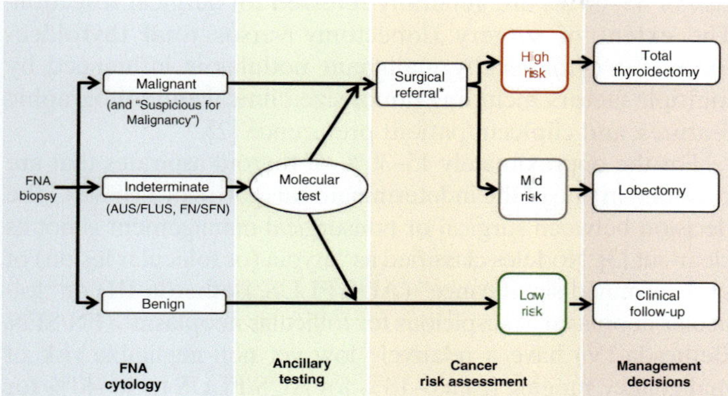

FIGURE 12.1 Simplified flowchart illustrating how cytologic and molecular testing results can guide management of thyroid nodules. The molecular tests described in this chapter are primarily indicated for aspirates classified in the "low-risk" indeterminate categories of the Bethesda System for Reporting Thyroid Cytopathology (atypia of undetermined significance/follicular lesion of undetermined significance [AUS/FLUS], follicular neoplasm/suspicious for follicular neoplasm [FN/SFN]). In this setting, ancillary molecular testing helps direct patients toward either surgical referral or clinical follow-up. Decisions regarding the extent of surgical resection (indicated by [*]) are determined by multiple factors, including (1) clinical/radiographic assessment of tumor size, extrathyroidal spread, nodal metastasis, and distant metastasis; (2) ultrasonographic and cytologic findings in the contralateral lobe; (3) patient/clinician preference; and (4) cytomorphologic or molecular features that may distinguish indolent/precancerous neoplasms from more aggressive disease. Regarding the latter, molecular tests that can detect genetic alterations characteristic of classical papillary thyroid carcinoma (e.g., *BRAF* V600E mutations, *RET-PTC1/3* fusions) could also be considered for aspirates in the higher-risk indeterminate category ("suspicious for malignancy") to help guide the extent of initial surgical resection. Abbreviations: *AUS/FLUS*, atypia of undetermined significance/follicular lesion of undetermined significance; *FN/SFN*, follicular neoplasm/suspicious for follicular neoplasm; *FNA*, fine-needle aspiration

(0–3%) and are typically followed by clinical and/or ultrasonographic observation. In contrast, nodules classified as cytologically "malignant" (Bethesda-VI, cancer risk of 94–96%) or "suspicious for malignancy" (Bethesda-V, cancer risk of 45–60%) are generally referred for surgical resection. The extent of surgery (lobectomy versus total thyroidectomy) for cytologically malignant nodules is influenced by multiple factors, including tumor size, clinical and sonographic features, and clinician/patient preference [2].

For the approximately 15–30% of thyroid aspirates that are classified in one of the indeterminate categories of TBSRTC, the decision between surgical or nonsurgical management is not as clear-cut [3]. Nodules classified as "atypia (or follicular lesion) of undetermined significance" (AUS/FLUS, Bethesda-III) or "follicular neoplasm"/"suspicious for follicular neoplasm" (FN/SFN, Bethesda-IV) have a relatively low yet non-negligible risk of malignancy, ranging from 6–18% for AUS/FLUS to 10–40% for FN/SFN [1]. Historically, surveillance by repeat FNA was an option for nodules classified as AUS/FLUS, with diagnostic lobectomy recommended for nodules that remained cytologically indeterminate on repeat FNA and/or otherwise showed worrisome clinical or sonographic features. Similarly, diagnostic lobectomy has traditionally been recommended for nodules classified as FN/SFN. However, the majority of AUS/FLUS and FN/SFN nodules that undergo surgical resection are ultimately found to be histologically benign. For these cases, surgery may be justified for diagnostic purposes but considered unnecessary from a therapeutic standpoint.

Ancillary molecular testing has emerged as a promising tool to improve risk stratification among thyroid nodules placed in these low-risk indeterminate categories of TBSRTC (Fig. 12.1). Molecular testing has dual aims in this context: (1) to identify biologically benign nodules that can be followed clinically rather than surgically and (2), for nodules that warrant resection, to help guide the extent of initial surgery (lobectomy versus total thyroidectomy). Of note, the primary indication for each of the molecular tests described herein is a cytologically indeterminate FNA. Therefore, routine microscopic evaluation of cytology slides is an essential step in determining whether ancillary molecular testing is appropriate for a thyroid nodule.

DNA, microRNA, mRNA, and proteins have all been investigated as analytes for ancillary testing on thyroid cytology specimens (Fig. 12.2). The four molecular tests that are currently offered by commercial laboratories for cytologically indeterminate thyroid FNAs are all nucleic acid-based tests and form the focus of this chapter: **Afirma Gene Expression Classifier** (Veracyte, Inc., South San Francisco, California), **RosettaGX Reveal** (Rosetta Genomics, Inc., Philadelphia, Pennsylvania), **ThyGenX/ThyraMIR** (Interpace Diagnostics, Parsippany, New Jersey), and **ThyroSeq** (University of Pittsburgh Medical Center, Pittsburgh, Pennsylvania, and CBLPath, Inc., Rye Brook, New York). These tests can be categorized by their general testing approach: (1) expression profiling for a panel of genes (mRNAs) or microRNAs, (2) genotyping for tumor-associated driver mutations and gene fusions, or (3) a combination of these methodologies (Table 12.2). Several immunohistochemical stains including HBME1, CK19, galectin-3, and *BRAF* VE1 (mutation-specific

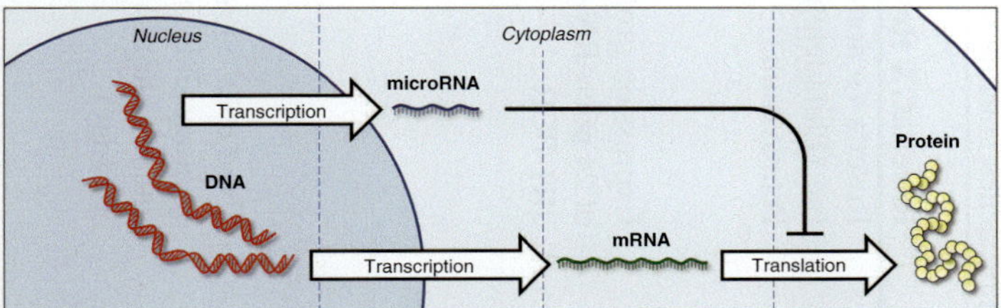

Analyte	DNA	microRNA	mRNA	Protein
Testing approach (and examples of tests)	NGS for point mutations, small insertion/deletions (ThyGenX, ThyroSeq)	RT-PCR to examine expression pattern of panel of microRNAs (ThyraMIR, RosettaGX Reveal)	DNA microarray to examine expression pattern of panel of mRNAs (Afirma GEC) NGS for gene fusions (ThyGenX, ThyroSeq)	Immunocytochemistry to examine expression pattern of various proteins (e.g., antibodies to BRAF VE1, HBME1, CK19, Galectin-3)

Figure 12.2 Analytes used in ancillary testing for thyroid cytology specimens. DNA, microRNA, mRNA, and proteins have all been explored as analytes to help risk-stratify thyroid nodules with indeterminate cytology. Examples of testing approaches using each of these analytes are shown. Abbreviations: *DNA*, deoxyribonucleic acid; *RNA*, ribonucleic acid; *mRNA*, messenger RNA; *PCR*, polymerase chain reaction

Table 12.2 Comparison of testing approaches, starting materials, sample collection, and concurrent cytology review

	Afirma GEC	**RosettaGX Reveal**	**ThyGenX/ ThyraMIR**	**ThyroSeq**
Company (Location)	Veracyte, Inc. (South San Francisco, California)	Rosetta Genomics, Inc. (Philadelphia, Pennsylvania)	Interpace Diagnostics, Inc. (Parsippany, New Jersey)	University of Pittsburgh Medical Center (Pittsburgh, Pennsylvania) and CBLPath, Inc. (Rye Brook, New York)
Testing approach	Expression profiles of 142 mRNAs by DNA microarray	Expression profiles of 24 microRNAs by qRT-PCR	ThyGenX: Hotspot mutations in 5 genes and 3 gene fusions by targeted NGS ThyraMIR: Expression profiles of 10 microRNAs by qRT-PCR	Hotspot mutations in 14 genes and 42 gene fusions by targeted NGS
Substrate for molecular testing	Fresh cells collected into nucleic acid preservative	Fixed cells on routine cytology slides (direct smear or liquid-based cytology)	Fresh cells collected into nucleic acid preservative	Fresh cells collected into nucleic acid preservative

Minimum quantity of material required for molecular testing	2 dedicated FNA passes	1 cytology slide with sufficient cellularity for cytologic interpretation	1 dedicated FNA pass containing at least 50 ng of cellular material	1–2 drops of FNA material
Sample collection/ shipping kits provided by vendor	Yes	Yes	Yes	Yes
Cytology review	Centralized[a]	Local or centralized	Local or centralized	Local or centralized

[a]Selected centers have been authorized to submit samples for Afirma testing based on cytologic review by local cytopathologists

antibody for the *BRAF* V600E mutation) have also been explored as markers of malignancy in thyroid resection specimens. The potential utility of these antibodies in thyroid cytology specimens has been explored in a variety of studies, but they will not be discussed further in this chapter [4–11].

When evaluating the performance of these ancillary molecular tests for cytologically indeterminate thyroid FNAs, readers should be aware of several caveats:

- Test performance is often extrapolated from its positive predictive value (PPV; corresponding to the posttest cancer risk associated with a positive test result) and negative predictive value (NPV; corresponding to the posttest probability of benignity associated with a negative test result). Importantly, PPV and NPV are not fixed properties of a test. Instead, these predictive values vary with the pretest probability of cancer in the tested population, which may differ from institution to institution [12, 13]. The prevalence of cancer among thyroid nodules classified as AUS/FLUS or FN/SFN is one estimate of the pretest cancer risk and can serve as a useful measure for determining whether the targeted test population for a particular institution is comparable to the population that was studied in the clinical validation of a molecular test.
- In clinical validation studies, the histopathologic reference diagnosis of resected thyroid nodules is typically classified in a binary manner (i.e., benign or malignant) to facilitate statistical analysis. However, this practice runs counter to evolving concepts of thyroid neoplasia as a continuum rather than a dichotomous process [2, 14].
- Similarly, clinical validation studies also confine the results of molecular tests into binary outcomes (negative or positive) to simplify statistical analysis. This approach may be apt for tests that report binary outcomes, such as the Afirma Gene Expression Classifier and Rosetta GX Reveal. However, for genotyping-based tests such as ThyroSeq or ThyGenX/ThyraMIR that offer a wide range of test results, the reduction of test results into either a "negative" or "positive" outcome for statistical purposes does not fully capture the gradation of risk estimates offered by these tests.

Expression Profiling to Risk-Stratify Indeterminate Thyroid FNAs

Histologically benign and malignant tumors show differential expression patterns of selected genes [15–18] and microRNAs [19–23]. These studies have formed the basis of ancillary tests that use proprietary algorithms to risk-stratify cytologically indeterminate thyroid FNAs based on either mRNA expression patterns (Afirma Gene Expression Classifier) or microRNA expression patterns (RosettaGX Reveal and ThyraMIR). The algorithms for these expression profiling-based tests have been optimized for high sensitivity and NPV to help "rule out" cancer among cytologically indeterminate thyroid nodules.

Afirma Gene Expression Classifier

The Afirma Gene Expression Classifier (GEC) analyzes the expression pattern of a large group of target genes using DNA microarrays (Fig. 12.3) [24]. The starting material for Afirma consists of two dedicated FNA passes collected into a vial of proprietary nucleic acid preservative solution, in addition to the FNA passes collected for microscopic cytology evaluation. If the cytology is classified as indeterminate (AUS/FLUS or FN/SFN), the concurrent sample collected for molecular testing is processed for microarray analysis. As a quality control step, the sample is first screened for the gene expression profiles of lesions that are not suited for analysis by the main GEC, including metastatic tumors (melanoma, breast carcinoma, renal cell carcinoma), parathyroid, and medullary thyroid carcinomas (MTC) (Table 12.3) [25, 26]. This screening step also includes gene expression analysis to identify samples concerning for malignant oncocytic (Hürthle-cell) thyroid tumors. Samples that trigger one of these six screening cassettes are reported as having a "suspicious" Afirma result, without subsequent analysis by the main 142-gene expression classifier. A sample that shows the expression pattern of MTC is additionally reported as "positive" for the

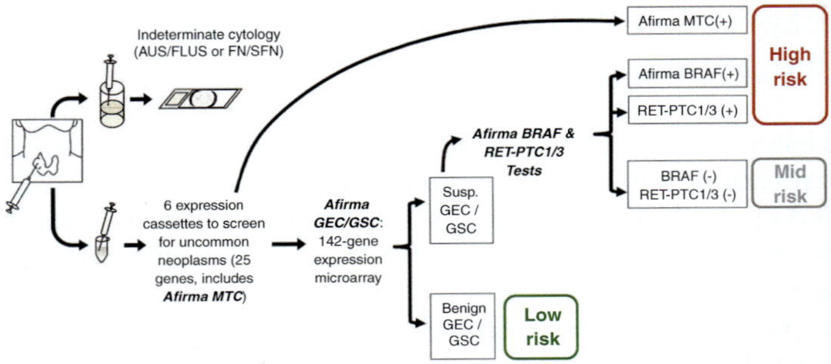

FIGURE 12.3 Afirma GEC/GSC and Malignancy Classifiers. See text for details. Abbreviations: *GEC*, Gene Expression Classifier; *GSC*, Gene Sequencing Classifier; *AUS/FLUS*, atypia of undetermined significance/follicular lesion of undetermined significance; *FN/SFN*, follicular neoplasm/suspicious for follicular neoplasm; *MTC*, medullary thyroid carcinoma. (Figure adapted from Nishino and Nikiforova [24] with permission from Archives of Pathology & Laboratory Medicine. Copyright 2018 College of American Pathologists)

Afirma MTC test, described further below. Specimens that pass this screening step advance to the main GEC, where the expression pattern of 142 genes is analyzed by a proprietary algorithm that classifies each FNA sample in a binary manner, as having either a "benign" or "suspicious" gene expression profile. The algorithm was trained using the gene expression profiles of histologically benign and malignant nodules.

The Afirma GEC was clinically validated in a prospective, multi-institutional study involving 129 AUS/FLUS (24% cancer prevalence), 81 FN/SFN (25% cancer prevalence), and 55 "suspicious for malignancy" (62% cancer prevalence) cases [27]. Among aspirates in the lower-risk cytologically indeterminate categories (AUS/FLUS or FN/SFN), Afirma demonstrated 90% sensitivity and ~50% specificity for cancer, corresponding to a high NPV (94–95%) for "benign" GEC results and a modest PPV (37–38%) for "suspicious" GEC results (Table 12.4) [25, 28–30]. Thus, for clinical practices where the prevalence of malignancy among AUS/FLUS and

TABLE 12.3 Quality controls to determine cellular composition of sample undergoing molecular analysis

	Afirma GEC	**RosettaGX Reveal**	**ThyGenX/ThyraMIR**	**ThyroSeq**
Confirmation of thyroid follicular cell sampling?	Yes: gene expression analysis for follicular cell adequacy [26]	Yes: nucleic acid extracted directly from follicular cells present on the cytology slide	Yes: gene expression analysis for thyroid follicular cells[a]	Yes: gene expression analysis for *TG*, *TTF1*, *NIS*, *KRT7* mRNAs [25]
Markers for C-cells and/or medullary carcinoma assessed?	Afirma MTC (gene expression analysis for *CALCA*, *CEACAM5*, *SCG3*, *SCN9A*, *SYT4*)	*miR-375*	*miR-375*	Gene expression analysis for *CALCA* mRNA
Markers for parathyroid assessed?	Gene expression analysis for *DMRT2*, *GCM2*, *KIDINS220*, *KL*, *PTH*, *SYCP2L*, *TMEM14B*	Unknown	Yes	Gene expression analysis for *PTH* mRNA
Others	Gene expression analysis for metastatic breast carcinoma, renal cell carcinoma, and melanoma	Unknown	Gene expression analysis for hematolymphoid markers	Gene expression analysis for *KRT20* mRNA (metastatic tumors)

[a]Personal communication from Dr. Sydney Finkelstein (Interpace Diagnostics)

Table 12.4 Performance characteristics of commercially available tests for indeterminate thyroid FNAs based on published validation studies[a]

	Afirma GEC [27]	RosettaGX Reveal [29]		ThyGenX/ ThyraMIR [28]	ThyroSeq (v2) [25, 30]
		Retrospective, multicenter			
Validation study design	**Prospective, multicenter**	**Entire validation set[b]**	**Agreement set[b]**	**Prospective, multicenter**	**Prospective and retrospective, single center**
Number of indeterminate FNAs	210	150	116	109	239
Prevalence of cancer (%)	24	21	12	32	26
Sensitivity (%)	90	74	100	89	90
Specificity (%)	52	74	80	85	93
NPV (%)	94	92	100	94	96
PPV (%)	37	43	41	74	81

[a]Only nodules classified as atypia/follicular lesion of undetermined significance (AUS/FLUS, Bethesda-III) or follicular neoplasm/suspicious for follicular neoplasm (FN/SFN, Bethesda-IV) are included in this table

[b]For comparison with the other tests in this table, only nodules with AUS/FLUS or FN/SFN cytology are included from RosettaGX Reveal's validation cohort. "Agreement Set" refers to subset of cases for which all three pathologists reviewing the resection specimen agreed on the reference histopathologic diagnosis

FN/SFN are similar to that of the Afirma validation cohort, the risk of cancer for a cytologically indeterminate nodule with a "benign" GEC result is ~5–6% (equivalent to 1-NPV). This low level of cancer risk is comparable to that of cytologically benign nodules, for which clinical/ultrasonographic monitoring is considered appropriate. In general, approximately 40% of patients with cytologically indeterminate thyroid nodules can avoid diagnostic surgery based on a "benign" Afirma GEC result [27, 31–36]. The remaining nodules with "suspicious" GEC results have a modest cancer risk (37–38%, corresponding to the PPV), for which a diagnostic lobectomy is generally advised. Of note, subset analyses in both the Afirma clinical validation study as well as independent post-validation studies suggest reduced specificity of the Afirma test among oncocytic (Hürthle-cell) lesions, raising concern that the test may overcall a larger proportion of histologically benign oncocytic neoplasms as having a "suspicious" GEC result relative to non-oncocytic thyroid lesions [32–34, 36].

To address the modest specificity and PPV of a "suspicious" Afirma GEC result, Veracyte offers additional tests known collectively as the Afirma Malignancy Classifiers. Afirma MTC and Afirma BRAF tests were introduced in 2014; RNA sequencing for *RET-PTC1/3* gene fusions was added to the Afirma Malignancy Classifier panel in 2017. As described above, the **Afirma MTC** is included among the screening cassettes used for quality control for the Afirma test. Afirma MTC identifies medullary thyroid carcinoma in FNA samples with high sensitivity and specificity by evaluating the expression levels of five genes: *CALCA*, *CEACAM5*, *SCG3*, *SCN9A*, and *SYT4* [37, 38]. Preoperative detection of MTC by FNA can facilitate surgical planning (total thyroidectomy with central lymph node dissection) in addition to prompting germline *RET* mutation analysis for multiple endocrine neoplasia type 2, as well as laboratory and imaging studies for metastatic disease, pheochromocytoma, and hyperparathyroidism. Patients with pheochromocytoma should undergo adrenergic blockade and adrenalectomy prior to thyroid surgery, while patients with hyperparathyroidism can undergo parathyroid surgery at the time of thyroidectomy [39].

The other two tests that comprise the Afirma Malignancy Classifiers evaluate samples for genetic changes associated with papillary thyroid carcinoma. The **Afirma BRAF** test analyzes samples for the gene expression profile associated with the *BRAF* V600E mutation [40], while the ***RET-PTC1/3*** assay uses RNA sequencing to identify oncogenic gene fusions involving the *RET* proto-oncogene. In the context of thyroid nodules, detection of *BRAF* V600E mutation, *RET-PTC1* gene fusion, or *RET-PTC3* gene fusion has high specificity for papillary thyroid carcinoma, whereby a positive test result can help establish a malignant diagnosis preoperatively and can influence decisions regarding the extent of the initial surgical procedure.

In 2017, Veracyte released an updated version of the Afirma test known as the Gene Sequencing Classifier (GSC). In addition to the incorporation of *RET-PTC1/3* gene fusion analysis to the Malignancy Classifiers, the new Afirma GSC uses an enhanced classification algorithm with reportedly superior specificity compared to the GEC, particularly among oncocytic nodules.

Taken together, the Afirma GSC (or GEC) and Malignancy Classifiers may help stratify cytologically indeterminate aspirates into three risk levels (Fig. 12.3):

- *Low risk* for cancer based on a "benign" Afirma GSC/GEC result, for which clinical and ultrasonographic monitoring of the nodule may be sufficient
- *Intermediate risk* for cancer based on a "suspicious" Afirma GSC/GEC result (with negative Afirma Malignancy Classifier results), for which diagnostic lobectomy is generally indicated
- *High risk* for cancer based on a "suspicious" Afirma GSC/GEC result with positive Afirma Malignancy Classifier results, for which surgical resection (lobectomy versus total thyroidectomy, depending on tumor size and clinical/ultrasonographic features) is indicated

RosettaGX Reveal

MicroRNAs are small (~22 nucleotide) noncoding RNAs that regulate gene expression at the posttranscriptional level by influencing the stability and translation of mRNA. The differential expression of selected microRNAs between benign and malignant thyroid nodules [19–23, 41], together with the stability of microRNAs and their ability to be isolated from routine formalin-fixed histology or alcohol-fixed cytology samples [19, 42–44], has encouraged the development of two microRNA-based commercial assays for risk-stratifying cytologically indeterminate thyroid FNA specimens: RosettaGX Reveal and ThyraMIR. The latter is a complementary test to ThyGenX and will be discussed in more detail in the next section.

RosettaGX Reveal uses cells harvested from routinely stained direct smears or liquid-based cytology slides as the starting material for molecular testing (Table 12.2, Fig. 12.4). There are two main advantages of using routine cytology slides as the substrate for molecular testing: (1) decreased need for dedicated FNA passes to collect cells specifically for molecular testing, as the diagnostic cytology slides can be repurposed for nucleic acid extraction, and (2) decreased potential for sampling error (as can occur when separate FNA passes are performed for microscopic and molecular analysis), since nucleic acid is extracted from the same cells that are considered indeterminate by microscopic evaluation (Table 12.3). One potential drawback to this approach is the need to sacrifice a diagnostic cytology slide for molecular testing; Rosetta Genomics offers digital slide-scanning services to maintain a digital archive of the cytomorphology.

Following nucleic acid extraction, the test analyzes the expression pattern of 24 microRNAs (Table 12.5) by RT-PCR to classify each sample as "benign" or "suspicious" by microRNA profiling. The inclusion of hsa-miR-375 in the 24-microRNA panel helps identify MTC among cytologically indeterminate FNAs. In a retrospective multicenter clinical validation study involving 189 AUS/FLUS, FN/SFN, and

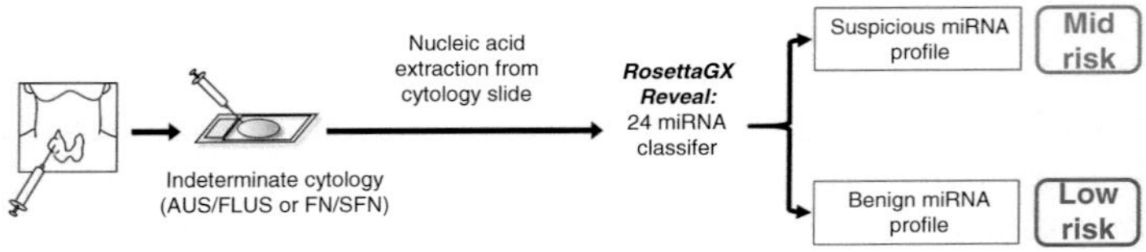

FIGURE 12.4 RosettaGX Reveal. See text for details. Abbreviations: *AUS/FLUS*, atypia of undetermined significance/follicular lesion of undetermined significance; *FN/SFN*, follicular neoplasm/suspicious for follicular neoplasm. (Figure adapted from Nishino and Nikiforova [24] with permission from Archives of Pathology & Laboratory Medicine. Copyright 2018 College of American Pathologists)

suspicious for malignancy aspirates (combined cancer prevalence of 32%), RosettaGX Reveal had 85% sensitivity, 72% specificity, 91% NPV, and 59% PPV for cancer [29].

Two caveats should be considered when reviewing the validation study for RosettaGX Reveal. First, the validation study reported higher test sensitivity (98%) and NPV (99%) among an "Agreement Set" comprised of a subset of 150 cases (27% prevalence of cancer) in which all three pathologists evaluating the resection specimen (two study pathologists, in addition to the original pathologist rendering the clinical diagnosis) concurred on the reference histopathologic diagnosis. The post-unblinding exclusion of 14 encapsulated follicular variant of papillary carcinomas from the "Agreement Set" (five of which were misclassified as having a "benign" microRNA profile by RosettaGX Reveal) likely accounts for the superior test sensitivity and NPV. Secondly, the advertised performance characteristics of RosettaGX Reveal are based on a validation cohort that includes "suspicious for malignancy" FNAs. In contrast, the performance characteristics of the other three commercial molecular tests for thyroid FNAs are based on validation cases classified cytologically as AUS/FLUS or FN/SFN. For the purposes of comparison with the other tests, we provide sensitivity, specificity, NPV, and PPV calculations for RosettaGX Reveal based only on AUS/FLUS and FN/SFN cases from their validation study:

Table 12.5 List of microRNAs included in RosettaGX Reveal and ThyraMIR tests

RosettaGX Reveal	ThyraMIR
hsa-miR-31-5p	hsa-miR-31-5p
hsa-miR-222-3p	hsa-miR-222-3p
hsa-miR-146b-5p	hsa-miR-146b-5p
hsa-miR-375	hsa-miR-375
hsa-miR-551b-3p	hsa-miR-551b-3p
hsa-miR-138-5p	hsa-miR-138-1-3p
hsa-miR-486-5p	hsa-miR-139-5p
hsa-miR-23a-3p	hsa-miR-29b-1-5p
hsa-miR-574-3p	hsa-miR-155
hsa-miR-152-3p	hsa-miR-204-5p
hsa-miR-200c-3p	
hsa-miR-345-5p	
hsa-miR-5701	
hsa-miR-424-3p	
hsa-miR-3074-5p	
hsa-miR-346	
hsa-miR-342-3p	
hsa-miR-181c-5p	
hsa-miR-125b-5p	
MID-50971	
MID-20094	
MID-50976	
MID-50969	
MID-16582	

- Total AUS/FLUS and FN/SFN cases ($n = 150$, 21% cancer prevalence): 74% sensitivity, 74% specificity, 92% NPV, and 43% PPV
- "Agreement Set" AUS/FLUS and FN/SFN cases ($n = 116$, 12% cancer prevalence): 100% sensitivity, 80% specificity, 100% NPV, and 41% PPV

Thus, RosettaGX Reveal's microRNA classifier shows performance characteristics that parallel that of the Afirma GEC. Among AUS/FLUS and FN/SFN nodules, a "benign" microRNA profile is associated with a low cancer risk (0–8%, depending on which of the above subset analyses are used) and may be safe to follow by clinical observation. On the other hand, AUS/FLUS and FN/SFN nodules with "suspicious" microRNA profiles are associated with an intermediate cancer risk (41–43%), for which surgical referral should be considered (Table 12.4).

Genotyping-Based Testing Approaches

A variety of mutations and gene rearrangements in the mitogen-activated protein kinase (*MAPK*) and phosphoinositide 3-kinase (PI3K) signaling pathways have been identified in thyroid cancer [45]. Oncogenic alterations in papillary thyroid carcinomas (PTC) include mutations in *BRAF* (40–50% of PTCs) or *RAS* (10–20% of PTCs), as well as *RET-PTC1* or *RET-PTC3* gene fusions (10–20% of PTCs). Similarly, genetic alterations in follicular thyroid carcinomas (FTC) include *RAS* mutations (40–50% of FTCs) and *PAX8-PPARG* gene fusions (30% of FTCs).

Testing FNA specimens for the *BRAF* V600E mutation alone may be useful as a predictive biomarker in specific situations. In patients with advanced thyroid cancer refractory to radioactive iodine treatment, detection of the *BRAF* V600E mutation can help identify patients who may benefit from clinical trials using selective BRAF inhibitors [46–49]. Cytology specimens may be a useful substrate for *BRAF* testing in this setting, since such patients typically have recurrent/

metastatic disease or surgically unresectable thyroid cancer (e.g., undifferentiated [anaplastic] thyroid carcinoma) amenable to FNA biopsy.

From a diagnostic standpoint, a single-gene testing approach for thyroid FNAs is limited in two ways. While detection of the *BRAF* V600E mutation in a thyroid FNA can secure a diagnosis of PTC with near-100% certainty (reviewed in [50]), this mutation is infrequent (~5%) among cytologically indeterminate thyroid FNAs, for which a positive molecular testing result would have the greatest impact on management decisions [51, 52]. Secondly, testing for *BRAF* V600E alone is insufficiently sensitive for malignancy because only 40–50% of PTCs harbor this mutation; the absence of this mutation does not exclude malignancy among cytologically indeterminate nodules. Taken together, the cost-effectiveness and utility of routine *BRAF* V600E testing as a sole marker for "ruling in" or "ruling out" cancer are dubious.

Given the limitations in this single-gene testing approach, the clinical application of mutational analysis for cytologically indeterminate thyroid FNAs has largely focused on multiplexed genotyping methods. An early genotyping panel for thyroid FNAs consisted of hotspot mutations in four genes (*BRAF*, *HRAS*, *KRAS*, *NRAS*) and three gene fusions (*RET-PTC1*, *RET-PTC3*, and *PAX8-PPARG*) to help risk-stratify thyroid FNAs with indeterminate cytology. Numerous studies have evaluated the performance of this seven-marker panel for thyroid FNAs [28, 53–58]. The largest clinical validation of this panel was a single-institution prospective study involving 247 AUS/FLUS (14% prevalence of cancer) and 214 FN/SFN (27% prevalence of cancer) aspirates. In this study, the seven-marker genotyping panel was reported to have high specificity (97–99%) and PPV (87–88%) for cancer [57]. Based on these results, commercial versions of this seven-marker panel were initially marketed as tests for "ruling in" malignancy among cytologically indeterminate thyroid nodules, whereby the detection of a mutation or gene fusion could direct a patient to definitive treatment with total thyroidectomy.

However, two caveats must be considered regarding the clinical utility of this seven-marker panel. First, for genotyping-based tests such as the seven-marker panel and the others described below, the PPV reported in clinical validation studies does not capture the gradation of cancer risk estimates associated with positive test results. For instance, the *BRAF* V600E mutation and *RET-PTC1/3* gene fusions are associated with near-100% risk for papillary carcinoma in the context of thyroid FNAs. In contrast, *RAS* mutations and *PAX8-PPARG* gene fusions have been identified in a broad spectrum of benign, premalignant, and malignant follicular-patterned neoplasms (e.g., follicular adenoma, follicular carcinoma, noninvasive follicular thyroid neoplasm with papillary-like nuclear features [NIFTP], encapsulated follicular variant of papillary thyroid carcinoma) and may be best considered markers of neoplasia rather than malignancy per se [14, 45, 56, 57, 59–66]. In other words, genotyping tests offer more granular estimates of cancer risk than can be conveyed by the test's reported PPV.

Secondly, in the aforementioned validation study, the seven-marker panel demonstrated a modest sensitivity (57%–63%) for malignancy, corresponding to 86–94% NPV among AUS/FLUS and FN/SFN cases [57]. Because of the 6–14% residual cancer risk (1-NPV) associated with a negative test result, this seven-marker panel was considered clinically inadequate as a test for "ruling out" cancer for patients with cytologically indeterminate thyroid nodules. Two commercially available tests have adopted different strategies to overcome the low NPV of the seven-marker genotyping panel. **ThyGenX/ThyraMIR** combines a limited genotyping panel with a microRNA-based expression classifier to improve sensitivity and NPV for malignancy. Alternatively, **ThyroSeq** tests for a vastly expanded panel of genetic alterations to improve the sensitivity and NPV of the genotyping approach for risk-stratifying cytologically indeterminate thyroid aspirates.

ThyGenX/ThyraMIR

Interpace Diagnostics combines microRNA expression profiling (ThyraMIR) with a limited genotyping panel (ThyGenX) to improve the risk stratification of cytologically indeterminate thyroid aspirates (Table 12.2). This testing approach requires a dedicated FNA pass collected into a vial of proprietary nucleic acid preservative, in addition to the FNA passes required for visual cytopathology interpretation (Fig. 12.5). For nodules with indeterminate cytology, the sample collected for molecular testing is processed as follows:

- Assessment of the expression levels of genes associated with thyroid follicular cells for quality control purposes (Table 12.3).
- ThyGenX tests thyroid FNA samples for oncogenic mutations in five genes (*BRAF*, *HRAS*, *KRAS*, *NRAS*, *PIK3CA*) and three gene fusions (*RET-PTC1*, *RET-PTC3*, *PAX8-PPARG*) using a next-generation sequencing platform.
  - The detection of a *BRAF* V600E mutation or *RET-PTC1/3* gene fusion is considered virtually diagnostic of malignancy in a thyroid FNA due to the strong

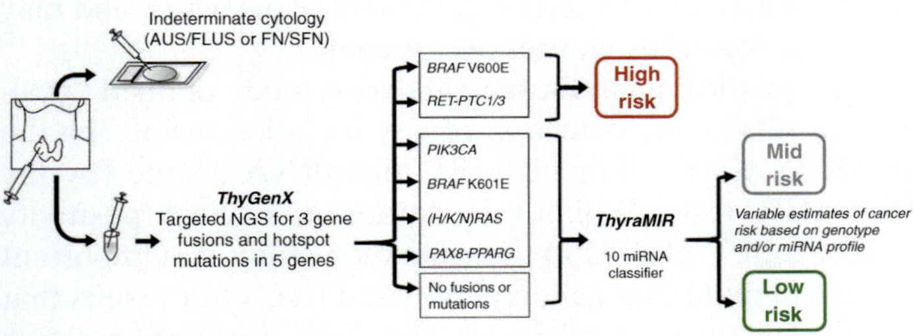

FIGURE 12.5 ThyGenX/ThyraMIR. See text for details. Abbreviations: *AUS/FLUS*, atypia of undetermined significance/follicular lesion of undetermined significance; *FN/SFN*, follicular neoplasm/suspicious for follicular neoplasm; *NGS*, next-generation sequencing; *miRNA*, microRNA. (Figure adapted from Nishino and Nikiforova [24] with permission from Archives of Pathology & Laboratory Medicine. Copyright 2018 College of American Pathologists)

  association of these genetic alterations with papillary thyroid carcinoma.
  - For the remaining ThyGenX results (i.e., no mutation/fusion, *H-/K-/N-RAS* mutations, *BRAF* K601E mutation, *PIK3CA* mutations, or *PAX8-PPARG* fusion), further refinement of cancer risk is accomplished with the ThyraMIR test.

- ThyraMIR assays for the expression patterns of ten microRNAs using quantitative RT-PCR to classify samples as having either a low-risk/benign versus high-risk/positive microRNA profile. ThyraMIR's test panel includes six microRNA sequences that closely overlap with RosettaGX Reveal's panel of 24 microRNAs (Table 12.5).

In a prospective multicenter validation study of 109 AUS/FLUS and FN/SFN aspirates, the combined ThyGenX/ThyraMIR tests demonstrated 89% sensitivity and 85% specificity for malignancy [28]. The cancer prevalence in this cohort of cytologically indeterminate nodules was 32%; at this prevalence of malignancy, the NPV of the combined ThyGenX/ThyraMIR tests was 94% (Table 12.4). In other words, "double-negative" samples with negative ThyGenX results and a low-risk microRNA profile by ThyraMIR testing have an approximately 6% (1-NPV) cancer risk and may be safe to follow by clinical observation.

For statistical analysis, the validation study defined "positive" results as the detection of any mutation/fusion (by the ThyGenX test) and/or high-risk microRNA profile (by the ThyraMIR test). While this definition of test positivity yielded a PPV of 74% in the validation study, it is important to keep in mind that genotyping-based tests offer results that span a wide range of risk levels. Therefore, in clinical practice, ThyGenX/ThyraMIR may help risk-stratify cytologically indeterminate FNA samples as follows:

- *Low risk* for cancer based on the absence of a mutation or gene fusion (negative ThyGenX test) and low-risk microRNA profile (negative ThyraMIR test). Clinical and ultrasonographic monitoring of the nodule may be sufficient.

- *Intermediate risks* for cancer based on other permutations of ThyGenX results (no mutation/fusion, *H-/K-/N-RAS* mutations, *BRAF* K601E mutation, *PAX8-PPARG* fusion) and ThyraMIR results (low- versus high-risk microRNA expression patterns). For samples in this category, Interpace Diagnostics uses laboratory data to refine estimates of cancer risk, which in turn typically warrant diagnostic lobectomy.
- *High risk* for cancer based on detection of *BRAF* V600E mutation or *RET-PTC1/3* fusions by the ThyGenX test. Surgical resection (lobectomy versus total thyroidectomy, depending on tumor size and clinical/ultrasonographic features) is indicated.

ThyroSeq

In 2014, The Cancer Genome Atlas (TCGA) project published its analysis of genomic alterations of nearly 500 PTCs [67]. This comprehensive approach identified novel oncogenic alterations associated with PTC, effectively reducing the fraction of PTCs with unknown driver mutations from 25% to 3.5% [67]. Nikiforov et al. capitalized on these large-scale genomic studies to develop **ThyroSeq**, which uses targeted next-generation sequencing to assay for a broad panel of single nucleotide variants, insertions/deletions, and gene fusions associated with thyroid neoplasia (Table 12.2).

ThyroSeq requires 1–2 drops of FNA material (collected into a vial of proprietary nucleic acid preservative solution) as the substrate for molecular testing (Fig. 12.6). Gene expression analysis serves as a quality control measure to monitor the cellular makeup of the sample (Table 12.3). Expression of genes such as *TTF1*, thyroglobulin (*TG*), sodium/iodide symporter (*SLC5A5/NIS*), and cytokeratin 7 (*KRT7*) are used to confirm adequate sampling of thyroid follicular cells in the aspirate. Conversely, aspirates with expression of genes associated with parafollicular/C cells (calcitonin-related peptide alpha [*CALCA*]) or parathyroid cells (parathyroid hormone [*PTH*]) can be flagged as

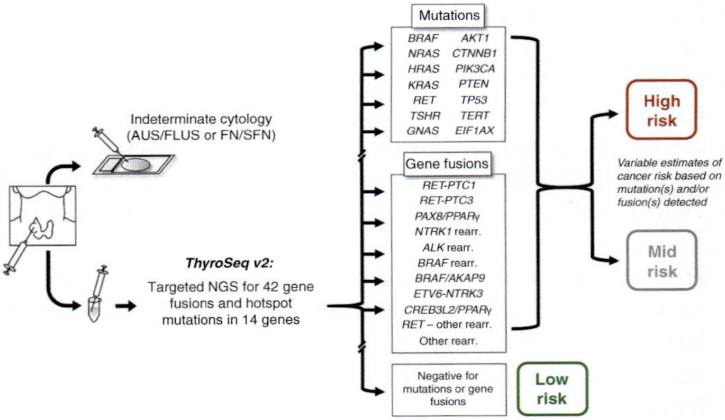

FIGURE 12.6 ThyroSeq. See text for details. Abbreviations: *AUS/FLUS*, atypia of undetermined significance/follicular lesion of undetermined significance; *FN/SFN*, follicular neoplasm/suspicious for follicular neoplasm; *NGS*, next-generation sequencing. (Figure adapted from Nishino and Nikiforova [24] with permission from Archives of Pathology & Laboratory Medicine. Copyright 2018 College of American Pathologists)

suspicious for medullary thyroid carcinoma or parathyroid sampling, respectively.

The list of genetic alterations included in the ThyroSeq test panel has evolved with updated versions of the test. The most comprehensive clinical validation of ThyroSeq to date has involved single-center studies using ThyroSeq v2, which includes 42 types of gene fusions and mutational hotspots in 14 different genes in its test panel [25, 30]. These validation studies have included a combination of prospectively and retrospectively analyzed thyroid FNA samples. Among 239 nodules with indeterminate cytology (96 AUS/FLUS and 143 FN/SFN, with a combined cancer prevalence of 26%), ThyroSeq v2 had high sensitivity (~90%) and specificity (~93%) for malignancy, corresponding to a NPV of 96% and PPV of 81% (Table 12.4). Independent reports of ThyroSeq v2 performance in actual clinical practice support the high NPV of the test [68–70]. At the same time, these post-validation studies indicate that the test's PPV for cancer may be lower (22–63%) than the 81% PPV that was initially reported in the clinical validation study. The lower PPV of a "mutation-positive" ThyroSeq v2 result in these studies may be explained in part by the prevalence of histologically benign or premalignant neoplasms that harbor *RAS*, *RAS*-like, and *EIF1AX* mutations [68–71].

As discussed above, interpretation of PPV is challenging for genotyping-based tests because the type of mutation factors heavily into posttest cancer risk. Mutations in *RAS* and related ("*RAS*-like") pathways may be considered a marker of neoplasia but appear to be less specific for malignancy, given the detection of these genetic changes in a range of benign, premalignant, and malignant follicular-patterned neoplasms. In contrast, *BRAF* V600E mutations and related ("*BRAF*-like") genetic alterations help rule in malignancy with near-100% specificity among indeterminate thyroid FNAs due to their strong association with papillary thyroid carcinoma. Additionally, *TERT* promoter mutations and *TP53* mutations – particularly when they co-occur with *BRAF*-like or *RAS*-like driver alterations – have been associated with clinically aggressive thyroid cancers, including undifferentiated (anaplastic) thyroid carcinoma and poorly differentiated thyroid carcinoma [72–79]. Finally, the allelic frequency with which a mutation/fusion is detected in a FNA sample may also inform posttest cancer risk, to the extent that a genetic alteration present at a low level implies an early step in the clonal evolution of a neoplasm.

Taken together, broad targeted genotyping panels like ThyroSeq v2 can help triage thyroid nodules by risk level, as follows:

- *Low risk*: Nodules that are negative for all mutations/fusions in the test panel or positive for a marker associated with benignity may be safe to monitor by clinical observation due to a very low (3–4%) risk of cancer.
- *Intermediate risks*: For nodules with isolated *RAS*, *RAS*-like, or *EIF1AX* mutations, diagnostic lobectomy may be suitable as the initial surgical approach, given the moderate risk of cancer in this setting.

- *High risk*: For nodules with *BRAF* V600E mutation or *RET-PTC1/3* gene fusion, surgical resection (lobectomy versus total thyroidectomy, depending on tumor size and clinical/sonographic features) is indicated due to the virtually 100% risk of papillary thyroid cancer associated with these alterations. The detection of *TP53* or *TERT* promoter mutations, particularly in concert with other alterations in the panel, may indicate a biologically aggressive cancer.

ThyroSeq v3, offered commercially since in 2017, makes two major updates to the test: (a) expansion of the number of genes in the test panel to 112 (compared to 56 genes in ThyroSeq v2) and (b) analysis of several genomic regions for copy-number alterations that are associated with thyroid cancer [67].The thyroidectomy specimens used for the training set for ThyroSeq v3 were also enriched for oncocytic (Hürthle-cell) nodules, with the goal of improving the preoperative distinction between nonneoplastic, benign neoplastic, and malignant Hürthle-cell tumors.

Each type of genetic alteration in the test panel is assigned a point value commensurate to its association with malignancy, as determined from review of the published literature as well as from analysis of internal and publically searchable databases. This weighted point-based system allows for the integration of all genetic alterations in a sample (or lack thereof) into a single "Genomic Classifier" (GC) score [80]. In the analytic validation study for ThyroSeq v3, authors used receiver operating curve (ROC) analysis to establish a GC cutoff for optimal sensitivity and specificity for malignancy. GC scores below this threshold are reported as "negative" (favoring benignity), while samples at or beyond the cutoff are reported as "positive." Using this GC cutoff, ThyroSeq v3 demonstrated 98.0% specificity and 90.9% sensitivity for malignancy among an analytic validation cohort of 175 thyroid FNA samples that was enriched for cancer (52.6% prevalence of cancer). As with previous versions of ThyroSeq, the genotype and allelic frequency of genetic alterations should provide additional risk stratification among GC "positive" cases. Clinical validation of ThyroSeq v3 in a prospective, blinded, multicenter study is in progress at this time.

Is One Ancillary Molecular Test Superior to the Others?

There is no evidence to date that one of the commercially available tests described in this chapter is superior to any of the others. On the one hand, direct head-to-head comparisons between these tests using a common validation cohort are currently lacking, due in part to the prohibitive costs associated with such a study. While the NPV and PPV reported by the clinical validation studies for each test reflect test performance to a degree, the differences in test design as well as differences in the composition of their respective validation cohorts limit meaningful comparison across studies. For these reasons, the latest management guidelines from the American Thyroid Association (ATA) do not endorse a specific molecular test for thyroid FNAs with indeterminate cytology [2].

With these caveats in mind, one emerging viewpoint is that the various approaches for molecular testing of thyroid FNA samples may be fundamentally similar from the standpoint of patient care. A high NPV for ruling out cancer remains a shared and vital goal for all four molecular tests reviewed in this chapter: the ability to identify biologically benign nodules preoperatively can triage appropriate patients toward clinical observation, thereby avoiding thyroid lobectomy for purely diagnostic purposes.

Genotyping tests offer a high degree of granularity in their results compared to the binary outcomes of gene expression-based tests; yet, for clinical decision-making, the granular genotyping results are typically binned into broader risk categories to help patients and clinicians choose between clinical observation and surgical management (and for the latter, to guide the extent of initial thyroid surgery). As a case in point, the detection of *RAS* and *RAS*-like mutations in FNA samples by genotyping tests such as ThyroSeq – while providing insight into the phenotype and molecular biology of a patient's thyroid nodule – generally leads to similar risk-based management recommendations (diagnostic lobectomy) as a "suspicious" Afirma GEC result.

The addition of markers that help "rule in" malignancy such as the *BRAF* V600E mutation (in the form of the Afirma BRAF test) and *RET-PTC1/3* gene fusions to Afirma's test panel further supports the notion that the different molecular tests for thyroid FNAs appear to converge with respect to their ability to stratify cytologically indeterminate aspirates as being either high, intermediate, or low risk for cancer (Fig. 12.1).

Ancillary Molecular Testing for Thyroid FNAs in the NIFTP Era

In recent years, there has been a trend toward more conservative treatment options for carefully selected low-risk thyroid neoplasms [2]. The recent nomenclature revision regarding noninvasive follicular thyroid neoplasm with papillary-like nuclear features (NIFTP) underscores ongoing efforts to classify and manage thyroid neoplasms commensurate to their risk of recurrence and/or metastasis [14].

Historically, thyroid tumors demonstrating a follicular architecture and the nuclear atypia of papillary carcinoma were classified as the "follicular variant" of papillary thyroid carcinoma (FV-PTC). However, the term "FV-PTC" itself encompasses tumors with diverse biologic and clinical characteristics; subclassification of these tumors relies mainly on histopathologic evaluation of tumor circumscription and invasion (Fig. 12.7). FV-PTCs with diffuse, infiltrative growth into the adjacent thyroid parenchyma (**Infiltrative FV-PTC**, Fig. 12.7a) are similar to classical papillary thyroid carcinoma (cPTC), with a tendency to be driven by *BRAF*-like alterations and a predilection for local recurrence and cervical lymph node metastasis [81–84].

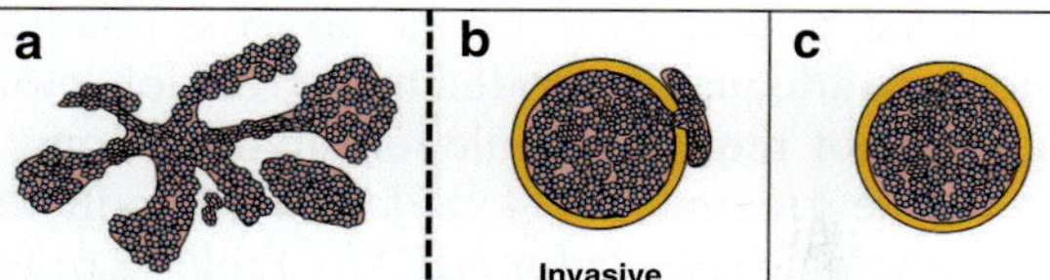

	a Infiltrative FV-PTC	b Invasive Encapsulated FV-PTC	c NIFTP
Intranuclear pseudoinclusions	Relatively frequent	None to rare	
Molecular alterations	"BRAF-like"	"RAS-like"	
Low-magnification appearance	Infiltrative; no encapsulation	Well-circumscribed and/or encapsulated	
Invasion	Parenchymal infiltration ± vascular invasion	Capsular and/or vascular invasion	No
Clinical behavior	Similar to classical-type PTC	Similar to FTC	Indolent

FIGURE 12.7 Follicular-patterned thyroid neoplasms with the nuclear atypia of papillary carcinoma: a comparison of pathologic, molecular, and clinical features. In the past, the term "follicular variant of papillary thyroid carcinoma" (FV-PTC) has been applied to each of these three tumors. Studies over the past decade have identified pathologically, molecularly, and clinically distinctive subcategories among these tumors: (**a**) infiltrative FV-PTC, (**b**) invasive encapsulated FV-PTC, and (**c**) NIFTP. Abbreviations: *NIFTP*, noninvasive follicular thyroid neoplasm with papillary-like nuclear features; *PTC*, papillary thyroid carcinoma; *FTC*, follicular thyroid carcinoma

In contrast, FV-PTCs that are encapsulated or otherwise well-demarcated from the surrounding thyroid parenchyma bear more molecular and clinical resemblance to follicular adenoma/carcinoma rather than cPTC. Encapsulated/well-demarcated FV-PTCs with capsular or vascular invasion (**Invasive Encapsulated FV-PTC**, Fig. 12.7b) have a predilection for distant metastasis via hematogenous spread, similar to follicular carcinomas [85]. On the other hand, encapsulated/well-demarcated FV-PTCs with no evidence of capsular or vascular invasion have an exceptionally indolent clinical course, akin to follicular adenomas [14, 83, 85–91]. Given the very low malignant potential of these tumors, the noninvasive subset of encapsulated/well-demarcated FV-PTC was recently reclassified as "noninvasive follicular thyroid neoplasm with papillary-like nuclear features" (Fig. 12.7c). NIFTP may be considered a precursor to its invasive counterpart. Such tumors are adequately treated by thyroid lobectomy and generally do not require completion thyroidectomy or radioactive iodine treatment [14, 85]. Careful adherence to the histopathologic criteria for NIFTP (Table 12.6) is essential to maintain the reproducibility and very low malignant potential of the NIFTP diagnosis [14, 92].

Genotyping studies of NIFTP have identified mutations in *RAS*, *BRAF* (K601E), and *EIF1AX*, as well as chromosomal rearrangements involving *THADA* or *PAX8-PPARG* [14, 93]. These alterations are similar to those of other follicular-patterned thyroid tumors such as follicular adenoma, follicular carcinoma, and invasive encapsulated FV-PTC and distinct from the "*BRAF*-like" genetic alterations characteristic of

Table 12.6 Histopathologic inclusion and exclusion criteria for the diagnosis of noninvasive follicular thyroid neoplasm with papillary-like nuclear features (NIFTP)

Inclusion criteria for NIFTP	**Exclusion criteria for NIFTP**
Encapsulation or clear demarcation	Capsular or vascular invasion
Predominantly follicular growth pattern	True papillary architecture
Nuclear score of 2 or 3[a]	>30% solid, insular, or trabecular architecture
	Psammoma bodies
	Features of tall cell or columnar cell variant of PTC
	Tumor necrosis
	>3 mitoses per 10 high-power (400x) fields

[a]Nuclear score refers to a three-point scoring system for assessing the nuclear atypia. One point is assigned for each of the following: (a) nuclear size and shape [enlargement, elongation, overlapping], (b) nuclear membrane irregularities [irregular contours, grooves, pseudoinclusions], and (c) chromatin changes [pallor/clearing, margination of chromatin to membrane]

cPTC and infiltrative FV-PTC [50, 67, 81, 84, 88, 94, 95]. Importantly, NIFTP and invasive encapsulated FV-PTC have overlapping molecular features, and the only distinguishing feature between NIFTP and invasive encapsulated FV-PTC to date is the histologic detection of capsular or vascular invasion in the latter (similar to the distinction between follicular adenoma and follicular carcinoma). Consequently, the diagnosis of NIFTP can only be made on resection specimens following histologic examination of the entire tumor periphery to exclude invasive growth [14, 92]. For these reasons, lobectomy is considered diagnostically necessary but therapeutically sufficient for NIFTP.

What Are the Cytologic Features of NIFTP?

As its name suggests, NIFTP is characterized by a follicular growth pattern and the presence of "papillary-like nuclear features," both of which can be seen to varying degrees in FNA cytology specimens. Retrospective studies have shown that nuclear atypia (nuclear enlargement and crowding, nuclear contour irregularity, nuclear molding, and chromatin pallor) can help distinguish aspirates of NIFTP from those of benign follicular nodules (i.e., follicular adenomas or adenomatous/hyperplastic nodules) [96–98]. Cytoarchitectural and/or nuclear features may also help distinguish aspirates of NIFTP from cPTC and infiltrative FV-PTC. Architecturally, aspirates of NIFTP yield a predominantly microfollicular cellular arrangement, in contrast to the papillary architecture or sheetlike groups characteristic of cPTC [99, 100]. Furthermore, nuclear contour irregularity is generally limited in NIFTP compared to cPTC or infiltrative FV-PTC, with most cases of NIFTP showing rare or no intranuclear cytoplasmic pseudoinclusions [84, 100–103]. These observations are in keeping with retrospective analyses showing that aspirates of NIFTPs (or equivalent tumors with their former name, noninvasive encapsulated FV-PTC) are usually classified in one of the indeterminate categories of TBSRTC (AUS/FLUS, FN/SFN, or suspicious for malignancy) rather than as "malignant" [97, 101, 104–111]. Thus, for aspirates with microfollicular architecture and modest nuclear atypia, recognition of the possibility of NIFTP and judicious use of these indeterminate categories for such cases may help encourage lobectomy rather than total thyroidectomy as the initial surgical approach.

Of note, reliable cytologic distinction between NIFTP and invasive encapsulated FV-PTC is not possible due to overlapping architectural and nuclear features [82, 84, 97, 99, 100]. As described above, the only distinguishing feature between these two tumors to date remains the histologic detection of capsular and/or vascular invasion.

What Are the Implications of the NIFTP Nomenclature Change on Thyroid FNA Molecular Testing?

The four commercially available molecular tests for thyroid FNAs discussed in this chapter were developed and clinically validated prior to the NIFTP nomenclature revision, at a time when noninvasive encapsulated FV-PTCs were by and large considered malignant tumors. Not surprisingly, these ancillary molecular tests often classify aspirates of NIFTPs as abnormal. Retrospective studies have reported NIFTPs among tumors identified as having "suspicious" Afirma GEC results [111–115] or *RAS*/"*RAS*-like" genetic alterations by genotyping tests such as ThyroSeq [60, 70, 111, 113].

Some authors have suggested that these molecular testing results should be considered false-positive outcomes when detected in NIFTPs and have recommended revalidation of these tests in view of the NIFTP reclassification [116]. However, there are counterarguments to conflating NIFTP with nodules demonstrating overtly benign histology. In contrast to most benign follicular nodules, NIFTPs currently require surgical management (i.e., lobectomy) for diagnostic and therapeutic purposes [14, 117]. In this light, the detection of NIFTPs as abnormal by molecular testing seems to be well-suited with current recommendations for diagnostic lobectomy for nodules with "suspicious" Afirma GEC results or *RAS*/"*RAS-like*" genotyping results.

Conclusions

Molecular and clinicopathologic studies have contributed to an increasingly nuanced model of thyroid neoplasia in recent years. The emergence of molecular diagnostics for thyroid FNAs reflects a larger trend toward a more risk-stratified approach to the diagnosis and management of thyroid neoplasms.

References

1. Baloch ZW, Cooper DS, Gharib H, Alexander EK. Overview of diagnostic terminology and reporting. In: Ali S, Cibas E, editors. The Bethesda system for reporting thyroid cytopathology. Cham: Springer; 2018. p. 1–6.
2. Haugen BR, Alexander EK, Bible KC, Doherty GM, Mandel SJ, Nikiforov YE, et al. 2015 American Thyroid Association Management guidelines for adult patients with thyroid nodules and differentiated thyroid cancer: the American Thyroid Association guidelines task force on thyroid nodules and differentiated thyroid cancer. Thyroid. 2016;26(1):1–133.
3. Bongiovanni M, Spitale A, Faquin WC, Mazzucchelli L, Baloch ZW. The Bethesda system for reporting thyroid cytopathology: a meta-analysis. Acta Cytol. 2012;56(4):333–9.
4. Das DK, Al-Waheeb SK, George SS, Haji BI, Mallik MK. Contribution of immunocytochemical stainings for galectin-3, CD44, and HBME1 to fine-needle aspiration cytology diagnosis of papillary thyroid carcinoma. Diagn Cytopathol. 2014;42(6):498–505.
5. Wobker SE, Kim LT, Hackman TG, Dodd LG. Use of BRAF v600e immunocytochemistry on FNA direct smears of papillary thyroid carcinoma. Cancer Cytopathol. 2015;123(9):531–9.

6. Ratour J, Polivka M, Dahan H, Hamzi L, Kania R, Dumuis ML, et al. Diagnosis of follicular lesions of undetermined significance in fine-needle aspirations of thyroid nodules. J Thyroid Res. 2013;2013:250347.
7. Cochand-Priollet B, Dahan H, Laloi-Michelin M, Polivka M, Saada M, Herman P, et al. Immunocytochemistry with cytokeratin 19 and anti-human mesothelial cell antibody (HBME1) increases the diagnostic accuracy of thyroid fine-needle aspirations: preliminary report of 150 liquid-based fine-needle aspirations with histological control. Thyroid. 2011;21(10):1067–73.
8. Lacoste-Collin L, d'Aure D, Berard E, Rouquette I, Delisle MB, Courtade-Saidi M. Improvement of the cytological diagnostic accuracy of follicular thyroid lesions by the use of the Ki-67 proliferative index in addition to cytokeratin-19 and HBME-1 immunomarkers: a study of 61 cases of liquid-based FNA cytology with histological controls. Cytopathology. 2014;25(3):160–9.
9. Bartolazzi A, Bellotti C, Sciacchitano S. Methodology and technical requirements of the galectin-3 test for the preoperative characterization of thyroid nodules. Appl Immunohistochem Mol Morphol. 2012;20(1):2–7.
10. Bartolazzi A, Orlandi F, Saggiorato E, Volante M, Arecco F, Rossetto R, et al. Galectin-3-expression analysis in the surgical selection of follicular thyroid nodules with indeterminate fine-needle aspiration cytology: a prospective multicentre study. Lancet Oncol. 2008;9(6):543–9.
11. Smith AL, Williams MD, Stewart J, Wang WL, Krishnamurthy S, Cabanillas ME, et al. Utility of the BRAF p.V600E immunoperoxidase stain in FNA direct smears and cell block preparations from patients with thyroid carcinoma. Cancer Cytopathol. 2018;126:406–13.
12. Ferris RL, Baloch Z, Bernet V, Chen A, Fahey TJ 3rd, Ganly I, et al. American Thyroid Association statement on surgical application of molecular profiling for thyroid nodules: current impact on perioperative decision making. Thyroid. 2015;25(7):760–8.
13. Valderrabano P, Leon ME, Centeno BA, Otto KJ, Khazai L, McCaffrey JC, et al. Institutional prevalence of malignancy of indeterminate thyroid cytology is necessary but insufficient to accurately interpret molecular marker tests. Eur J Endocrinol. 2016;174(5):621–9.
14. Nikiforov YE, Seethala RR, Tallini G, Baloch ZW, Basolo F, Thompson LD, et al. Nomenclature revision for encapsulated follicular variant of papillary thyroid carcinoma: a paradigm

shift to reduce overtreatment of indolent tumors. JAMA Oncol. 2016;2(8):1023–9.
15. Chudova D, Wilde JI, Wang ET, Wang H, Rabbee N, Egidio CM, et al. Molecular classification of thyroid nodules using high-dimensionality genomic data. J Clin Endocrinol Metab. 2010;95(12):5296–304.
16. Eszlinger M, Krohn K, Frenzel R, Kropf S, Tonjes A, Paschke R. Gene expression analysis reveals evidence for inactivation of the TGF-beta signaling cascade in autonomously functioning thyroid nodules. Oncogene. 2004;23(3):795–804.
17. Eszlinger M, Wiench M, Jarzab B, Krohn K, Beck M, Lauter J, et al. Meta- and reanalysis of gene expression profiles of hot and cold thyroid nodules and papillary thyroid carcinoma for gene groups. J Clin Endocrinol Metab. 2006;91(5):1934–42.
18. Mazzanti C, Zeiger MA, Costouros NG, Umbricht C, Westra WH, Smith D, et al. Using gene expression profiling to differentiate benign versus malignant thyroid tumors. Cancer Res. 2004;64(8):2898–903.
19. Rossi ED, Bizzarro T, Martini M, Capodimonti S, Sarti D, Cenci T, et al. The evaluation of miRNAs on thyroid FNAC: the promising role of miR-375 in follicular neoplasms. Endocrine. 2016;54(3):723–32.
20. Dettmer M, Perren A, Moch H, Komminoth P, Nikiforov YE, Nikiforova MN. Comprehensive MicroRNA expression profiling identifies novel markers in follicular variant of papillary thyroid carcinoma. Thyroid. 2013;23(11):1383–9.
21. Dettmer M, Vogetseder A, Durso MB, Moch H, Komminoth P, Perren A, et al. MicroRNA expression array identifies novel diagnostic markers for conventional and oncocytic follicular thyroid carcinomas. J Clin Endocrinol Metab. 2013;98(1):E1–7.
22. Nikiforova MN, Tseng GC, Steward D, Diorio D, Nikiforov YE. MicroRNA expression profiling of thyroid tumors: biological significance and diagnostic utility. J Clin Endocrinol Metab. 2008;93(5):1600–8.
23. Yip L, Kelly L, Shuai Y, Armstrong MJ, Nikiforov YE, Carty SE, et al. MicroRNA signature distinguishes the degree of aggressiveness of papillary thyroid carcinoma. Ann Surg Oncol. 2011;18(7):2035–41.
24. Nishino M, Nikiforova M. Update on molecular testing for cytologically indeterminate thyroid nodules. Arch Pathol Lab Med. 2018;142(4):446–57.

25. Nikiforov YE, Carty SE, Chiosea SI, Coyne C, Duvvuri U, Ferris RL, et al. Highly accurate diagnosis of cancer in thyroid nodules with follicular neoplasm/suspicious for a follicular neoplasm cytology by ThyroSeq v2 next-generation sequencing assay. Cancer. 2014;120(23):3627–34.
26. Patel KN, Angell TE, Barbiarz J, Barth NM, Blevins TC, Duh Q, et al. Clinical validation of an improved genomic classifier for cytologically indeterminate thyroid nodules using an NGS platform and machine learning algorithms in an independent prospective multicenter blinded cohort demonstrates improved performance (conference abstract). World Congress on Thyroid Cancer. Boston, Massachusetts; 2017.
27. Alexander EK, Kennedy GC, Baloch ZW, Cibas ES, Chudova D, Diggans J, et al. Preoperative diagnosis of benign thyroid nodules with indeterminate cytology. N Engl J Med. 2012;367(8):705–15.
28. Labourier E, Shifrin A, Busseniers AE, Lupo MA, Manganelli ML, Andruss B, et al. Molecular testing for miRNA, mRNA, and DNA on fine-needle aspiration improves the preoperative diagnosis of thyroid nodules with indeterminate cytology. J Clin Endocrinol Metab. 2015;100(7):2743–50.
29. Lithwick-Yanai G, Dromi N, Shtabsky A, Morgenstern S, Strenov Y, Feinmesser M, et al. Multicentre validation of a microRNA-based assay for diagnosing indeterminate thyroid nodules utilising fine needle aspirate smears. J Clin Pathol. 2017;70(6):500–7.
30. Nikiforov YE, Carty SE, Chiosea SI, Coyne C, Duvvuri U, Ferris RL, et al. Impact of the multi-gene ThyroSeq next-generation sequencing assay on cancer diagnosis in thyroid nodules with atypia of undetermined significance/follicular lesion of undetermined significance cytology. Thyroid. 2015;25(11):1217–23.
31. Alexander EK, Schorr M, Klopper J, Kim C, Sipos J, Nabhan F, et al. Multicenter clinical experience with the Afirma gene expression classifier. J Clin Endocrinol Metab. 2014;99(1):119–25.
32. Harrell RM, Bimston DN. Surgical utility of Afirma: effects of high cancer prevalence and oncocytic cell types in patients with indeterminate thyroid cytology. Endocr Pract. 2014;20(4):364–9.
33. Lastra RR, Pramick MR, Crammer CJ, LiVolsi VA, Baloch ZW. Implications of a suspicious afirma test result in thyroid fine-needle aspiration cytology: an institutional experience. Cancer Cytopathol. 2014;122(10):737–44.
34. McIver B, Castro MR, Morris JC, Bernet V, Smallridge R, Henry M, et al. An independent study of a gene expression classifier

(Afirma) in the evaluation of cytologically indeterminate thyroid nodules. J Clin Endocrinol Metab. 2014;99(11):4069–77.
35. Marti JL, Avadhani V, Donatelli LA, Niyogi S, Wang B, Wong RJ, et al. Wide inter-institutional variation in performance of a molecular classifier for indeterminate thyroid nodules. Ann Surg Oncol. 2015;22(12):3996–4001.
36. Brauner E, Holmes BJ, Krane JF, Nishino M, Zurakowski D, Hennessey JV, et al. Performance of the Afirma gene expression classifier in Hurthle cell thyroid nodules differs from other indeterminate thyroid nodules. Thyroid. 2015;25(7):789–96.
37. Kloos RT, Monroe RJ, Traweek ST, Lanman RB, Kennedy GC. A genomic alternative to identify medullary thyroid cancer preoperatively in thyroid nodules with indeterminate cytology. Thyroid. 2016;26(6):785–93.
38. Pankratz DG, Hu Z, Kim SY, Monroe RJ, Wong MG, Traweek ST, et al. Analytical performance of a gene expression classifier for medullary thyroid carcinoma. Thyroid. 2016;26(11):1573–80.
39. Wells SA Jr, Asa SL, Dralle H, Elisei R, Evans DB, Gagel RF, et al. Revised american thyroid association guidelines for the management of medullary thyroid carcinoma. Thyroid. 2015;25(6):567–610.
40. Diggans J, Kim SY, Hu Z, Pankratz D, Wong M, Reynolds J, et al. Machine learning from concept to clinic: reliable detection of BRAF V600e DNA mutations in thyroid nodules using high-dimensional RNA expression data. Pac Symp Biocomput. 2015:371–82.
41. Dettmer MS, Perren A, Moch H, Komminoth P, Nikiforov YE, Nikiforova MN. MicroRNA profile of poorly differentiated thyroid carcinomas: new diagnostic and prognostic insights. J Mol Endocrinol. 2014;52(2):181–9.
42. Gustafson D, Tyryshkin K, Renwick N. microRNA-guided diagnostics in clinical samples. Best Pract Res Clin Endocrinol Metab. 2016;30(5):563–75.
43. Jung M, Schaefer A, Steiner I, Kempkensteffen C, Stephan C, Erbersdobler A, et al. Robust microRNA stability in degraded RNA preparations from human tissue and cell samples. Clin Chem. 2010;56(6):998–1006.
44. Petriella D, Galetta D, Rubini V, Savino E, Paradiso A, Simone G, et al. Molecular profiling of thin-prep FNA samples in assisting clinical management of non-small-cell lung cancer. Mol Biotechnol. 2013;54(3):913–9.
45. Nikiforov YE. Role of molecular markers in thyroid nodule management: then and now. Endocr Pract. 2017;23(8):979–88.

46. Cabanillas ME, Patel A, Danysh BP, Dadu R, Kopetz S, Falchook G. BRAF inhibitors: experience in thyroid cancer and general review of toxicity. Horm Cancer. 2015;6(1):21–36.
47. Brose MS, Cabanillas ME, Cohen EE, Wirth LJ, Riehl T, Yue H, et al. Vemurafenib in patients with BRAF(V600E)-positive metastatic or unresectable papillary thyroid cancer refractory to radioactive iodine: a non-randomised, multicentre, open-label, phase 2 trial. Lancet Oncol. 2016;17(9):1272–82.
48. Falchook GS, Millward M, Hong D, Naing A, Piha-Paul S, Waguespack SG, et al. BRAF inhibitor dabrafenib in patients with metastatic BRAF-mutant thyroid cancer. Thyroid. 2015;25(1):71–7.
49. Rothenberg SM, McFadden DG, Palmer EL, Daniels GH, Wirth LJ. Redifferentiation of iodine-refractory BRAF V600E-mutant metastatic papillary thyroid cancer with dabrafenib. Clin Cancer Res. 2015;21(5):1028–35.
50. Nikiforov YE, Nikiforova MN. Molecular genetics and diagnosis of thyroid cancer. Nat Rev Endocrinol. 2011;7(10):569–80.
51. Trimboli P, Treglia G, Condorelli E, Romanelli F, Crescenzi A, Bongiovanni M, et al. BRAF-mutated carcinomas among thyroid nodules with prior indeterminate FNA report: a systematic review and meta-analysis. Clin Endocrinol. 2016;84(3):315–20.
52. Pusztaszeri MP, Krane JF, Faquin WC. BRAF testing and thyroid FNA. Cancer Cytopathol. 2015;123(12):689–95.
53. Beaudenon-Huibregtse S, Alexander EK, Guttler RB, Hershman JM, Babu V, Blevins TC, et al. Centralized molecular testing for oncogenic gene mutations complements the local cytopathologic diagnosis of thyroid nodules. Thyroid. 2014;24(10):1479–87.
54. Cantara S, Capezzone M, Marchisotta S, Capuano S, Busonero G, Toti P, et al. Impact of proto-oncogene mutation detection in cytological specimens from thyroid nodules improves the diagnostic accuracy of cytology. J Clin Endocrinol Metab. 2010;95(3):1365–9.
55. Eszlinger M, Krogdahl A, Munz S, Rehfeld C, Precht Jensen EM, Ferraz C, et al. Impact of molecular screening for point mutations and rearrangements in routine air-dried fine-needle aspiration samples of thyroid nodules. Thyroid. 2014;24(2):305–13.
56. Eszlinger M, Piana S, Moll A, Bosenberg E, Bisagni A, Ciarrocchi A, et al. Molecular testing of thyroid fine-needle aspirations improves presurgical diagnosis and supports the histologic identification of minimally invasive follicular thyroid carcinomas. Thyroid. 2015;25(4):401–9.

57. Nikiforov YE, Ohori NP, Hodak SP, Carty SE, LeBeau SO, Ferris RL, et al. Impact of mutational testing on the diagnosis and management of patients with cytologically indeterminate thyroid nodules: a prospective analysis of 1056 FNA samples. J Clin Endocrinol Metab. 2011;96(11):3390–7.
58. Nikiforov YE, Steward DL, Robinson-Smith TM, Haugen BR, Klopper JP, Zhu Z, et al. Molecular testing for mutations in improving the fine-needle aspiration diagnosis of thyroid nodules. J Clin Endocrinol Metab. 2009;94(6):2092–8.
59. Medici M, Kwong N, Angell TE, Marqusee E, Kim MI, Frates MC, et al. The variable phenotype and low-risk nature of RAS-positive thyroid nodules. BMC Med. 2015;13:184.
60. Paulson VA, Shivdasani P, Angell TE, Cibas ES, Krane JF, Lindeman NI, et al. Noninvasive follicular thyroid neoplasm with papillary-like nuclear features accounts for more than half of "carcinomas" harboring ras mutations. Thyroid. 2017;27(4):506–11.
61. Armstrong MJ, Yang H, Yip L, Ohori NP, McCoy KL, Stang MT, et al. PAX8/PPARgamma rearrangement in thyroid nodules predicts follicular-pattern carcinomas, in particular the encapsulated follicular variant of papillary carcinoma. Thyroid. 2014;24(9):1369–74.
62. Eberhardt NL, Grebe SK, McIver B, Reddi HV. The role of the PAX8/PPARgamma fusion oncogene in the pathogenesis of follicular thyroid cancer. Mol Cell Endocrinol. 2010;321(1):50–6.
63. Giordano TJ, Beaudenon-Huibregtse S, Shinde R, Langfield L, Vinco M, Laosinchai-Wolf W, et al. Molecular testing for oncogenic gene mutations in thyroid lesions: a case-control validation study in 413 postsurgical specimens. Hum Pathol. 2014;45(7):1339–47.
64. Krane JF, Cibas ES, Alexander EK, Paschke R, Eszlinger M. Molecular analysis of residual ThinPrep material from thyroid FNAs increases diagnostic sensitivity. Cancer Cytopathol. 2015;123(6):356–61.
65. Najafian A, Noureldine S, Azar F, Atallah C, Trinh G, Schneider EB, et al. RAS mutations, and RET/PTC and PAX8/PPAR-gamma chromosomal rearrangements are also prevalent in Benign thyroid lesions: implications thereof and a systematic review. Thyroid. 2017;27(1):39–48.
66. Nikiforova MN, Lynch RA, Biddinger PW, Alexander EK, Dorn GW 2nd, Tallini G, et al. RAS point mutations and PAX8-PPAR gamma rearrangement in thyroid tumors: evidence for distinct

molecular pathways in thyroid follicular carcinoma. J Clin Endocrinol Metab. 2003;88(5):2318–26.
67. Cancer Genome Atlas Research Network. Integrated genomic characterization of papillary thyroid carcinoma. Cell. 2014;159(3):676–90.
68. Shrestha RT, Evasovich MR, Amin K, Radulescu A, Sanghvi TS, Nelson AC, et al. Correlation between histological diagnosis and mutational panel testing of thyroid nodules: a two-year institutional experience. Thyroid. 2016;26(8):1068–76.
69. Taye A, Gurciullo D, Miles BA, Gupta A, Owen RP, Inabnet WB 3rd, et al. Clinical performance of a next-generation sequencing assay (ThyroSeq v2) in the evaluation of indeterminate thyroid nodules. Surgery. 2018;163(1):97–103.
70. Valderrabano P, Khazai L, Leon ME, Thompson ZJ, Ma Z, Chung CH, et al. Evaluation of ThyroSeq v2 performance in thyroid nodules with indeterminate cytology. Endocr Relat Cancer. 2017;24(3):127–36.
71. Karunamurthy A, Panebianco F, J Hsiao S, Vorhauer J, Nikiforova MN, Chiosea S, et al. Prevalence and phenotypic correlations of EIF1AX mutations in thyroid nodules. Endocr Relat Cancer. 2016;23(4):295–301.
72. Landa I, Ganly I, Chan TA, Mitsutake N, Matsuse M, Ibrahimpasic T, et al. Frequent somatic TERT promoter mutations in thyroid cancer: higher prevalence in advanced forms of the disease. J Clin Endocrinol Metab. 2013;98(9):E1562–6.
73. Xu B, Ghossein R. Genomic landscape of poorly differentiated and anaplastic thyroid carcinoma. Endocr Pathol. 2016;27(3):205–12.
74. Landa I, Ibrahimpasic T, Boucai L, Sinha R, Knauf JA, Shah RH, et al. Genomic and transcriptomic hallmarks of poorly differentiated and anaplastic thyroid cancers. J Clin Invest. 2016;126(3):1052–66.
75. Liu T, Wang N, Cao J, Sofiadis A, Dinets A, Zedenius J, et al. The age- and shorter telomere-dependent TERT promoter mutation in follicular thyroid cell-derived carcinomas. Oncogene. 2014;33(42):4978–84.
76. Melo M, da Rocha AG, Vinagre J, Batista R, Peixoto J, Tavares C, et al. TERT promoter mutations are a major indicator of poor outcome in differentiated thyroid carcinomas. J Clin Endocrinol Metab. 2014;99(5):E754–65.
77. Song YS, Lim JA, Choi H, Won JK, Moon JH, Cho SW, et al. Prognostic effects of TERT promoter mutations are

enhanced by coexistence with BRAF or RAS mutations and strengthen the risk prediction by the ATA or TNM staging system in differentiated thyroid cancer patients. Cancer. 2016;122(9):1370–9.
78. Vuong HG, Duong UN, Altibi AM, Ngo HT, Pham TQ, Tran HM, et al. A meta-analysis of prognostic roles of molecular markers in papillary thyroid carcinoma. Endocr Connect. 2017;6(3):R8–R17.
79. Xu B, Tuttle RM, Sabra MM, Ganly I, Ghossein R. Primary thyroid carcinoma with low-risk histology and distant metastases: clinicopathologic and molecular characteristics. Thyroid. 2017;27(5):632–40.
80. Nikiforova MN, Mercurio S, Wald AI, Barbi de Moura M, Callenberg K, Santana-Santos L, et al. Analytical performance of the ThyroSeq v3 genomic classifier for cancer diagnosis in thyroid nodules. Cancer. 2018;124(8):1682–90.
81. Rivera M, Ricarte-Filho J, Knauf J, Shaha A, Tuttle M, Fagin JA, et al. Molecular genotyping of papillary thyroid carcinoma follicular variant according to its histological subtypes (encapsulated vs infiltrative) reveals distinct BRAF and RAS mutation patterns. Mod Pathol. 2010;23(9):1191–200.
82. Zhao L, Dias-Santagata D, Sadow PM, Faquin WC. Cytological, molecular, and clinical features of noninvasive follicular thyroid neoplasm with papillary-like nuclear features versus invasive forms of follicular variant of papillary thyroid carcinoma. Cancer Cytopathol. 2017;125:323–31.
83. Finnerty BM, Kleiman DA, Scognamiglio T, Aronova A, Beninato T, Fahey TJ 3rd, et al. Navigating the management of follicular variant papillary thyroid carcinoma subtypes: a classic PTC comparison. Ann Surg Oncol. 2015;22(4):1200–6.
84. Kim TH, Lee M, Kwon AY, Choe JH, Kim JH, Kim JS, et al. Molecular genotyping of the non-invasive encapsulated follicular variant of papillary thyroid carcinoma. Histopathology. 2018;72(4):648–61.
85. Ganly I, Wang L, Tuttle RM, Katabi N, Ceballos GA, Harach HR, et al. Invasion rather than nuclear features correlates with outcome in encapsulated follicular tumors: further evidence for the reclassification of the encapsulated papillary thyroid carcinoma follicular variant. Hum Pathol. 2015;46(5):657–64.
86. Rivera M, Tuttle RM, Patel S, Shaha A, Shah JP, Ghossein RA. Encapsulated papillary thyroid carcinoma: a clinico-

pathologic study of 106 cases with emphasis on its morphologic subtypes (histologic growth pattern). Thyroid. 2009;19(2):119–27.
87. Gupta S, Ajise O, Dultz L, Wang B, Nonaka D, Ogilvie J, et al. Follicular variant of papillary thyroid cancer: encapsulated, non-encapsulated, and diffuse: distinct biologic and clinical entities. Arch Otolaryngol Head Neck Surg. 2012;138(3):227–33.
88. Howitt BE, Jia Y, Sholl LM, Barletta JA. Molecular alterations in partially-encapsulated or well-circumscribed follicular variant of papillary thyroid carcinoma. Thyroid. 2013;23(10):1256–62.
89. Liu J, Singh B, Tallini G, Carlson DL, Katabi N, Shaha A, et al. Follicular variant of papillary thyroid carcinoma: a clinicopathologic study of a problematic entity. Cancer. 2006;107(6):1255–64.
90. Thompson LD. Ninety-four cases of encapsulated follicular variant of papillary thyroid carcinoma: A name change to Noninvasive Follicular Thyroid Neoplasm with Papillary-like Nuclear Features would help prevent overtreatment. Mod Pathol. 2016;29(7):698–707.
91. Vivero M, Kraft S, Barletta JA. Risk stratification of follicular variant of papillary thyroid carcinoma. Thyroid. 2013;23(3):273–9.
92. Seethala RR, Baloch ZW, Barletta JA, Khanafshar E, Mete O, Sadow PM, et al. Noninvasive follicular thyroid neoplasm with papillary-like nuclear features: a review for pathologists. Mod Pathol. 2018;31(1):39–55.
93. Panebianco F, Kelly LM, Liu P, Zhong S, Dacic S, Wang X, et al. THADA fusion is a mechanism of IGF2BP3 activation and IGF1R signaling in thyroid cancer. Proc Natl Acad Sci U S A. 2017;114(9):2307–12.
94. Ghossein R. Encapsulated malignant follicular cell-derived thyroid tumors. Endocr Pathol. 2010;21(4):212–8.
95. Yoo SK, Lee S, Kim SJ, Jee HG, Kim BA, Cho H, et al. Comprehensive analysis of the transcriptional and mutational landscape of follicular and papillary thyroid cancers. PLoS Genet. 2016;12(8):e1006239.
96. Maletta F, Massa F, Torregrossa L, Duregon E, Casadei GP, Basolo F, et al. Cytological features of "noninvasive follicular thyroid neoplasm with papillary-like nuclear features" and their correlation with tumor histology. Hum Pathol. 2016;54:134–42.
97. Brandler TC, Zhou F, Liu CZ, Cho M, Lau RP, Simsir A, et al. Can noninvasive follicular thyroid neoplasm with papillary-like nuclear features be distinguished from classic papillary thyroid

carcinoma and follicular adenomas by fine-needle aspiration? Cancer Cytopathol. 2017;125(6):378–88.
98. Strickland KC, Howitt BE, Barletta JA, Cibas ES, Krane JF. Suggesting the cytologic diagnosis of noninvasive follicular thyroid neoplasm with papillary-like nuclear features (NIFTP): A retrospective analysis of atypical and suspicious nodules. Cancer Cytopathol. 2018;126(2):86–93.
99. Bizzarro T, Martini M, Capodimonti S, Straccia P, Lombardi CP, Pontecorvi A, et al. Young investigator challenge: The morphologic analysis of noninvasive follicular thyroid neoplasm with papillary-like nuclear features on liquid-based cytology: Some insights into their identification. Cancer. 2016;124(10):699–710.
100. Strickland KC, Vivero M, Jo VY, Lowe AC, Hollowell M, Qian X, et al. Preoperative cytologic diagnosis of noninvasive follicular thyroid neoplasm with papillary-like nuclear features: a prospective analysis. Thyroid. 2016;26(10):1466–71.
101. Howitt BE, Chang S, Eszlinger M, Paschke R, Drage MG, Krane JF, et al. Fine-needle aspiration diagnoses of noninvasive follicular variant of papillary thyroid carcinoma. Am J Clin Pathol. 2015;144(6):850–7.
102. Mito JK, Alexander EK, Angell TE, Barletta JA, Nehs MA, Cibas ES, et al. A modified reporting approach for thyroid FNA in the NIFTP era: A 1-year institutional experience. Cancer Cytopathol. 2017;125(11):854–64.
103. Ibrahim AA, Wu HH. Fine-needle aspiration cytology of noninvasive follicular variant of papillary thyroid carcinoma is cytomorphologically distinct from the invasive counterpart. Am J Clin Pathol. 2016;146(3):373–7.
104. Canberk S, Gunes P, Onenerk M, Erkan M, Kilinc E, Kocak Gursan N, et al. New concept of the encapsulated follicular variant of papillary thyroid carcinoma and its impact on the Bethesda System for Reporting Thyroid Cytopathology: a single-institute experience. Acta Cytol. 2016;60(3):198–204.
105. Layfield LJ, Baloch ZW, Esebua M, Kannuswamy R, Schmidt RL. Impact of the reclassification of the non-invasive follicular variant of papillary carcinoma as benign on the malignancy risk of the Bethesda System for Reporting Thyroid Cytopathology: a meta-analysis study. Acta Cytol. 2017;61(3):187–93.
106. Zhou H, Baloch ZW, Nayar R, Bizzarro T, Fadda G, Adhikari-Guragain D, et al. Noninvasive follicular thyroid neoplasm with papillary-like nuclear features (NIFTP): implications for the risk of malignancy (ROM) in the Bethesda System

for Reporting Thyroid Cytopathology (TBSRTC). Cancer Cytopathol. 2018;126(1):20–6.
107. Strickland KC, Howitt BE, Marqusee E, Alexander EK, Cibas ES, Krane JF, et al. The impact of noninvasive Follicular variant of papillary thyroid carcinoma on rates of malignancy for Fine-needle aspiration diagnostic categories. Thyroid. 2015;25(9):987–92.
108. Faquin WC, Wong LQ, Afrogheh AH, Ali SZ, Bishop JA, Bongiovanni M, et al. Impact of reclassifying noninvasive follicular variant of papillary thyroid carcinoma on the risk of malignancy in The Bethesda System for Reporting Thyroid Cytopathology. Cancer Cytopathol. 2016;124(3):181–7.
109. Ohori NP, Wolfe J, Carty SE, Yip L, LeBeau SO, Berg AN, et al. The influence of the noninvasive follicular thyroid neoplasm with papillary-like nuclear features (NIFTP) resection diagnosis on the false-positive thyroid cytology rate relates to quality assurance thresholds and the application of NIFTP criteria. Cancer Cytopathol. 2017;125(9):692–700.
110. Valderrabano P, Khazai L, Thompson ZJ, Sharpe SC, Tarasova VD, Otto KJ, et al. Cancer risk associated with nuclear atypia in cytologically indeterminate thyroid nodules: a systematic review and meta-analysis. Thyroid. 2018;28(2):210–9.
111. Lastra RR, Birdsong G, Hwang DH, Jorda M, Kerr DA, McGrath C, et al. Preoperative cytologic interpretation of noninvasive follicular thyroid neoplasm with papillary-like nuclear features: a 1-year multi-institutional experience. J Am Soc Cytopathol. 2018;7(2):79–85.
112. Samulski TD, LiVolsi VA, Wong LQ, Baloch Z. Usage trends and performance characteristics of a "gene expression classifier" in the management of thyroid nodules: an institutional experience. Diagn Cytopathol. 2016;44(11):867–73.
113. Jiang XS, Harrison GP, Datto MB. Young investigator challenge: molecular testing in noninvasive follicular thyroid neoplasm with papillary-like nuclear features. Cancer. 2016;124(12):893–900.
114. Hang JF, Westra WH, Cooper DS, Ali SZ. The impact of noninvasive follicular thyroid neoplasm with papillary-like nuclear features on the performance of the Afirma gene expression classifier. Cancer Cytopathol. 2017;125(9):683–91.
115. Wong KS, Angell TE, Strickland KC, Alexander EK, Cibas ES, Krane JF, et al. Noninvasive follicular variant of papillary thyroid carcinoma and the Afirma gene-expression classifier. Thyroid. 2016;26(7):911–5.

116. Sahli ZT, Umbricht CB, Schneider EB, Zeiger MA. Thyroid nodule diagnostic markers in the face of the new NIFTP category: time for a reset? Thyroid. 2017;27(11):1393–9.
117. Cho U, Mete O, Kim MH, Bae JS, Jung CK. Molecular correlates and rate of lymph node metastasis of non-invasive follicular thyroid neoplasm with papillary-like nuclear features and invasive follicular variant papillary thyroid carcinoma: the impact of rigid criteria to distinguish non-invasive follicular thyroid neoplasm with papillary-like nuclear features. Mod Pathol. 2017;30(6):810–25.

Chapter 13
Molecular Diagnostics in Breast Cytology

Liza M. Quintana

Abbreviations

AJCC	American Joint Committee on Cancer
ASCO	American Society of Clinical Oncology
ATM	Ataxia telangiectasia mutated
BRCA1	Breast cancer 1, early onset
BRCA2	Breast cancer 2, early onset
CAP	College of American Pathologists
CB	Cellblock
CDH1	E-cadherin
CEP17	Centromere enumeration probe 17
cfDNA	Cell-free circulating DNA
CHEK2	Checkpoint kinase 2
CNB	Core needle biopsy
CTC	Circulating tumor cell
ctDNA	Circulating tumor DNA
CTLA-4	Cytotoxic T-lymphocyte-associated protein 4

L. M. Quintana
Department of Pathology, Beth Israel Deaconess Medical Center, Boston, MA, USA
e-mail: lmquinta@bidmc.harvard.edu

S. Roy-Chowdhuri et al. (eds.), *Molecular Diagnostics in Cytopathology*, https://doi.org/10.1007/978-3-319-97397-5_13

DCIS	Ductal carcinoma *in situ*
DNA	Deoxyribonucleic acid
EGFR	Epidermal growth factor receptor
ER	Estrogen receptor
ERBB2	erb-b2 receptor tyrosine kinase 2 (HER2)
ETV6	ETS variant 6
FFPE	Formalin-fixed paraffin-embedded
FISH	Fluorescence *in situ* hybridization
FNA	Fine needle aspiration
GI	Gastrointestinal
HER2	Human epidermal growth factor receptor 2 (ERBB2)
ICC	Immunocytochemistry
IHC	Immunohistochemistry
ISH	*In situ* hybridization
MAML2	Mastermind-like protein 2
MECT1	Mucoepidermoid carcinoma translocated 1
MYB	MYB proto-oncogene
NCCN	National Comprehensive Cancer Network
NFIB	Nuclear factor 1 B-type
NGS	Next generation sequencing
NST	No special type (breast carcinoma of no special type; also referred to as invasive ductal carcinoma)
NTRK	Neurotrophic tyrosine kinase, receptor
PALB2	Partner and localizer of BRCA2
PARP	Poly (ADP-ribose) polymerase
PD-1	Programmed cell death protein 1 (CD279)
PD-L1	Programmed death-ligand 1 (CD274)
PIK3CA	Phosphatidylinositol 4,5-bisphosphate 3-kinase catalytic subunit alpha
PR	Progesterone receptor
PTEN	Phosphatase and tensin homolog
ROR	Risk of recurrence
RS	Recurrence score
RT-PCR	Reverse transcription-polymerase chain reaction
STK11	Serine/threonine kinase 11
TP53	Tumor protein 53
WHO	World Health Organization

Key Points

- Breast cancer is heterogeneous in terms of histologic appearance, molecular features, biology, and response to therapy
- Gene expression profiling studies have established a molecular classification identifying four major subtypes: luminal A, luminal B, HER2 enriched, and basal-like
- ER, PR, and HER2 are the most important markers that are routinely part of diagnostic workup of all breast cancers because of their prognostic and predictive value
- ER and PR testing is routinely performed by IHC
- HER2 testing can be evaluated by IHC and/or ISH
- Rare special subtypes of breast carcinoma have pathognomonic translocations that can be identified by FISH
- Several molecular assays can be used to estimate the risk of recurrence and potential benefit of adjuvant chemotherapy
- CTCs and ctDNA show promise as prognostic biomarkers and as ways to monitor disease and predict treatment
- Immunotherapy is being investigated in breast cancer, and immune checkpoint inhibitors show promise in its treatment
- Approximately 10% of breast cancer is hereditary; germline mutations in *BRCA1* and *BRCA2* account for half of these

Breast cancer refers to a heterogeneous group of tumors that together comprise the most common type of cancer in women, accounting for 30% of all new cancer diagnoses [1].

The diagnosis and management of breast cancer relies on the evaluation of clinicopathological features such as histological subtype, grade, tumor size, presence of lymphovascular invasion, and axillary lymph node involvement [2–4]. The choice of treatment largely relies on these factors and the presence or absence of three key biomarkers, ER, PR, and HER2, which also carry prognostic significance. Currently, these are the only biomarkers recommended by ASCO and CAP for routine clinical management of patients with primary, recurrent, and metastatic breast carcinoma [5–7]. In addition, a handful of well-known translocations in rare subtypes are recognized and assayed by FISH.

Studies, initially using gene expression arrays and subsequently using an RT-PCR assay, have demonstrated that most breast cancers can be classified into one of the four molecular subtypes based on their gene expression signatures: luminal A, luminal B, HER2-enriched, and basal-like. Recently, molecular testing has gained prominence in breast cancer management. A number of gene expression-based tests are now available in early breast cancer to assess prognosis and identify patients with ER-positive breast cancer who may benefit from chemotherapy in addition to endocrine therapy. Next generation sequencing has also begun to be used to search for unexpected potential drug targets. CTCs and ctDNA are also under investigation for clinical utility. As our understanding of the immune landscape of breast cancer evolves, immunotherapy and the role of the immune microenvironment are being investigated as well.

In this chapter, we review the main biomarkers and molecular tests used in breast cancer, beginning with ER, PR, HER2, and Ki-67; describe the role of FISH in identifying recurrent translocations in some breast cancer subtypes; discuss molecular classification of breast cancer and molecular prognostic tests; describe some molecular tests and treatments that show promise for future management of breast cancer; and discuss common germline mutations seen in hereditary breast cancer.

Biomarkers ER, PR, HER2, and Ki-67

The biomarkers used in routine clinical management of patients with primary, recurrent, and metastatic breast carcinoma are ER, PR, and HER2 [5–7]. A minority of invasive breast carcinomas, approximately 15%, do not express any of these markers and are classified as triple negative [8]. The role of the proliferation marker Ki-67 has been extensively studied, but its use in routine clinical practice varies among institutions.

Hormone Receptors ER and PR

The majority of breast carcinomas, approximately 70%, are ER positive. ER status predicts the likelihood of response to endocrine therapy such as tamoxifen and aromatase inhibitors. ER and PR testing is routinely performed in the evaluation of patients with invasive breast carcinoma to determine which patients should be treated with antiestrogen therapy. ER testing, with or without PR testing, is performed in cases of DCIS.

Proper specimen handling is required to obtain the most accurate results for ER/PR assays. ASCO and CAP provide best practice guidelines on how to handle specimens, with their most recent updates being in 2010 [5]. Specimens used for testing (cytology specimens, CNB, or resection specimens) should have an ischemic time (i.e., time to fixation) of ≤ 1 h and be fixed in 10% neutral buffered formalin for 6–72 h. The guideline mentions that cytology specimens fixed in alcohol may result in uninterpretable results [5]. Correlation with morphology and clinical information or repeating the assay in a different sample may be of use. However, studies evaluating the performance of ER assays performed on cytology samples collected into an alcohol fixative which is then formalin fixed, or samples collected directly into formalin, show good correlation with those performed on histologic tissue samples fixed per ASCO/CAP guidelines [9, 10]. ICC analysis of ER can also be successfully performed on alcohol-fixed direct smears; the use of air-dried direct smears show less concordance [11–13]. PR results, on the other hand, show variable concordance and may be falsely negative.

Hormone receptor status is determined by the nuclear expression of ER and PR in accordance with the ASCO/CAP guidelines [5]. The guidelines require that reports include percentage/proportion of tumor cells with nuclear staining, the intensity of staining, and an interpretation. The percentage of tumor cells is determined by evaluating all tumor cells on the slide and can be performed by estimation or quantification. The intensity of staining is an estimate of the average staining in the positive cells and is reported as weak, moderate, or strong. The interpretations reported include positive, negative, and uninterpretable. A positive result requires that a minimum of 1% of the tumor cells are positive at any intensity (Fig. 13.1a–d). For cytology samples with limited tumor cellularity or scant tumor staining, the guidelines state that 100 cells should be counted or used to estimate percentage.

Carcinomas that have low-level expression of ER (1–10%) may have outcomes more similar to patients that are ER negative and may not benefit from endocrine therapies [14]. Further, many of these carcinomas are of non-luminal subtypes by gene expression profiling. As we learn more about tumor heterogeneity and better understand tumor biology and clinical implications, we can better define which patient population will best benefit from endocrine therapy.

HER2

Approximately 10–15% of breast cancers are clinically HER2 positive [15]. HER2 expression identifies patients who are likely to benefit from HER2-targeted therapy such as trastuzumab, lapatinib, and others. These targeted therapies have

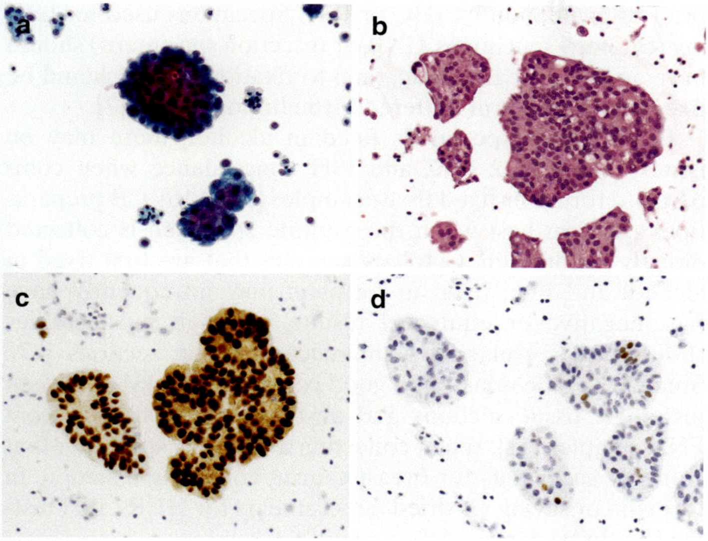

FIGURE 13.1 Metastatic breast carcinoma to pleural fluid. Papanicolaou-stained ThinPrep (**a**) and H&E-stained cellblock slide (**b**) with corresponding ER IHC (**c**) and PR IHC (**d**). The ER is positive with > 95% of tumor nuclei staining with strong intensity. The PR is positive with approximately 5–10% of tumor nuclei showing medium intensity staining. The primary breast carcinoma, from a year prior, was a grade 2 invasive ductal carcinoma that was ER positive (> 95% of cells with strong staining), PR positive (1–5% of cells with medium staining), and HER2 negative (by IHC and FISH)

been shown to improve disease free and overall survival [5]. However, because of the side effects of this therapy, only patients who are expected to benefit should be treated. HER2 is evaluated in early-stage invasive carcinoma and in recurrent or metastatic breast cancer; HER2 testing is not routinely performed on DCIS. The test may be repeated if there is a histopathologic discrepancy such as a high-grade tumor that is HER2 negative.

As with ER and PR assays, the ASCO and CAP guidelines have specific criteria about how tissue should be handled prior to evaluation by IHC or ISH. Specimens used for testing (cytology specimens, CNB, or resection specimens) should have an ischemic time (i.e., time to fixation) of ≤ 1 h and be fixed in 10% neutral buffered formalin for 6–72 h [7].

For cytology specimens fixed in alcohol, there may be issues with HER2 IHC and ISH concordance when compared to formalin-fixed tissue samples [9, 10, 16]. CB preparations perform best when the aspirate specimen is collected directly in formalin. Cytology samples that are first fixed in alcohol and then fixed in formalin may infrequently have false-negative or equivocal results, although most studies show good correlation with matched tissue sections [17]. Studies have demonstrated good correlation of ISH between histologic tissue sections and air-dried direct smears from FNA samples [18]. When collecting a cytology specimen that is highly suspicious for breast cancer, collecting a sample in formalin or saving air-dried direct smears for HER2 ISH testing should be considered.

HER2 status is determined by protein expression (IHC) and/or *HER2* gene amplification (ISH). (Table 13.1, Fig. 13.2a, b) HER2 guidelines were updated in 2018 based on feedback from pathologists [7, 19–21].

The IHC definition for positive and negative did not change from the 2013 guidelines [7, 22]. The update clarified the definition of equivocal HER2 IHC (2+); it is now defined as weak to moderate complete membrane staining in > 10% of invasive tumor cells. The panel also recognized that there may be some unusual staining patterns that may not have incomplete staining but are *HER2* amplified (i.e., micropapillary carcinoma).

HER2 ISH can be performed by either a single-probe assay or dual-probe assay; however, in the updated guideline, the panel prefers dual-probe testing. *HER2* is considered amplified when the assay shows ≥ 6.0 *HER2* signals/cell using a single-probe system. By dual-probe testing, it is positive if there is a *HER2/CEP17* ratio of ≥ 2.0 with an average *HER2* copy number of ≥ 4.0 (Fig. 13.3).

Table 13.1 HER2 testing. It is recommended that the uncommon dual-probe ISH groups undergo concomitant review with the IHC slide. The IHC result, if positive or negative, is the result used for clinical management. If the IHC result is equivocal (2+), then the result is as indicated in the table [7]

	IHC	Dual-probe ISH
Negative	0: no staining or membrane staining that is faint or incomplete in ≤ 10% of tumor cells 1+: incomplete faint membrane staining in > 10% of tumor cells	*HER2/CEP17* < 2.0, *HER2* copies < 4.0
Equivocal	2+: weak to moderate complete membrane staining in > 10% of tumor cells	NA
ISH groups requiring review	NA	Result for these uncommon groups is based on IHC if IHC is negative (0 or 1+) or positive (3+) However, if IHC is 2+, the following would be considered negative: *HER2/CEP17* ≥ 2.0, *HER2* copies <4.0 *HER2/CEP17* < 2.0, *HER2* copies ≥ 4.0 but <6.0 If IHC is 2+, the following would be considered positive: *HER2/CEP17* < 2.0, *HER2* copies ≥ 6.0
Positive	3+: intense complete circumferential membrane staining in > 10% of tumor cells	*HER2/CEP17* ≥ 2.0, *HER2* copies ≥ 4.0

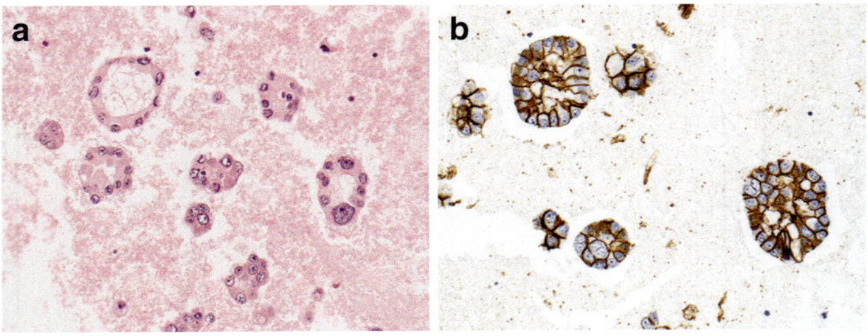

FIGURE 13.2 Metastatic breast carcinoma to pleural fluid. H&E-stained cellblock slide (**a**) with corresponding HER2 IHC (**b**). The HER2 IHC shows 3+ strong membranous staining. The FISH is amplified with a *HER2/CEP17* ratio of 3.1. The primary breast carcinoma, from 3 years prior, was a grade 3 invasive ductal that was ER positive, PR negative, and HER2 positive by IHC (3+) and FISH (*HER2/CEP17* ratio of 3.9)

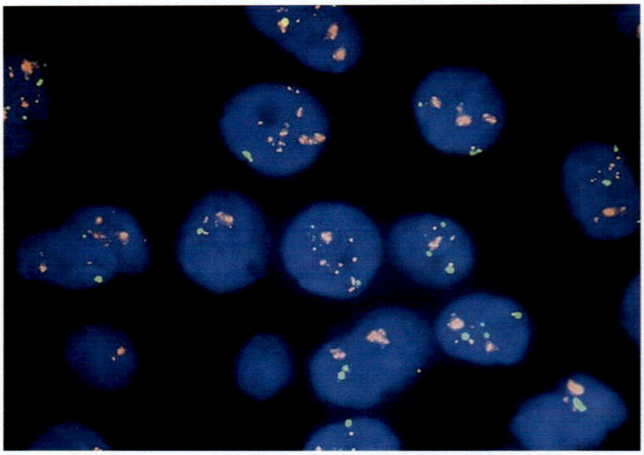

FIGURE 13.3 HER2-positive breast cancer. FISH using a dual-probe system – red signal denotes *HER2* gene copies and green denotes copies of chromosome 17. This tumor shows *HER2* gene amplification. (Image courtesy of Christine Bryke, MD, Beth Israel Deaconess Medical Center, Boston, MA)

There are uncommon dual-probe ISH groups (referred to as groups 2, 3, and 4) for which review of the IHC and ISH is recommended (see Table 13.1). These groups are estimated to account for about 5% of cases. If the corresponding IHC is

3+, then the HER2 result is positive; conversely, if the IHC is 0 or 1+, then the HER2 result is negative. For cases with equivocal IHC (2+), then the ISH slide must undergo additional review. If review does not result in an unequivocal positive or negative, then the diagnosis is as listed in Table 13.1. The guidelines provide example comments to be included in the report for these uncommon situations [7].

As previously mentioned, HER2 testing is performed by IHC and/or ISH. Some institutions perform one assay or the other and reflex to a second assay only if results are equivocal; others perform both IHC and ISH concurrently. For example, many institutions initially perform IHC and reflex equivocal (2+) results for ISH testing.

Some laboratories have used an alternative chromosome 17 probe in double-equivocal cases – cases that were equivocal by IHC and ISH. Using the alternative probe resulted in a minor increase in breast cancers classified as HER2 positive. There was not sufficient data to determine if this population of patients benefit from HER2-targeted therapy. Therefore, the 2018 guidelines do not recommend routine use of alternative chromosome 17 probes [7]. While not part of the current guidelines, there are data to suggest that perhaps utilizing molecular assays, such as determining the molecular subtype or use of next-generation sequencing, may be a better predictor of response to HER2-targeted therapy [23–26].

Ki-67

The Ki-67 proliferation index is important to mention because it has been investigated as a prognostic and predictive factor [27–29]. In routine practice it is evaluated by IHC on cytologic or tissue samples [30]. However, there are no uniformly accepted standards for pre-analytic processing, staining methodology, or interpretation, and there is considerable interobserver variability in its evaluation [14, 31, 32]. In a proportion of cases, the interpretation of Ki-67 labeling differs from FNA (or core-needle biopsy) when compared with the resected primary breast tumor resulting in both falsely high and low results [13, 30, 33].

While high and low values are clinically reproducible and can be clinically useful, there are no universally agreed upon cutoffs. Currently a Ki-67 labeling index by IHC is not recommended by the AJCC or NCCN to guide adjuvant endocrine therapy or chemotherapy decisions [34–38].

The evaluation of proliferation by Ki-67, along with ER, PR, and HER2, can be used to determine the IHC4 score and has been shown to provide prognostic information in patients with ER-positive breast cancer that have been treated endocrine therapy [39]. The IHC4 score utilizes levels of ER, PR, HER2, and Ki-67 and a complex weighted algorithm [39, 40].

Evaluation of proliferation is useful in determining prognosis, and genes involved in proliferation are utilized in the multi-gene signatures discussed below [14].

Molecular Classification of Breast Cancer

Knowledge gained over the past few decades has provided us with alternate ways to categorize breast cancer. The molecular classification system was initially proposed by Perou and colleagues in 2000 [41, 42].

Initial gene expression profiling identified four intrinsic subtypes of breast carcinoma: luminal-like, HER2 enriched, basal-like, and normal breast-like. Further analysis refined characterization of the subtypes, including division of the luminal category into luminal A and luminal B subtypes. Subsequent studies have identified additional subgroups including claudin low and molecular apocrine [29]. Currently, the most widely accepted and reproducible subtypes have been designated luminal A, luminal B, HER2-enriched, and basal-like [27, 29, 43] (Table 13.2).

The luminal group is so named because it has expression profiles similar to the normal luminal epithelial component of the breast and comprises approximately 70% of all breast carcinomas [43]. Carcinomas that cluster in this group express hormone receptors ER and PR [29]. Luminal A carcinomas have high expression of ER and low expression of proliferation markers and have a good prognosis. Luminal B carcinomas tend to have a higher histologic grade, a higher proliferation

TABLE 13.2 Molecular subtypes of breast cancer

Intrinsic Subtype	Gene Expression	IHC Surrogate	Prognosis	Treatment
Luminal A	Hormone receptors, luminal genes	ER/PR positive, HER2 negative Ki-67 low	Good	Endocrine therapy Chemotherapy for selected patients
Luminal B	Hormone receptors, luminal genes	ER/PR positive HER2 negative with high Ki-67 or HER positive with low Ki-67	Intermediate	Endocrine therapy, +/– chemotherapy Anti-HER2 therapy if HER2 positive
HER2-enriched	Genes in the HER2 amplicon	ER/PR negative HER2 positive	Poor	Anti-HER2 therapy and chemotherapy
Basal-like	High-molecular weight cytokeratins, EGFR	ER/PR negative HER2 negative Basal-like marker (CK5/6, EGFR)	Poor	Chemotherapy PARP inhibitor (select patients with *BRCA* mutation)

rate, and a subset of them overexpresses HER2. Luminal A carcinomas have a more favorable prognosis compared to luminal B carcinomas.

The HER2-enriched group, comprising approximately 15% of breast cancers, is composed of carcinomas that generally have high expression of *HER2* and other genes in that amplicon [44]. These carcinomas have a low expression of hormone receptor-associated genes and are clinically hormone receptor negative [29]. Not all clinically HER2-positive carcinomas are HER2-enriched by gene expression profiling; half of HER2-positive carcinomas detected by IHC and/or ISH have this molecular phenotype, but the rest clusters with the luminal groups [44]. HER2-enriched carcinomas overall have a poor prognosis; however, the introduction of HER2-targeted therapies has improved the survival of this patient population [22].

The basal-like group is a heterogeneous group of carcinomas [43]. A majority of these carcinomas, approximately 55–85%, are triple negative (i.e., negative for ER, PR, and HER2); conversely, approximately 75–85% of triple-negative carcinomas are basal-like by gene expression profiling [45, 46]. Tumors in the basal-like group express high-molecular weight cytokeratins as seen in normal myoepithelial cells ("basal cells") of the breast, have low expression of ER-related genes, and do not overexpress *HER2* [43, 45]. Treatment is based on chemotherapeutic agents because triple-negative carcinomas do not respond to endocrine or HER2-targeted therapies. Approximately 80% of breast cancers that occur in women with germline mutations in *BRCA1* are basal-like. Drugs targeting poly (ADP-ribose) polymerase (PARP) have been evaluated for use in these patients. The FDA recently approved a PARP inhibitor for use in certain types of BRCA-mutated carcinomas. The majority of basal-like carcinomas have a poor prognosis; however, there are special subtypes of breast carcinoma, including adenoid cystic carcinoma and secretory carcinoma (discussed below) and acinic cell carcinoma that are basal-like by gene expression profiling but have a good prognosis [47].

Attempts at using immunohistochemistry as surrogates for approximation of molecular subtype have been proposed but are imperfect [31, 43, 48–50]. (Table 13.2) The carcinomas that cluster in the luminal group are generally hormone receptor positive by gene expression and IHC. Luminal A carcinomas are ER and PR positive and HER2 negative and have a low proliferation by Ki-67 labeling. Luminal B carcinomas are ER positive but may show a lower expression of PR both clinically and by gene expression. Luminal B carcinomas can be either HER2 negative with high proliferation by Ki-67 labeling or HER2 positive with low proliferation. HER2-enriched carcinomas are hormone receptor negative and are clinically HER2 positive (IHC or ISH). A majority of basal-like carcinomas are triple negative and show expression of high-molecular weight cytokeratin CK5/6 and EGFR [48].

These developments have helped provide a better understanding of the tumor biology and reinforce the heterogeneity the disease. The intrinsic molecular subtypes may be a better representation of the tumor biology, but currently they are not used clinically. The main factors that drive treatment decisions are knowledge of the tumor hormone receptor status and HER2 status because this predicts who will benefit from endocrine and anti-HER2 therapy [14, 43].

Special Subtypes of Breast Carcinomas with Associated Translocations

There are a few special histologic subtypes of breast cancer that resemble their counterparts in the salivary gland and harbor the same pathognomonic translocations which can be evaluated in the workup of these lesions. These include adenoid cystic carcinoma, secretory carcinoma, and mucoepidermoid carcinoma (Table 13.3). It is important to correctly identify these special subtypes; while adenoid cystic carcinoma and secretory carcinoma are triple negative and cluster in the basal-like group by gene expression profiling, they generally have a good prognosis.

TABLE 13.3 Special subtypes of breast carcinoma with associated translocations

Special subtype	Genes involved	Translocation	Comment
Adenoid cystic carcinoma	*MYB* (MYB proto-oncogene, transcription factor) *NFIB* (nuclear factor I-B)	t(6;9)(q22–23;p23–24)	A single case has shown *MYB* amplification
Secretory carcinoma	*ETV6* (ETS variant 6) *NTRK3* (neurotrophic tropomyosin receptor kinase)	t(12;15)(p13;q25)	The translocation is also present in congenital fibrosarcoma and mesoblastic nephroma
Mucoepidermoid carcinoma	*MECT1* (mucoepidermoid carcinoma translocated-1) *MAML2* (mastermind-like 2)	t(11;19)(q21;p13)	

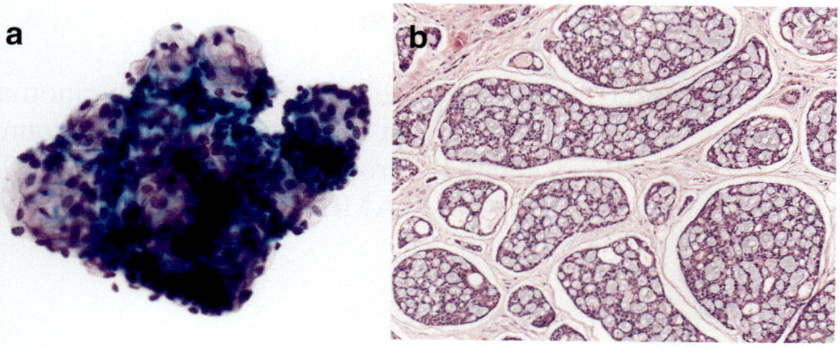

FIGURE 13.4 Adenoid cystic carcinoma. Papanicolaou-stained ThinPrep (**a**) shows basaloid cells that surround variably sized spheres of matrix material. The corresponding surgical excision (**b**) shows the infiltrating nests with a cribriform architecture

Adenoid Cystic Carcinoma

Adenoid cystic carcinomas of the breast and salivary gland have rearrangement of the *MYB* gene, most frequently a recurrent translocation involving the *MYB* and *NFIB* genes [47] (Fig. 13.4a, b). This translocation is seen in 23–100% of cases of adenoid cystic carcinoma in the breast; a single case with *MYB* amplification has been reported [47, 51]. This translocation, t(6;9)(q22–23;p23–24), leads to a *MYB-NFIB* fusion gene which results in overexpression of the MYB protein [51, 52]. The use of IHC for MYB can be utilized as a surrogate to FISH [53]. When evaluating MYB IHC, in the context of the appropriate morphology and immunoprofile, strong and diffuse nuclear staining is needed to support a diagnosis of adenoid cystic carcinoma.

Secretory Carcinoma

A majority of secretory carcinomas (> 90%), like the secretory carcinomas of the salivary gland, harbor a recurrent translocation. The translocation t(12;15)(p13;q25) results in the *ETV6-NTRK3* fusion gene encoding a chimeric tyrosine kinase protein [15, 47]. Therapies targeting the NTRK kinase have been utilized [26].

Mucoepidermoid Carcinoma

Mucoepidermoid is another rare primary breast carcinoma, accounting for 0.3% of all breast cancers, similar to its counterpart in the salivary gland. It harbors a translocation, t(11;19)(q21;p13), creating a MECT1-MAML2 fusion protein [29, 54].

Multi-gene Prognostic Tests

Multi-gene prognostic tests for breast cancer have been developed and employed in clinical practice to provide information about how carcinomas will respond to systemic therapy as well as prognostic information regarding patient outcome. Many of the genes evaluated in these assays are associated with hormone receptors, HER2, and proliferation. Since most ER-negative carcinomas are considered high-risk, the prognostic value of these multi-gene assays is in ER-positive carcinomas [51].

While most of these tests are used in the adjuvant setting after definitive surgical resection, use in the neoadjuvant setting is being studied [55]. These assays are performed on FFPE tissue sections and are important to be aware of since they are utilized in clinical practice. The most common tests are Oncotype DX, MammaPrint, the Prosigna Breast Cancer Prognostic Gene Signature Assay, EndoPredict, and Breast Cancer Index. The Prosigna assay and EndoPredict assay can be set up in a local laboratory, whereas the others are performed at a central laboratory. In the eighth edition of the AJCC staging manual, the Oncotype DX score can be incorporated into the staging of ER-positive and HER2-negative breast cancer [36].

Oncotype DX

Oncotype DX (Genomic Health, Redwood, CA) is a 21-gene RT-PCR assay that measures gene expression in FFPE carcinoma samples (CNB or surgical resection specimen). The 21 genes include 16 cancer-related and 5 control genes [27, 40, 56]. The 16 cancer-related genes are those involved in proliferation, ER expression, HER2, and invasion.

This assay estimates the risk of relapse in patients with ER-positive, HER2-negative, and lymph node-negative breast cancer and provides information about value of chemotherapy in addition to endocrine therapy in this patient subgroup [56, 57]. Patients are divided into three groups based on a calculated recurrence score (RS) that is reported as a continuous variable between 0 and 100. This score estimates the likelihood of distant recurrence within 10 years. The RS is also predictive of locoregional recurrence in patients treated with endocrine therapy [58, 59]. Initially validated in patients with lymph node-negative disease, it also predicts chemotherapy benefit in patients with lymph node-positive breast cancer [57, 60–62]. Results of the Rx for Positive Node, Endocrine-Responsive Breast Cancer Trial (RxPonder) will provide information about whether the addition of chemotherapy to endocrine therapy in patients with node-positive breast cancer and low-to-intermediate RS provides any benefit [57, 62].

Based on the RS, patients are stratified into low- (< 18), intermediate- (18–30), and high- (31–100) risk groups. Patients with low RS have a low risk of locoregional or distant recurrence and do not benefit from chemotherapy [57, 59]. Patients with high-risk RS have a high risk of recurrence and do benefit from the addition of chemotherapy to endocrine therapy. Initially it was unclear if the addition of chemotherapy would benefit the patients in the intermediate-risk group. The results of Trial Assigning Individualized Options for Treatment (TAILORx) showed that hormone receptor-positive, HER2-negative, axillary lymph node-negative patients in the intermediate group had similar outcomes when treated with adjuvant endocrine and chemoendocrine therapy; however, in some women 50 years of age or younger, there was some benefit of adjuvant chemotherapy [63].

Oncotype DX is the most widely used genomic assay in the USA and is currently performed on FFPE breast cancer tissue. Oncotype DX is performed on early-stage invasive breast cancer that is ER positive and HER2 negative. The lymph node status is incorporated into the results so that information is necessary for appropriate interpretation. The NCCN guidelines suggest utilizing this assay to help determine if patients should receive chemotherapy in addition to endocrine therapy in carcinomas that are hormone receptor positive, HER2 negative, > 0.5 cm, and lymph node negative or with a micrometastasis (≤ 2 mm) [64]. A separate assay for patients with DCIS is also available (the Oncotype DCIS score).

MammaPrint

The MammaPrint assay (Agendia NV, Amsterdam, Netherlands) is a microarray-based assay that was cleared by the FDA in 2007. The initial limitation of this assay was that it required fresh tissue, but it is now validated for use on FFPE tissue samples. The basis for this assay was a prognostic signature based on expression of 70 genes [65]. The genes were initially identified in 78 tumors from a cohort of lymph node-negative breast cancers that were 5 cm or smaller in women under 55 years of age. Half the patients were ER positive. Genes were identified that portended either a good or bad prognosis.

The prognostic signature was later validated in large studies in patients with node-positive and node-negative disease. Early results from the prospective Microarray in Node-Negative and 1 to 3 Positive Lymph Node Disease May Avoid Chemotherapy (MINDACT) trial found that women who had high-risk breast cancer based on standard clinicopathologic features and who had 0–3 positive lymph nodes may not require chemotherapy based if they have a low-risk MammaPrint result [66].

MammaPrint results are reported as either low risk or high risk and are meant to help select patients who are likely to benefit from chemotherapy; however, it does not make recommendations about endocrine therapy. Based on results of the assay, a select group of patients who would have received chemotherapy as standard of care may be spared [35].

MammaPrint is performed on early-stage breast cancer that is < 5 cm and can be ER positive or negative. The assay has been validated in both lymph node-negative and lymph node-positive patients.

Prosigna Breast Cancer Prognostic Gene Signature Assay

The Prosigna Breast Cancer Prognostic Gene Signature Assay (NanoString Technologies, Seattle, WA) is a modification of the prediction analysis of microarray 50 (PAM50) assay and was approved by the FDA in 2013 [55]. The assay is validated for postmenopausal women with ER-positive breast carcinomas with either node-negative (stage I or II) or node-positive disease (stage II). It is performed on FFPE tissue sections. The initial studies that categorized the intrinsic subtypes measured the expression of thousands of genes. The PAM50 assay was designed to reproducibly identify the intrinsic subtypes based on a smaller set of genes – the expression of 50 genes and 5 reference genes [67].

The assay is a 50-gene RT-PCR microarray performed on postoperative FFPE tissue samples of invasive carcinoma. It assigns tumors to one of the following intrinsic subtypes: luminal A, luminal B, HER2-enriched, and basal-like. It also evaluates clinical variables and gene expression profiles to provide a risk of distant recurrence at 10 years in postmenopausal women with hormone receptor, node-negative or node-positive disease [27]. In patients with node-negative cancers, the risk of recurrence (ROR) is classified as low, intermediate, or high. In node-positive cancers, the score is reported as low-risk or high-risk.

EndoPredict

EndoPredict (Myriad Genetics, Inc., Salt Lake City, UT) is an RT-PCR-based assay [68]. Based on the evaluation of eight cancer-related genes and three reference genes, and relevant clinicopathologic factors (tumor size and nodal status), a score (EPclin) is calculated. This genomic test is for patients with early-stage, ER-positive, HER2-negative, and lymph node-negative breast cancer. It predicts the risk of metastases in patients being treated with endocrine therapy alone [69]. The results are binary – low-risk and high-risk.

Breast Cancer Index

Breast cancer index (bioTheranostics, San Diego, CA) is an RT-PCR-based assay [70, 71]. It uses a combination of two gene expression biomarkers, the H/I ratio (*HOXB23*, *IL17BR*) and the molecular grade index (MGI), to predict the risk of late recurrence (5–10 years after diagnosis). The MGI incorporates genes involved in proliferation. The prognostic utility of these biomarkers was validated in the Stockholm trial in a cohort of patients treated with tamoxifen [70, 72]. The assay is utilized in ER-positive, node-negative breast cancer. The results provide information about whether or not extending hormone therapy would be beneficial.

Next-Generation Sequencing

Breast cancer, as with all cancers, develops because of mutations and alterations in certain genes [73]. There are a limited number of genes for which more than 10% of breast tumors show alterations. The Tumor Cancer Genome Atlas (TCGA) reported that the most common mutations are in *TP53* (37%) and *PIK3CA* (36%); others have reported similar findings [45, 74].

The types of alterations vary depending on the hormone receptor and HER2 status and by the molecular subtype of the carcinoma. The luminal A and luminal B breast cancers show the most frequent number of and more diverse altera-

TABLE 13.4 Molecular subtype of primary breast carcinoma and commonly associated gene alterations [45, 75]

	Gene mutations	Other genes
Luminal A	*PIK3CA* (45%), *GATA3* (14%), *TP53* (12%), *MAP3K1* (13%), *CDH1* (9%), *MAP2K4* (7%), *AKT1* (4%)	
Luminal B	*PIK3CA* and *TP53* (29% each), *GATA3* (15%)	*ATM* loss, *MDM2* amplification
HER2-enriched	*TP53* (72%), *PIK3CA* (39%)	*HER2* amplification (80%)
Basal-like	*TP53* (80%), *PIK3CA* (9%)	*PTEN* loss; *RB1* mutation/loss (20%)

tions compared to HER2-enriched and basal-like [29, 45, 75] (Table 13.4). While primary and metastatic breast carcinomas often have a similar profile, they do not always [74, 75]. The Aiming to Understand the Molecular Aberrations in Metastatic Breast Cancer trial (AURORA) is a multinational study that will utilize NGS profiling in advanced breast cancer with the goal to provide insights into the genetic alterations in metastatic breast cancer and the response to targeted therapies [76, 77].

Clinically, patients who have relapsed or recurrent carcinoma that has been refractory to their current treatment regimen may benefit from having their carcinoma evaluated for mutations that have targetable treatments or for which a clinical trial is available. Sequencing a large panel of genes can identify which alterations drive a specific patient's disease [26]. The samples used for NGS in this context are the treated carcinoma sample. This technology is successfully performed on solid tumors. Appropriate samples include FFPE tissue samples, FFPE cellblock cytology samples from FNA or effusions, and other cytology specimens including the supernatant [26, 78].

Circulating Tumor Cells and Cell-Free Tumor DNA

Evaluations of CTCs and ctDNA are considered "liquid biopsies" (also see Chap. 20). These biomarkers may be useful for monitoring disease in patients with breast cancer.

CTCs are cancer cells that have entered the blood stream. Their presence, most often seen in patients with metastatic carcinoma, is a poor prognostic sign and is associated with shorter survival. There are multiple methods to evaluate CTCs, but there is currently only one FDA-approved assay – CellSearch (Menarini Silicon Biosystems, Inc., Florence, Italy). Studies performed in breast cancer patients have shown that for patients with metastatic breast carcinoma, CTC levels of ≥5 cells per 7.5 mL of blood is associated with a poor prognosis [79, 80]. The presence of CTCs in patients without metastatic breast carcinoma is a bad prognostic sign as they predict early recurrence and decreased overall survival [80, 81]. The DNA from CTCs can be evaluated by NGS to identify genomic alterations that may have targetable therapies.

Cell-free DNA (cfDNA) is shed into the circulation by both normal cells and carcinoma cells. NGS evaluation of the circulating tumor DNA (ctDNA) has been used to identify clinically relevant alterations without tumor biopsy and has been shown to have prognostic value in patient outcome [80, 82]. There is currently no identified cutoff that correlates with prognosis. The evaluation of ctDNA can capture many of the targetable mutations seen in tissue biopsies and therefore may spare patients from undergoing a biopsy.

Immunotherapy

The immune system plays a role in the development and progression of breast cancer [83]. Studies have shown that tumor-infiltrating lymphocytes (TILs) are prognostic and are predictive of response to certain therapies [84]. In particular, breast carcinomas that are HER2 positive and triple negative often have detectible TILs, which in some cases are prominent [84]. Based on the success of immunotherapy seen in many solid tumors, there is an interest in how breast cancer will respond. Immune checkpoint inhibitor therapy specific for *CTLA-4*, PD-1, and PD-L1 is being investigated in breast cancer [85]. Immunotherapy has shown promise for the treatment of breast carcinoma but is currently not a standard of care.

Hereditary Breast Cancer

Approximately 10% of breast cancer cases are hereditary [27, 51, 64, 86, 87]. About half of these are due to germline mutations in *BRCA1* or *BRCA2*. Other genes associated with increased risk for development of breast cancer, some of which are associated with clinical syndromes, include *TP53*, *ATM*, *CDH1*, *CHEK2*, *PALB2*, *PTEN*, and *STK11* (Table 13.5). After appropriate screening and genetic counseling, evaluation may be appropriate for patients who are suspected of harboring a high-risk germline mutation [64, 88]. There are different options when selecting an appropriate test and include syndrome or gene-specific tests, high-penetrance gene panels, high and moderate panels, and comprehensive panels that include genes in multiple different cancers and syndromes [89].

Table 13.5 Common genes associated with hereditary breast cancers [51, 64, 87]

Gene	Chromosome	Lifetime risk of developing breast cancer	Associated syndrome (if applicable)	Other associated carcinomas	Comment
BRCA1	17q21	70–85%	Hereditary breast and ovarian cancer syndrome	Ovarian, prostatic	Histology: basal-like carcinomas with pushing boarders, lymphocytic infiltrate, and central scar/necrosis; triple negative. DCIS less frequent in this population
BRCA2	13q12.3	50–70%	Hereditary breast and ovarian cancer syndrome	Ovarian, prostatic, melanoma	Histology: most are carcinomas of NST; more frequently ER+ than controls
TP53	17p13.1	25–50%	Li-Fraumeni syndrome	Bone and soft tissue sarcomas, CNS tumors, leukemia, adrenocortical	

ATM	11q22.3	20–30%	Ataxia-telangiectasia (a.k.a. Louis-Bar) syndrome	Lymphoma, gastric, CNS	
CDH1	16q22.1	39–52%	Hereditary diffuse gastric cancer (linitis plastica) syndrome	Diffuse gastric carcinoma	Histology: lobular carcinoma
CHEK2	22q12.1	29–37%		Colonic, prostate	
PALB2	16p12.2	~ 20%	Fanconi anemia	Pancreatic	
PTEN	10q23.31	25–85%	Cowden syndrome	Thyroid, endometrial	The syndrome is also associated with benign skin lesions and GI hamartomatous polyps
STK11	19p13.3	~ 30%	Peutz-Jeghers syndrome	Gastrointestinal (colonic, rectal, pancreatic), ovarian	The syndrome is also associated with macules on lips and buccal mucosa and GI hamartomatous polyps

Conclusion

Advances in molecular pathology have broadened our understanding of the biology of breast cancer and changed the way we classify it. The assay options that impact how we manage and treat patients with breast cancer are growing. However, practical considerations when determining utility of these assays include cost and availability: they are expensive, may not be available to everyone, and do not always provide necessary additional information [4, 14]. While the addition of molecular assays can help guide treatment decisions, microscopy remains essential in management of breast cancer [90]. The most critical information that pathologists can provide to ensure their patients receive appropriate care is a careful gross and microscopic evaluation, accurate diagnosis, and information about the hormone receptor status and the HER2 status [5, 14, 22, 43].

References

1. Siegel RL, Miller KD, Jemal A. Cancer statistics, 2017. CA Cancer J Clin. 2017;67(1):7–30.
2. Lester SC, Bose S, Chen YY, Connolly JL, de Baca ME, Fitzgibbons PL, et al. Protocol for the examination of specimens from patients with ductal carcinoma in situ of the breast. Arch Pathol Lab Med. 2009;133(1):15–25.
3. Lester SC, Connolly JL, Amin MB. College of American Pathologists protocol for the reporting of ductal carcinoma in situ. Arch Pathol Lab Med. 2009;133(1):13–4.
4. Rakha EA, Reis-Filho JS, Baehner F, Dabbs DJ, Decker T, Eusebi V, et al. Breast cancer prognostic classification in the molecular era: the role of histological grade. Breast Cancer Res. 2010;12(4):207.
5. Hammond ME, Hayes DF, Dowsett M, Allred DC, Hagerty KL, Badve S, et al. American Society of Clinical Oncology/College of American Pathologists guideline recommendations for immunohistochemical testing of estrogen and progesterone receptors in breast cancer. Arch Pathol Lab Med. 2010;134(6):907–22.

6. Van Poznak C, Somerfield MR, Bast RC, Cristofanilli M, Goetz MP, Gonzalez-Angulo AM, et al. Use of biomarkers to guide decisions on systemic therapy for women with metastatic breast Cancer: American Society of Clinical Oncology clinical practice guideline. J Clin Oncol. 2015;33(24):2695–704.
7. Wolff AC, Hammond MEH, Allison KH, Harvey BE, Mangu PB, Bartlett JMS, et al. Human epidermal growth factor receptor 2 testing in breast cancer: American Society of Clinical Oncology/College of American Pathologists clinical practice guideline focused update. J Clin Oncol. 2018;36(20):2105–22.
8. Badve S, Dabbs DJ, Schnitt SJ, Baehner FL, Decker T, Eusebi V, et al. Basal-like and triple-negative breast cancers: a critical review with an emphasis on the implications for pathologists and oncologists. Mod Pathol. 2011;24(2):157–67.
9. Hanley KZ, Birdsong GG, Cohen C, Siddiqui MT. Immunohistochemical detection of estrogen receptor, progesterone receptor, and human epidermal growth factor receptor 2 expression in breast carcinomas: comparison on cell block, needle-core, and tissue block preparations. Cancer. 2009;117(4):279–88.
10. Kinsella MD, Birdsong GG, Siddiqui MT, Cohen C, Hanley KZ. Immunohistochemical detection of estrogen receptor, progesterone receptor and human epidermal growth factor receptor 2 in formalin-fixed breast carcinoma cell block preparations: correlation of results to corresponding tissue block (needle core and excision) samples. Diagn Cytopathol. 2013;41(3):192–8.
11. Cano G, Milanezi F, Leitao D, Ricardo S, Brito MJ, Schmitt FC. Estimation of hormone receptor status in fine-needle aspirates and paraffin-embedded sections from breast cancer using the novel rabbit monoclonal antibodies SP1 and SP2. Diagn Cytopathol. 2003;29(4):207–11.
12. Gong Y, Symmans WF, Krishnamurthy S, Patel S, Sneige N. Optimal fixation conditions for immunocytochemical analysis of estrogen receptor in cytologic specimens of breast carcinoma. Cancer. 2004;102(1):34–40.
13. Stalhammar G, Rosin G, Fredriksson I, Bergh J, Hartman J. Low concordance of biomarkers in histopathological and cytological material from breast cancer. Histopathology. 2014;64(7):971–80.
14. Coates AS, Winer EP, Goldhirsch A, Gelber RD, Gnant M, Piccart-Gebhart M, et al. Tailoring therapies–improving the management of early breast cancer: St Gallen International

Expert Consensus on the Primary Therapy of Early Breast Cancer 2015. Ann Oncol. 2015;26(8):1533–46.
15. Schnitt SJ, Collins LC. Biopsy interpretation of the breast. 3rd ed. Philadelphia: Wolters Kluwer Health; 2018.
16. Nishimura R, Okamoto N, Satou M, Kojima K, Tanaka S. HER 2 immunohistochemistry for breast cancer cell blocks can be used in the same way as that used for histological specimens. Diagn Cytopathol. 2016;44(4):274–9.
17. Doxtader EE, Calhoun BC, Sturgis CD, Booth CN. HER2 FISH concordance in breast cancer patients with both cytology and surgical pathology specimens. J Am Soc Cytopathol. 2018;7(1):31–6.
18. Krishnamurthy S. Applications of molecular techniques to fine-needle aspiration biopsy. Cancer. 2007;111(2):106–22.
19. Wolff AC, Hammond ME, Hicks DG, Allison KH, Bartlett JM, Bilous M, et al. Reply to E.A. Rakha et al. J Clin Oncol. 2015;33(11):1302–4.
20. Rakha EA, Pigera M, Shaaban A, Shin SJ, D'Alfonso T, Ellis IO, et al. National guidelines and level of evidence: comments on some of the new recommendations in the American Society of Clinical Oncology and the College of American Pathologists human epidermal growth factor receptor 2 guidelines for breast cancer. J Clin Oncol. 2015;33(11):1301–2.
21. Hammond ME, Hicks DG. American Society of Clinical Oncology/College of American Pathologists human epidermal growth factor receptor 2 testing clinical practice guideline upcoming modifications: proof that clinical practice guidelines are living documents. Arch Pathol Lab Med. 2015;139(8):970–1.
22. Wolff AC, Hammond ME, Hicks DG, Dowsett M, McShane LM, Allison KH, et al. Recommendations for human epidermal growth factor receptor 2 testing in breast cancer: American Society of Clinical Oncology/College of American Pathologists clinical practice guideline update. J Clin Oncol. 2013;31(31):3997–4013.
23. Ali SM, Alpaugh RK, Buell JK, Stephens PJ, Yu JQ, Wu H, et al. Antitumor response of an ERBB2 amplified inflammatory breast carcinoma with EGFR mutation to the EGFR-TKI erlotinib. Clin Breast Cancer. 2014;14(1):e14–6.
24. Donaldson AR, Shetty S, Wang Z, Rivera CL, Portier BP, Budd GT, et al. Impact of an alternative chromosome 17 probe and the 2013 American Society of Clinical Oncology and College of American Pathologists guidelines on fluorescence in situ hybrid-

ization for the determination of HER2 gene amplification in breast cancer. Cancer. 2017;123(12):2230–9.

25. Llombart-Cussac A, Cortés J, Paré L, Galván P, Bermejo B, Martínez N, et al. HER2-enriched subtype as a predictor of pathological complete response following trastuzumab and lapatinib without chemotherapy in early-stage HER2-positive breast cancer (PAMELA): an open-label, single-group, multicentre, phase 2 trial. Lancet Oncol. 2017;18(4):545–54.
26. Ross JS, Gay LM. Comprehensive genomic sequencing and the molecular profiles of clinically advanced breast cancer. Pathology. 2017;49(2):120–32.
27. Hagemann IS. Molecular testing in breast cancer: a guide to current practices. Arch Pathol Lab Med. 2016;140(8):815–24.
28. Penault-Llorca F, Radosevic-Robin N. Ki67 assessment in breast cancer: an update. Pathology. 2017;49(2):166–71.
29. Rakha EA, Green AR. Molecular classification of breast cancer: what the pathologist needs to know. Pathology. 2017;49(2):111–9.
30. Robertson S, Stalhammar G, Darai-Ramqvist E, Rantalainen M, Tobin NP, Bergh J, et al. Prognostic value of Ki67 analysed by cytology or histology in primary breast cancer. J Clin Pathol. 2018;71(9):787–94.
31. Tang P, Tse GM. Immunohistochemical surrogates for molecular classification of breast carcinoma: a 2015 update. Arch Pathol Lab Med. 2016;140(8):806–14.
32. Giuliano AE, Connolly JL, Edge SB, Mittendorf EA, Rugo HS, Solin LJ, et al. Breast cancer-major changes in the American Joint Committee on Cancer eighth edition cancer staging manual. CA Cancer J Clin. 2017;67(4):290–303.
33. Ahn S, Lee J, Cho MS, Park S, Sung SH. Evaluation of Ki-67 index in core needle biopsies and matched breast cancer surgical specimens. Arch Pathol Lab Med. 2018;142(3):364–8.
34. Harris LN, Ismaila N, McShane LM, Andre F, Collyar DE, Gonzalez-Angulo AM, et al. Use of biomarkers to guide decisions on adjuvant systemic therapy for women with early-stage invasive breast cancer: American Society of Clinical Oncology clinical practice guideline. J Clin Oncol. 2016;34(10):1134–50.
35. Krop I, Ismaila N, Andre F, Bast RC, Barlow W, Collyar DE, et al. Use of biomarkers to guide decisions on adjuvant systemic therapy for women with early-stage invasive breast cancer: American Society of Clinical Oncology clinical practice guideline focused update. J Clin Oncol. 2017;35(24):2838–47.

36. Amin MB, American Joint Committee on Cancer, American Cancer Society. AJCC cancer staging manual. Eight edition/ editor-in-chief, Mahul B. Amin editors, Stephen B. Edge, MD, FACS and 16 others; Donna M. Gress, RHIT, CTR – Technical editor ; Laura R. Meyer, CAPM – Managing editor. Chicago: American Joint Committee on Cancer, Springer; 2017. xvii, 1024p.
37. Gnant M, Harbeck N, Thomssen C. St. Gallen/Vienna 2017: a brief summary of the consensus discussion about escalation and de-escalation of primary breast cancer treatment. Breast Care (Basel). 2017;12(2):102–7.
38. NCCN Guidelines Version 1.2018 Breast Cancer. https://www.nccn.org/professionals/physician_gls/pdf/breast.pdf. Accessed 16 May 2018.
39. Cuzick J, Dowsett M, Pineda S, Wale C, Salter J, Quinn E, et al. Prognostic value of a combined estrogen receptor, progesterone receptor, Ki-67, and human epidermal growth factor receptor 2 immunohistochemical score and comparison with the Genomic Health recurrence score in early breast cancer. J Clin Oncol. 2011;29(32):4273–8.
40. Paoletti C, Hayes DF. Molecular testing in breast cancer. Annu Rev Med. 2014;65:95–110.
41. Perou CM, Sorlie T, Eisen MB, van de Rijn M, Jeffrey SS, Rees CA, et al. Molecular portraits of human breast tumours. Nature. 2000;406(6797):747–52.
42. Sorlie T, Perou CM, Tibshirani R, Aas T, Geisler S, Johnsen H, et al. Gene expression patterns of breast carcinomas distinguish tumor subclasses with clinical implications. Proc Natl Acad Sci U S A. 2001;98(19):10869–74.
43. Schnitt SJ. Classification and prognosis of invasive breast cancer: from morphology to molecular taxonomy. Mod Pathol. 2010;23(Suppl 2):S60–4.
44. Toss A, Cristofanilli M. Molecular characterization and targeted therapeutic approaches in breast cancer. Breast Cancer Res. 2015;17:60.
45. Cancer Genome Atlas N. Comprehensive molecular portraits of human breast tumours. Nature. 2012;490(7418):61–70.
46. Rakha EA, Reis-Filho JS, Ellis IO. Basal-like breast cancer: a critical review. J Clin Oncol. 2008;26(15):2568–81.
47. Pareja F, Geyer FC, Marchio C, Burke KA, Weigelt B, Reis-Filho JS. Triple-negative breast cancer: the importance of molecular and histologic subtyping, and recognition of low-grade variants. NPJ Breast Cancer. 2016;2:16036.

48. Cheang MC, Voduc D, Bajdik C, Leung S, McKinney S, Chia SK, et al. Basal-like breast cancer defined by five biomarkers has superior prognostic value than triple-negative phenotype. Clin Cancer Res. 2008;14(5):1368–76.
49. Guiu S, Michiels S, Andre F, Cortes J, Denkert C, Di Leo A, et al. Molecular subclasses of breast cancer: how do we define them? The IMPAKT 2012 Working Group Statement. Ann Oncol. 2012;23(12):2997–3006.
50. Cheang MC, Martin M, Nielsen TO, Prat A, Voduc D, Rodriguez-Lescure A, et al. Defining breast cancer intrinsic subtypes by quantitative receptor expression. Oncologist. 2015;20(5):474–82.
51. Pareja F, Marchiò C, Reis-Filho JS. Molecular diagnosis in breast cancer. Diagn Histopathol. 2018;24(2):71–82.
52. D'Alfonso TM, Mosquera JM, MacDonald TY, Padilla J, Liu YF, Rubin MA, et al. MYB-NFIB gene fusion in adenoid cystic carcinoma of the breast with special focus paid to the solid variant with basaloid features. Hum Pathol. 2014;45(11):2270–80.
53. Poling JS, Yonescu R, Subhawong AP, Sharma R, Argani P, Ning Y, et al. MYB labeling by immunohistochemistry is more sensitive and specific for breast adenoid cystic carcinoma than MYB labeling by FISH. Am J Surg Pathol. 2017;41(7):973–9.
54. Lakhani SR, Ellis IO, Schnitt SJ, Tan PH, van de Vijver MJ. WHO classification of tumours of the breast. 4th ed. Lyon: International Agency for Research on Cancer; 2012.
55. Fayanju OM, Park KU, Lucci A. Molecular genomic testing for breast cancer: utility for surgeons. Ann Surg Oncol. 2018;25(2):512–9.
56. Paik S, Shak S, Tang G, Kim C, Baker J, Cronin M, et al. A multigene assay to predict recurrence of tamoxifen-treated, node-negative breast cancer. N Engl J Med. 2004;351(27):2817–26.
57. Sparano JA, Gray RJ, Makower DF, Pritchard KI, Albain KS, Hayes DF, et al. Prospective validation of a 21-gene expression assay in breast cancer. N Engl J Med. 2015;373(21):2005–14.
58. Mamounas EP, Tang G, Fisher B, Paik S, Shak S, Costantino JP, et al. Association between the 21-gene recurrence score assay and risk of locoregional recurrence in node-negative, estrogen receptor-positive breast cancer: results from NSABP B-14 and NSABP B-20. J Clin Oncol. 2010;28(10):1677–83.
59. Turashvili G, Brogi E, Morrow M, Dickler M, Norton L, Hudis C, et al. Breast carcinoma with 21-gene recurrence score lower than 18: rate of locoregional recurrence in a large series with clinical follow-up. BMC Cancer. 2018;18(1):42.

60. Dowsett M, Cuzick J, Wale C, Forbes J, Mallon EA, Salter J, et al. Prediction of risk of distant recurrence using the 21-gene recurrence score in node-negative and node-positive postmenopausal patients with breast cancer treated with anastrozole or tamoxifen: a TransATAC study. J Clin Oncol. 2010;28(11):1829–34.
61. Albain KS, Barlow WE, Ravdin PM, Farrar WB, Burton GV, Ketchel SJ, et al. Adjuvant chemotherapy and timing of tamoxifen in postmenopausal patients with endocrine-responsive, node-positive breast cancer: a phase 3, open-label, randomised controlled trial. Lancet. 2009;374(9707):2055–63.
62. Jasem J, Fisher CM, Amini A, Shagisultanova E, Rabinovitch R, Borges VF, et al. The 21-gene recurrence score assay for node-positive, early-stage breast cancer and impact of RxPONDER trial on chemotherapy decision-making: have clinicians already decided? J Natl Compr Cancer Netw. 2017;15(4):494–503.
63. Sparano JA, Gray RJ, Makower DF, Pritchard KI, Albain KS, Hayes DF, et al. Adjuvant chemotherapy guided by a 21-gene expression assay in breast cancer. N Engl J Med. 2018; 379(2):111–21.
64. NCCN Guidelines Version 1.2018 Genetic/Familial High-Risk Assessment: Breast and Ovarian. https://www.nccn.org/professionals/physician_gls/pdf/genetics_screening.pdf. Accessed 16 May 2018.
65. van't Veer LJ, Dai H, van de Vijver MJ, He YD, Hart AA, Mao M, et al. Gene expression profiling predicts clinical outcome of breast cancer. Nature. 2002;415(6871):530–6.
66. Cardoso F, van't Veer LJ, Bogaerts J, Slaets L, Viale G, Delaloge S, et al. 70-gene signature as an aid to treatment decisions in early-stage breast cancer. N Engl J Med. 2016;375(8):717–29.
67. Parker JS, Mullins M, Cheang MC, Leung S, Voduc D, Vickery T, et al. Supervised risk predictor of breast cancer based on intrinsic subtypes. J Clin Oncol. 2009;27(8):1160–7.
68. Filipits M, Rudas M, Jakesz R, Dubsky P, Fitzal F, Singer CF, et al. A new molecular predictor of distant recurrence in ER-positive, HER2-negative breast cancer adds independent information to conventional clinical risk factors. Clin Cancer Res. 2011;17(18):6012–20.
69. Muller BM, Keil E, Lehmann A, Winzer KJ, Richter-Ehrenstein C, Prinzler J, et al. The EndoPredict gene-expression assay in clinical practice – performance and impact on clinical decisions. PLoS One. 2013;8(6):e68252.
70. Zhang Y, Schnabel CA, Schroeder BE, Jerevall PL, Jankowitz RC, Fornander T, et al. Breast cancer index identifies

early-stage estrogen receptor-positive breast cancer patients at risk for early- and late-distant recurrence. Clin Cancer Res. 2013;19(15):4196–205.

71. Sgroi DC, Sestak I, Cuzick J, Zhang Y, Schnabel CA, Schroeder B, et al. Prediction of late distant recurrence in patients with oestrogen-receptor-positive breast cancer: a prospective comparison of the breast-cancer index (BCI) assay, 21-gene recurrence score, and IHC4 in the TransATAC study population. Lancet Oncol. 2013;14(11):1067–76.
72. Jerevall PL, Ma XJ, Li H, Salunga R, Kesty NC, Erlander MG, et al. Prognostic utility of HOXB13:IL17BR and molecular grade index in early-stage breast cancer patients from the Stockholm trial. Br J Cancer. 2011;104(11):1762–9.
73. Vogelstein B, Kinzler KW. The multistep nature of cancer. Trends Genet. 1993;9(4):138–41.
74. Roy-Chowdhuri S, de Melo GD, Routbort MJ, Patel KP, Singh RR, Broaddus R, et al. Multigene clinical mutational profiling of breast carcinoma using next-generation sequencing. Am J Clin Pathol. 2015;144(5):713–21.
75. Santarpia L, Bottai G, Kelly CM, Gyorffy B, Szekely B, Pusztai L. Deciphering and targeting oncogenic mutations and pathways in breast cancer. Oncologist. 2016;21(9):1063–78.
76. Zardavas D, Maetens M, Irrthum A, Goulioti T, Engelen K, Fumagalli D, et al. The AURORA initiative for metastatic breast cancer. Br J Cancer. 2014;111(10):1881–7.
77. Maetens M, Brown D, Irrthum A, Aftimos P, Viale G, Loibl S, et al. The AURORA pilot study for molecular screening of patients with advanced breast cancer-a study of the breast international group. NPJ Breast Cancer. 2017;3:23.
78. Roy-Chowdhuri S, Mehrotra M, Bolivar AM, Kanagal-Shamanna R, Barkoh BA, Hannigan B, et al. Salvaging the supernatant: next generation cytopathology for solid tumor mutation profiling. Mod Pathol. 2018;31(7):1036–45.
79. Cristofanilli M, Budd GT, Ellis MJ, Stopeck A, Matera J, Miller MC, et al. Circulating tumor cells, disease progression, and survival in metastatic breast cancer. N Engl J Med. 2004;351(8):781–91.
80. Rossi G, Mu Z, Rademaker AW, Austin LK, Strickland KS, Costa RLB, et al. Cell-free DNA and circulating tumor cells: comprehensive liquid biopsy analysis in advanced breast cancer. Clin Cancer Res. 2018;24(3):560–8.
81. Lucci A, Hall CS, Lodhi AK, Bhattacharyya A, Anderson AE, Xiao L, et al. Circulating tumour cells in non-metastatic breast cancer: a prospective study. Lancet Oncol. 2012;13(7):688–95.

82. Stover DG, Parsons HA, Ha G, Freeman SS, Barry WT, Guo H, et al. Association of Cell-Free DNA tumor fraction and somatic copy number alterations with survival in metastatic triple-negative breast cancer. J Clin Oncol. 2018;36(6):543–53.
83. Cimino-Mathews A, Foote JB, Emens LA. Immune targeting in breast cancer. Oncology (Williston Park). 2015;29(5):375–85.
84. Denkert C, Wienert S, Poterie A, Loibl S, Budczies J, Badve S, et al. Standardized evaluation of tumor-infiltrating lymphocytes in breast cancer: results of the ring studies of the international immuno-oncology biomarker working group. Mod Pathol. 2016;29(10):1155–64.
85. Emens LA. Breast cancer immunotherapy: facts and hopes. Clin Cancer Res. 2018;24(3):511–20.
86. Lalloo F, Evans DG. Familial breast cancer. Clin Genet. 2012;82(2):105–14.
87. Khan A, Ellis IO, Hanby AM, Cosar ER, Rakha EA, Kandil D. Precision molecular pathology of breast cancer. New York: Springer; 2015. x, 338p.
88. Robson ME, Storm CD, Weitzel J, Wollins DS, Offit K. American Society of Clinical O. American Society of Clinical Oncology policy statement update: genetic and genomic testing for cancer susceptibility. J Clin Oncol. 2010;28(5):893–901.
89. Hall MJ, Forman AD, Pilarski R, Wiesner G, Giri VN. Gene panel testing for inherited cancer risk. J Natl Compr Cancer Netw. 2014;12(9):1339–46.
90. Rosai J. Why microscopy will remain a cornerstone of surgical pathology. Lab Investig. 2007;87(5):403–8.

Chapter 14
Molecular Diagnostics in Salivary Gland Cytology

Esther Diana Rossi and Zubair W. Baloch

Abbreviations

ACC	Acinic cell carcinoma
AdCC	Adenoid cystic carcinoma
AR	Androgen receptor
BCA	Basal cell adenoma
BCAdc	Basal cell adenocarcinoma
Ca-ex-PA	Carcinoma ex pleomorphic adenoma
CAMSG	Cribriform adenocarcinoma of the minor salivary glands

E. D. Rossi (✉)
Division of Anatomic Pathology and Histology, Fondazione Policlinico Unviersitario "A. Gemelli", Catholic University of Sacred Heart, Rome, Italy
e-mail: esther.rossi@policlinicogemelli.it

Z. W. Baloch
Department of Pathology and Laboratory Medicine, Hospital of the University of Pennsylvania, Philadelphia, PA, USA
e-mail: baloch@pennmedicine.upenn.edu

S. Roy-Chowdhuri et al. (eds.), *Molecular Diagnostics in Cytopathology*, https://doi.org/10.1007/978-3-319-97397-5_14

EMC	Epithelial-myoepithelial carcinoma
FC	Flow cytometry
FFPE	Formalin-fixed paraffin-embedded
FISH	Fluorescence *in situ* hybridization
FNA	Fine-needle aspiration
GFAP	Glial fibrillary acidic protein
HCCC	Hyalinizing clear cell carcinoma
ICC	Immunocytochemistry
LEF-1	Lymphoid enhancer-binding factor 1
MEC	Mucoepidermoid carcinoma
NGS	Next-generation sequencing
PA	Pleomorphic adenoma
PLGA	Polymorphous (low-grade) adenocarcinoma
RT-PCR	Reverse transcription-polymerase chain reaction
SDC	Salivary duct carcinoma
SeCa	Secretory carcinoma
SGT	Salivary gland tumor
SMA	Smooth muscle actin
SQCC	Squamous cell carcinoma
STAT-5a	Signal transducer and activator of transcription 5a
WT	Warthin tumor

Key Terminology

Break-apart FISH probes	Break-apart FISH probes are designed to detect specific translocations. They are designed to flank on either side of a gene so that in the presence of a translocation, the two colors will lead to a split signal
Gene fusion	A *fusion gene* is a hybrid gene formed from two previously separate genes. It can occur as a result of translocation, interstitial deletion, or chromosomal inversion. Gene fusions are known in many

	cancers as driver or passenger mutations. They play an important role in both etiology and pathogenesis of cancer and are considered as potential diagnostic and prognostic markers and possible therapeutic targets
Mutation	Change in the nucleotide sequence of a gene or a chromosome. It may be classified into various ways. One of these classifications involves classifying mutations based on the effect on structure: (1) *small-scale mutations* and (2) *large-scale mutations*
Translocation	A rearrangement in which a segment of one chromosome is transferred to another nonhomologous chromosome or to a new position within the same chromosome

Key Points

- Salivary gland tumor (SGT) cytomorphology guides the application of ancillary techniques
- Ancillary techniques are needed in some cases of SGT in order to overcome the morphological limitations
- Recent discoveries of specific translocations and resulting fusion oncogenes in subsets of SGT may lead to a new paradigm in diagnosing FNAC samples
- Molecular results must be interpreted within the context of the clinical, radiologic, and cytologic findings
- Awareness of known advantages and limitation of specific molecular techniques is important for correlating molecular findings with a specific cytologic diagnosis

General Background

The role of fine-needle aspiration (FNA) in the evaluation and management of salivary gland lesions is well established [1–7]. However, salivary gland FNA remains one of the more challenging areas in diagnostic cytopathology for the following reasons: (a) the heterogeneous nature of salivary gland tumors (SGTs), with more than 40 different types of neoplasms described in the current WHO classification scheme; (b) the intratumoral heterogeneity of biphasic SGT; and (c) the morphologic components shared among SGTs, such as oncocytic cells, squamous metaplasia, clear cells, hyaline globules, and myoepithelial cells. Therefore, in some cases a specific diagnosis may not be rendered based on morphology alone, and the resulting diagnostic uncertainty can affect clinical management. Several authors have demonstrated that the use of ancillary techniques (including immunocytochemistry and molecular testing) can overcome the morphological limitations and refine the diagnostic practice of salivary gland cytology [1–20].

Recently, subsets of SGTs have been characterized cytogenetically by the presence of specific and recurrent translocations [1–13]. These translocations and the consequent fusion oncogenes and oncoproteins can serve as diagnostic markers in FNA specimens of salivary gland lesions. The interpretation of molecular test results also requires knowledge of the molecular pathology of the different entities and their clinical relevance. For example, a case of salivary gland adenocarcinoma not otherwise specified can be better subclassified as a hyalinizing clear cell adenocarcinoma (HCCC) based on the specific gene fusion (*EWSR1-ATF1*) [3, 4].

Ancillary techniques such as special histochemical stains, immunocytochemistry (ICC), fluorescence *in situ* hybridization (FISH), reverse transcriptase polymerase chain reaction (RT-PCR), next-generation sequencing (NGS), and flow cytometry (FC) can be successfully applied to FNA material to improve the diagnostic accuracy for many SGTs [3–23]. Several of these techniques can be easily introduced into the diagnostic workflow, particularly as they become more widely available, cost-effective, and efficient with shorter turnaround times [3, 4]. Although several publications have highlighted the feasibility and reliability of their use in a variety of cytology specimen preparations, the application of ancillary testing to formalin-fixed paraffin-embedded (FFPE) cellblock material is considered the most reliable [3, 4, 8] (Table 14.1). The reason can be attributed to the fact that the majority of biomarkers evaluated by immunoperoxidase (IPOX) staining have been validated using FFPE tissue blocks. Thus, cytology cellblocks have the advantage of being analogous to paraffin tissue blocks, with minimal need of standardization for ICC.

Although these ancillary techniques are carried out mostly on cellblocks, some authors have emphasized that they can also be performed on both conventional and liquid-based cytology (LBC) preparations (Table 14.1). Among the ancillary techniques, ICC, FC, and FISH are the tests most frequently used to rule out lymphomas and subclassify SGTs. Cytologic preparations (smears and cytospins) are generally considered superior to FFPE cellblock or tissue sections for FISH, since the whole nuclei of intact cells inherent to cytologic preparations

TABLE 14.1 Cytology material adequate for the application of molecular testing [13–23]

Technique/ methodology	***Conventional cytologic preparations***	***Liquid-based preparations***	***Cellblocks***
ICC	✓	✓	✓
Histochemistry	✓	✓	✓
DNA testing	✓	✓	✓
RNA testing	✓	✓	✓
FC	✓	✓	✗
FISH	✓	✓	✓

ICC immunocytochemistry, *FC* flow cytometry, *FISH* fluorescence *in situ* hybridization
✓ Yes; ✗No

lack the truncation artifacts of FFPE sections, and therefore provide optimal signal visualization and counting.

Translocations and Fusion Oncogenes in Salivary Gland Tumors

In recent years, several SGTs have been found to harbor recurrent genetic alterations. The major translocations and resulting fusion oncogenes are summarized in Table 14.2.

These genetic alterations are associated with a specific subset of well-defined benign and malignant salivary gland neoplasms; some can also occur in tumors from other organs. For example, the translocation t(12; 22) associated with HCCC is also found in four other neoplasms with different morphologies and clinical behaviors: angiomatoid fibrous histiocytoma, clear cell sarcoma of soft tissue, primary pulmonary myxoid sarcoma, and clear cell sarcoma-like tumor of the gastrointestinal tract [3, 4]. Also, the translocation t(6;9)(q22–23;p23–24) characteristic of salivary gland AdCC is commonly seen in AdCC of the breast and in benign dermal cylindromas. While these genomic alterations can provide powerful diagnostic markers for histological as well as FNA samples [24–28], none of them are pathognomonic or specific, and the absence of a genetic rearrangement does not exclude any particular SGT. These markers additionally may provide prognostic information and guide targeted therapy in some cases.

These translocations are usually found in both benign and malignant neoplasms, and, in SGTs with more than one cell type, they are not limited to a specific cell type [3, 4]. For example, 50–60% cases of pleomorphic adenoma (PA) are characterized by the translocation t(3;8)(p21;q12) involving *PLAG1* gene and one of several other fusion partners, the most common being *CTNNB1* (the gene encoding β-catenin) [16]. This translocation results in upregulation and overexpression of *PLAG1* protein and downregulation of its partners, which can be assessed by

Table 14.2 Specific translocations and gene fusions in salivary gland lesions

SGT	Translocations	Genes involved	Prevalence
Pleomorphic adenoma	t(3;8)(p21;q12) *HMGA2* rearrangement, *HMGA2 and MDM2* amplification	*PLAG1*, *CTNNB1*, and *LIFR* *HMGA2*, *MDM2*, and *WIFI*	60%
MEC	t(11;19)(q21–22;p13) *t(6; 22)(p21;q12)*	*MAML2-CRTC1* gene fusion *EWSR1-POU5F1* gene fusion	60–75%
AdCC	t(6;9)(q22–23;p23–24) *MYB* rearrangement	*MYB-NFIB* gene fusion	65%
SeCA	t(12;15)(p13;q25)	*ETV6-NTRK3* gene fusion	90–100%
HCCC	t(12;22)(q13;q12)	*EWSR1-ATF1* gene fusion	85%
Carcinoma ex-PA	t(3;8)(p21;q12)	*PLAG1*, *CTNNB1*, and *LIFR*	
CAMSG	*PRKD* rearrangement	*PRKD1*, *2*, *3*, *ARID1A*	80%
PAd	*PRKD1* mutation *PRKD* gene family rearrangements	*PRKD1* *PRKD1*, *PRKD2*, *PRKD3*, *ARID1A*, or *DDX3X*	73%

SGT salivary gland tumor, *PA* pleomorphic adenoma, *MEC* mucoepidermoid carcinoma, *AdCC* adenoid cystic carcinoma, *SeCa* secretory carcinoma, *HCCC* hyalinizing clear cell Ca, *CAMSG* cribriform adenocarcinoma of minor salivary gland, *ACC* acinic cell carcinoma, *PAd* polymorphous (low-grade) adenocarcinoma

ICC (Table 14.3). *PLAG1* expression is absent in AdCC, mucoepidermoid carcinoma (MEC), and acinic cell carcinoma (ACC) but can be seen in 20% cases of polymorphous low-grade adenocarcinoma (PLGA). A minor subset

Table 14.3 Other ancillary techniques in the different salivary gland tumors

SGT	ICC or special stains	Possible differential diagnoses
PA	PLAG1 positive	Basal cell adenoma/carcinoma (SMA, calponin, and S100 positive) AdCC Myoepithelioma
MEC	Mucicarmine positive	WT, mucocele, PA, chronic sialadenitis
AdCC	MYB and CD117 positive	PA, basaloid neoplasms, PLGA, epithelia-myoepithelial Ca
SeCa	Mammaglobin, GCDFP15 and S100 positive; DOG1 negative	ACC, PA, WT, MEC
HCCC	P63, HMW keratin positive; SMA, calponin, GFAP and S100 negative	Tumors with clear cell features (myoepithelioma, MEC, oncocytoma, metastatic renal cell, and melanoma)
CAMSG	CK7, CK8, CK18, S100, SMA, Calponin positive; TTF-1 and Thyroglobulin negative. Rarely positive for CD117 and p16	Metastatic papillary thyroid carcinoma

PA pleomorphic adenoma, *MEC* mucoepidermoid carcinoma, *AdCC* adenoid cystic carcinoma, *SeCa* secretory carcinoma, *HCCC* hyalinizing clear cell Ca, *CAMSG* cribriform adenocarcinoma of minor salivary gland, *WT* Warthin tumor, *ACC* acinic cell carcinoma, *PAd* polymorphous (low-grade) adenocarcinoma, *HMW* high molecular weight

of PAs (10%) shows chromosomal rearrangements in 12q13–15 involving *HMGA2* gene. Furthermore, *PLAG1* and *HMGA2* gene rearrangements are present only in PA and carcinoma-ex-PA and have not been found in any other SGTs. The application of ICC or FISH for *PLAG1* will likely be useful in those SGT cases in which it may be difficult to distinguish PA from other benign or malignant neoplasms with basaloid features.

MEC, in approximately 60–70% of cases, has been associated with a specific translocation t(11;19) (q14–21;p12–13) involving the *CRTC1* (*MECT1*) gene at 19p13 and the *MAML2* gene at 11q21 [1–5]. Studies on the human MEC cells have shown that *CRTC1-MAML2* fusion oncoprotein upregulates the epidermal growth factor receptor (*EGFR*) ligand amphiregulin (*AREG*) by co-activating the transcription factor CREB and AREG subsequently. This results in activation of the *EGFR* signaling and promotion of MEC cell growth and survival. The *CRTC1-MAML2* translocation is typically found in low- to intermediate-grade MEC and is associated with low-risk of tumor recurrences, metastases, and tumor-related mortality. However, this fusion has also been reported in some cases of high-grade MEC, suggesting that translocation status does not always supersede histologic grading and clinical staging as prognostic predictor. Since the presence of *CRTC1-MAML2* fusion is specific for MEC, it can be used to distinguish MEC from other SGTs. Specifically the detection of a *MAML2* rearrangement by FISH has the potential to be useful to confirm a diagnosis of MEC in cytology samples and small biopsies.

While most AdCCs show pathognomonic features which can be easily recognized and diagnosed on FNA samples, a subset share morphological features with other SGT with basaloid phenotype [3–5], such as PA, basal cell adenoma, basal cell adenocarcinoma, myoepithelioma, epi-myoepithelial carcinoma, and PLGA. Some authors have shown that expression of KIT (CD117), myoepithelial markers, and S100, while not entirely specific, can aid in the diagnosis of AdCC. In addition, the translocation t(6;9)(q21–24;p13–23) involving *MYB* and *NFIB* genes is found in up to 86% (range, 28–86%)

of AdCC cases. This translocation associated with *MYB* overexpression in most AdCC (89%) can therefore be used as a diagnostic marker [12].

Secretory carcinoma (SeCa), aka mammary analogue secretory carcinoma (MASC), was first introduced as a specific malignant SGT by Skalova et al. in a 2010 report of 16 cases [29]. The original designation MASC derived from the fact that its morphological, immunohistochemical, and molecular profile are identical to that of secretory carcinoma of the breast. It is characterized by the specific translocation t(12;15)(p13;q25), leading to a fusion between *ETV6* and *NTRK3* which is found in nearly 100% of cases and has not been reported in any other primary SGT [1–5]. Morphologically, salivary gland secretory carcinoma can resemble ACC, oncocytic neoplasms, and some cases of MEC, although it lacks coarse cytoplasmic zymogen granules or the presence of eosinophilic cells with intracytoplasmic mucin [23, 24]. The application of ICC (confirming positivity for S100, mammaglobin, GATA-3, GCDFP15 and negativity for DOG-1) and molecular testing for *ETV6* translocation will confirm the diagnosis of secretory carcinoma [23] (Table 14.3). The application of FISH probes for *ETV6* on FNA samples is especially useful to establish the diagnosis in difficult cases (Fig. 14.1).

The hyalinizing clear cell carcinoma (HCCC) is a rare SGT, which is usually diagnosed on FNA specimens as “adenocarcinoma, not otherwise specified (NOS)” [1–5, 25]. However, given its well-established low-grade nature, correct classification and distinction from other primary SGTs are important. HCCC is characterized by a specific translocation t(12;22)(q13;q12) generating an *EWSR1-ATF1* fusion gene, which is present in approximately 85% of cases [1–5]. In cases with this diagnostic suspicion, a conclusive diagnosis of HCCC can be established with the assessment for the specific *EWSR1* rearrangement, which is not present in other SGT with clear cell features, except for a subset (35%) of clear cell myoepithelial carcinomas and rare EMC (9%) that can be easily distinguished by their specific and different immunocytochemical profiles.

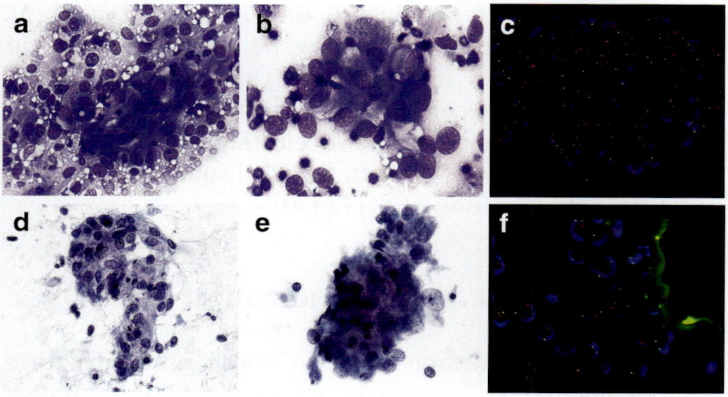

FIGURE 14.1 A case of fine-needle aspiration diagnosed as secretory carcinoma (previously known as mammary analogue secretory carcinoma) showing cohesive groups of neoplastic cells with finely vacuolated cytoplasm round to oval nuclei and few with prominent nucleoli (**a**, **b**, low- and high-power, air-dried smears stained with Diff-Quik® stain). The alcohol-fixed on-site smears stained with Papanicolaou stain highlight the delicate cytoplasm and nuclear pleomorphism (low and high power, **c**, **d**). The break-apart fluorescence *in situ* hybridization to evaluate for disruption of *ETV6* gene shows *ETV6* rearrangement (**e**, **f**, low and high power)

The polymorphous low-grade adenocarcinoma (PLGA), recently renamed as polymorphous adenocarcinoma (PAd), harbors a *PRKD1* p.E710D mutation or one of the *PRKD* gene family (*PRKD1*, *PRKD2*, or *PRKD3)* rearrangements, which have not been found in other SGTs [1–5, 27, 28, 30]. Since the morphology of PAd and AdCC overlap, molecular analysis can be extremely helpful. Furthermore, the *PRKD1* mutation has been significantly associated with metastasis-free clinical course.

Another low-grade carcinoma, related to PAd, is cribriform adenocarcinoma of minor salivary gland (CAMSG) [30]. It can be confused with PAd in minor salivary gland sites and with papillary thyroid carcinoma (PTC) in cervical lymph node metastases. The differential diagnoses of CAMSG also include salivary duct carcinoma, AdCC, PA, and other basaloid neoplasms. In 2014, Weinreb et al. described several novel *PRKD* gene rearrangements in CAMSG as well as in PAd [28]. This recent discovery emphasized the molecular overlap and the potential shared pathogenesis between these two entities and justifies the decision to leave CAMSG with the PAd subheading, as per new WHO classification of SGTs [30].

Fluorescence *In Situ* Hybridization (FISH)

The *in situ*-based detection of nucleic acids has the advantage of providing useful diagnostic information within the context of the cytomorphology [10, 11, 15, 31]. Currently there are two different methods commonly utilized: (1) fluorescence *in situ* hybridization (FISH) and (2) chromogenic *in situ* hybridization (CISH). In SGT, the majority of clinically relevant genetic alterations are rearrangements generating gene fusions, and FISH has been shown to be superior to other FISH techniques for demonstrating rearrangements. As previously mentioned, cytologic smears and cytospin preparations have the advantage of evaluating signals in whole nuclei without truncation artifact from sectioning; however, cell-blocks can also be used with the same adaptations and validations used for histological FFPE sections. It is recommended to use dual-observer scoring to circumvent intra- and inter-observer variability.

When positive, FISH analysis can confirm a diagnosis, even on salivary gland FNA samples with limited number of lesional cells. At present no set requirements have been established regarding the minimum number cell required for interpreting FISH studies in salivary gland FNA specimens. The overexpression of translocation-associated proteins and/or downstream target proteins can be assessed using ICC and can serve as a diagnostic surrogate for the molecular alterations discussed above [3–8, 11, 12]. Since ICC for the fusion protein is usually more sensitive but less specific than FISH analysis, it can be used as a triage tool before FISH testing.

Polymerase Chain Reaction (PCR)

Almost all cytologic preparations are an excellent source of material for PCR analysis, since samples with as few as 50 to 100 cells are adequate to obtain good PCR results. One of the most used applications of PCR is the study of gene expression, including the production of fusion transcripts using RT-PCR. PCR-based assay is more sensitive than FISH for detecting different translocations; however, it is not able to detect unknown molecular variants, which can be detected by FISH analysis.

Flow Cytometry (FC)

FC is used to evaluate lymphoproliferative lesions. The cytologic diagnosis of lymphoid lesions, especially of low-grade cytology, may be extremely difficult, and FC can be useful in distinguishing reactive proliferations from lymphoma. For B-cell lymphomas, the demonstration of a clonal population based upon the presence of kappa or lambda light chain restriction as well as expression of BCL2 is diagnostic. The presence of an altered T-cell immunophenotype also can be used to suggest a possible T-cell lymphoma. Some authors have demonstrated that the combination of morphology and FC could diagnose and classify lymphoid proliferations in salivary gland FNA with a sensitivity of 100% and specificity of 83% [14]. FC is also able to detect the presence of nonlymphoid neoplastic cells in an FNA [15].

Conclusions

Even though the diagnosis of salivary gland tumors is based mostly on cytomorphologic parameters, the recent advances in the application of ancillary techniques (ICC-, FISH-, and DNA-/RNA-based testing) have proven to be useful when a

Table 14.4 Main issues with the application of molecular testing on salivary gland cytology

Molecular test results	Correlation and resolution
Negative results which were expected to be positive	Review cytomorphology Review the sample sent for molecular testing for adequacy and other factors (tumor cell percentage, inflammatory cells, necrosis)
Molecular signature discrepancies between the primary tumor and metastasis of the assay failed in spite of adequate amount of cytology specimen submitted for molecular testing	Review and compare the cytomorphology between the primary tumor and metastases to exclude the possibility of second primary. Confirm that molecular techniques employed for primary and metastatic tumor are similar or working at similar assay sensitivity and specificity Review the sample sent for molecular testing for tumor cellularity and other pre-analytical variables such as fixation method, cellular degeneration, and tumor necrosis
Unreported genetic alteration	Review current genetics for all possible genetic alteration reported in SGTs

conclusive or specific diagnosis cannot be made on morphology alone. However, the use of ancillary techniques does have some inherent limitations, which need to be recognized and resolved (Table 14.4). Both cellblock and cytologic preparations (conventional and liquid-based preparations) can be used. It is likely that in the near future ancillary testing of SGT samples will not only help in establishing a specific diagnosis but also provide prognostic and therapeutic information to guide clinical management.

References

1. Andersson MK, Stenman G. The landscape of gene fusions and somatic mutations in salivary gland neoplasms – Implications for diagnosis and therapy. Oral Oncol. 2016;57:63–9.
2. Weinreb I. Translocation-associated salivary gland tumors: a review and update. Adv Anat Pathol. 2013;20:367–77.
3. Pusztaszeri MP, García JJ, Faquin WC. Salivary gland FNA: new markers and new opportunities for improved diagnosis. Cancer Cytopathol. 2016;124:307–16.
4. Pusztaszeri MP, Faquin WC. Update in salivary gland cytopathology: recent molecular advances and diagnostic applications. Semin Diagn Pathol. 2015;32:264–74.
5. Griffith CC, Schmitt AC, Little JL, Magliocca KR. New developments in salivary gland pathology: clinically useful ancillary testing and new potentially targetable molecular alterations. Arch Pathol Lab Med. 2017;141:381–95.
6. Griffith CC, Siddiqui MT, Schmitt AC. Ancillary testing strategies in salivary gland aspiration cytology: a practical pattern-based approach. Diagn Cytopathol. 2017;45:808–19.
7. Rossi ED, Wong LQ, Bizzarro T, et al. The impact of FNAC in the management of salivary gland lesions: Institutional experiences leading to a risk-based classification scheme. Cancer Cytopathol. 2016;124:388–96.
8. Wang H, Fundakowski C, Khurana JS, Jhala N. Fine-needle aspiration biopsy of salivary gland lesions. Arch Pathol Lab Med. 2015;139:1491–7.
9. Foo WC, Jo VY, Krane JF. Usefulness of translocation-associated immunohistochemical stains in the fine-needle aspiration diagnosis of salivary gland neoplasms. Cancer Cytopathol. 2016;124:397–405.
10. Evrard SM, Meilleroux J, Daniel G, Basset C, Lacoste-Collin L, Vergez S, et al. Use of fluorescent in-situ hybridisation in salivary gland cytology: a powerful diagnostic tool. Cytopathology. 2017;28:312–20.
11. Hudson JB, Collins BT. MYB gene abnormalities t(6;9) in adenoid cystic carcinoma fine-needle aspiration biopsy using fluo-

rescence in situ hybridization. Arch Pathol Lab Med. 2014;138:403–9.
12. Pusztaszeri MP, Sadow PM, Ushiku A, et al. MYB immunostaining is a useful ancillary test for distinguishing adenoid cystic carcinoma from pleomorphic adenoma in fine-needle aspiration biopsy specimens. Cancer Cytopathol. 2014;122:257–65.
13. Moon A, Cohen C, Siddiqui MT. MYB expression: potential role in separating adenoid cystic carcinoma (ACC) from pleomorphic adenoma (PA). Diagn Cytopathol. 2016;44:799–804.
14. MacCallum PL, Lampe HB, Cramer H, Matthews TW. Fine-needle aspiration cytology of lymphoid lesions of the salivary gland: a review of 35 cases. J Otolaryngol. 1996;25:300–4.
15. Stacchini A, Aliberti S, Pacchioni D, Demurtas A, Isolato G, Gazzera C, et al. Flow cytometry significantly improves the diagnostic value of fine needle aspiration cytology of lymphoproliferative lesions of salivary glands. Cytopathology. 2014;25:231–40.
16. Jo VY, Sholl LM, Krane JF. Distinctive patterns of CTNNB1 (β-Catenin) alterations in salivary gland basal cell adenoma and basal cell adenocarcinoma. Am J Surg Pathol. 2016;40:1143–50.
17. Bilodeau EA, Acquafondata M, Barnes EL, Seethala RR. A comparative analysis of LEF-1 in odontogenic and salivary tumors. Hum Pathol. 2015;46(2):255–9.
18. Mino M, Pilch BZ, Faquin WC. Expression of KIT (CD117) in neoplasms of the head and neck: an ancillary marker for adenoid cystic carcinoma. Mod Pathol. 2003;16:1224–31.
19. Wilson TC, Ma D, Tilak A, Tesdahl B, Robinson RA. Next-generation sequencing in salivary gland basal cell adenocarcinoma and basal cell adenoma. Head Neck Pathol. 2016 Dec;10(4):494–500.
20. Schmitt AC, McCormick R, Cohen C, Siddiqui MT. DOG1, p63, and S100 protein: a novel immunohistochemical panel in the differential diagnosis of oncocytic salivary gland neoplasms in fine-needle aspiration cell blocks. J Am Soc Cytopathol. 2014;3:303–8.
21. Schmitt AC, Cohen C, Siddiqui MT. Expression of SOX10 in salivary gland oncocytic neoplasms: a review and a comparative analysis with other immunohistochemical markers. Acta Cytol. 2015;59(5):384–90.
22. Schwartz LE, Begum S, Westra WH, Bishop JA. GATA3 immunohistochemical expression in salivary gland neoplasms. Head Neck Pathol. 2013;7:311–5.

23. Oza N, Sanghvi K, Shet T, et al. Mammary analogue secretory carcinoma of parotid: Is preoperative cytological diagnosis possible? Diagn Cytopathol. 2016;44:519–25.
24. Kawahara A, Taira T, Abe H, Takase Y, Kurita T, Sadashima E, et al. Diagnostic utility of phosphorylated signal transducer and activator of transcription 5 immunostaining in the diagnosis of mammary analogue secretory carcinoma of the salivary gland: a comparative study of salivary gland cancers. Cancer Cytopathol. 2015;123:603–11.
25. Milchgrub S, Vuitch F, Saboorian MH, et al. Hyalinizing clear cell carcinoma of salivary glands in fine needle aspiration. Diagn Cytopathol. 2000;23:333–7.
26. Kawahara A, Harada H, Akiba J, Kage M. Salivary duct carcinoma cytologically diagnosed distinctly from salivary gland carcinomas with squamous differentiation. Diagn Cytopathol. 2008;36:485–93.
27. Rooper L, Sharma R, Bishop JA. Polymorphous low grade adenocarcinoma has a consistent p63+/p40- immunophenotype that helps distinguish it from adenoid cystic carcinoma and cellular pleomorphic adenoma. Head Neck Pathol. 2015;9:79–84.
28. Weinreb I, Piscuoglio S, Martelotto LG, et al. Hotspot activating PRKD1 somatic mutations in polymorphous low-grade adenocarcinomas of the salivary glands. Nat Genet. 2014;46:1166–9.
29. Skalova A, Michal M, Simpson RH. Newly described salivary gland tumors. Mod Pathol. 2017;30:S27–43.
30. El-Naggar AK, Chan JKC, Grandis JR, Takata T, Slootweg PJ. WHO classification of head and neck tumours. 4th ed. Lyon: IARC Press; 2017.
31. MacCallum PL, Lampe HB, Cramer H, Matthews TW. Fine-needle aspiration cytology of lymphoid lesions of the salivary gland: a review of 35 cases. J Otolaryngol. 1996;25:300–4.

Chapter 15
Molecular Diagnostics in Pancreatic and Biliary Cytology

Mingjuan Lisa Zhang and Martha Bishop Pitman

Abbreviations

ACC	Acinar cell carcinoma
CEA	Carcinoembryonic antigen
DNA	Deoxyribonucleic acid
EUS	Endoscopic ultrasound
FISH	Fluorescence *in situ* hybridization
FNA	Fine-needle aspiration
GNAS	Guanine nucleotide-binding protein, alpha stimulating

M. L. Zhang
Department of Pathology, Massachusetts General Hospital, Boston, MA, USA
e-mail: mlzhang@mgh.harvard.edu

M. B. Pitman (✉)
Department of Pathology, Harvard Medical School, Massachusetts General Hospital, Boston, MA, USA
e-mail: mpitman@mgh.harvard.edu

S. Roy-Chowdhuri et al. (eds.), *Molecular Diagnostics in Cytopathology*, https://doi.org/10.1007/978-3-319-97397-5_15

IPMN	Intraductal papillary mucinous neoplasm
KRAS	Kirsten rat sarcoma viral oncogene homolog
MCN	Mucinous cystic neoplasm
NGS	Next-generation sequencing
PanNEC	Pancreatic neuroendocrine carcinoma
PanNET	Pancreatic neuroendocrine tumor
PCF	Pancreatic cyst fluid
PDAC	Pancreatic ductal adenocarcinoma
pRb	Retinoblastoma protein
SCA	Serous cystadenoma
SPN	Solid pseudopapillary neoplasm
VHL	von Hippel-Lindau

Key Terminology

Allele	Variant form of a gene. Each gene has two copies that are inherited from each parent and may differ from each other, resulting in a variant form or allele
Germline mutation	Inherited genetic alterations that occur in the reproductive/germ cells (i.e., sperm and eggs) and becomes incorporated into the DNA of every cell in the body. Germline mutations are passed from parents to offspring and are also referred to as hereditary mutations
Loss of heterozygosity	Loss of a gene and its surrounding chromosomal region on one of two paired chromosomes. The somatic loss of wild-type alleles is a common genetic event in cancer development

Mutant	Any form of an allele other than the wild type is a variant or mutant allele. While variants can represent polymorphisms common to the population (>1% of the population), mutant usually refers to variations that are detected in <1% of the population
Pancreatic cyst fluid	Fluid contained within a pancreatic cyst
Sensitivity	For a medical test with a binary classification system, sensitivity refers to the proportion of sick patients who are correctly identified with a positive test result. Tests with high sensitivity have low false-negative rates; consequently, a negative test result is helpful for excluding disease
Somatic mutation	Genetic alteration acquired by a tumor cell that can be passed to the progeny of the mutated tumor cell during cell division. Somatic mutations that cause cancer will be present only within the tumor where they occur
Specificity	For a medical test with a binary classification system, specificity refers to the proportion of healthy patients who are correctly identified with a negative test result. Tests with high specificity have low false-positive rates; a positive test result is thus helpful for "ruling in" disease

Key Points

- Molecular testing has limited diagnostic utility in pancreatic and biliary cytology but can be useful in certain settings, particularly for the diagnosis of pancreatic cysts
- *KRAS/GNAS* mutations are highly sensitive and specific for the detection of neoplastic mucinous cysts, and *GNAS* mutations are highly specific for the detection of intraductal papillary mucinous neoplasm (IPMN) versus other cystic lesions of the pancreas
- *TP53* mutation, loss of *SMAD4/DPC4*, or loss of p16 (*CDKN2A/INK4A)* detected in pancreatic cyst fluid supports a high-risk cyst warranting surgical resection
- Loss of *SMAD4* nuclear staining using immunohistochemistry, which is seen in ~55% of pancreatic ductal adenocarcinomas, supports malignancy
- Addition of fluorescence *in situ* hybridization (FISH) and/or next-generation sequencing (NGS) to cytology improves the diagnostic sensitivity of biliary duct brushings

In pancreatic and biliary cytology, molecular testing has overall limited diagnostic utility for solid lesions but can add significant value in the preoperative diagnosis of pancreatic cysts. As the detection of pancreatic cysts by radiologic imaging in asymptomatic patients has increased in recent years, differentiating between benign cystic lesions and those with malignant potential is essential for patient management. Currently, the standard of care for the preoperative diagnosis of pancreatic cysts is endoscopic ultrasound-guided fine-needle aspiration (EUS-FNA) with pancreatic cyst fluid (PCF) analysis [1–4]. PCF uses a combination of cytology and fluid chemistry (i.e., CEA/amylase levels) to distinguish mucinous from non-mucinous etiology and to assess for high-risk features of malignancy [5]. In some institutions, molecular testing is performed on all PCF with sufficient cyst fluid to improve the detection of mucinous cysts. With the addition of routine molecular analysis, where *KRAS/GNAS* mutations are highly specific for a mucinous etiology, the detection of mucinous cysts by PCF is reported to have a sensitivity of 90% and specificity >90% [6–9].

Despite developments in sampling technology, bile duct brushing cytology shows high specificity but low sensitivity for malignancy [10]. Fluorescence *in situ* hybridization (FISH) and molecular testing using next-generation sequencing (NGS) can be performed on aspiration or exfoliative cytological material and assist in the diagnosis of malignancy.

Cystic Pancreatic Lesions

Tissue Management

Fresh, unfixed, and undiluted PCF is required for accurate evaluation and analysis. PCF can be triaged using minimal cyst fluid volumes for cytology, CEA/amylase analysis, and molecular testing [11] (Table 15.1; Box 15.1).

Table 15.1 Practical pancreatic cyst fluid analysis of cystic pancreatic lesions

	Cytology	**Chemistry**	**Molecular mutations**
Pseudocyst	Amorphous cyst debris Yellow hematoidin-like pigment Variable inflammation No epithelial cells other than contaminating gastrointestinal epithelium	CEA < 192 ng/mL Amylase ≥ 250 U/L	None

(continued)

Table 15.1 (continued)

	Cytology	Chemistry	Molecular mutations
SCA	Scant cellularity Uniform non-mucinous cuboidal cells Hemosiderin-laden macrophages	CEA < 192 ng/mL Amylase < 5 ng/mL	*VHL* (3p25)
IPMN	Thick, colloid-like extracellular mucin Low-grade atypia: mucinous epithelium often indistinguishable from gastric epithelium High-grade atypia: small epithelial cells with increased nuclear-to-cytoplasmic ratio, irregular nuclear membranes, background cellular necrosis	CEA ≥ 192 ng/mL Amylase variable	*KRAS* *GNAS* *TP53*, p16 (*CDKN2A*), *SMAD4/DPC4* indicate high-risk cyst
MCN			*KRAS*

Box 15.1

Volume < 0.5 mL:

CEA (0.3 mL) or *KRAS/GNAS* (0.3 mL)

Volume > 0.5 mL:

1. *KRAS/GNAS* (vortexed, neat, 0.3 mL)
2. CEA (0.3 mL supernatant)
3. Amylase (0.3 mL supernatant)
4. Cytology (cell button; cytospin)
5. Bank (residual supernatant)

It has been demonstrated that using supernatant fluid for CEA/amylase testing is comparable to using neat fluid/cell-block preparation [11]. Furthermore, the added value of *KRAS* testing alone may be small if the combination of cytology and CEA levels are conclusive, as *KRAS* mutation status does not add to the determination of a mucinous cyst if CEA is ≥ 192 ng/mL and does not stratify the lesion by grade.

Nonneoplastic Cystic Lesions

Serous cystadenomas (SCAs) are the most common benign cystic neoplasm of the pancreas and account for 1–2% of pancreatic neoplasms [12, 13]. The goal of preoperative diagnosis is to distinguish these benign cysts from neoplastic mucinous cysts, thus allowing optimal triage of patients to conservative management versus surgical resection. However, the lack of specific cytomorphological features makes diagnosis extremely challenging on cytology alone, with a sensitivity of 10% in a recent case series [14]. Mutations in the von Hippel-Lindau (*VHL*) gene (3p25), loss of heterozygosity of chromosome 3 at the *VHL* gene locus, or aneuploidy of chromosome 3p were identified in 67% of sporadic and hereditary SCAs and not found in cystic mucinous neoplasms [15]. Thus, the detection of a *VHL* mutation on PCF supports a diagnosis of SCA. Of note, pancreatic neuroendocrine tumors (PanNETs), which may be cystic, can have *VHL* deletions in up to 25% of sporadic cases [16].

Neoplastic Cystic Lesions (Mucinous)

Mucinous cysts are diagnosed using the proposed standardized terminology system for pancreaticobiliary specimens from the Papanicolaou Society of Cytopathology based on having one of the following features: thick, colloid-like extracellular mucin, mucinous cyst lining epithelium, and/or elevated CEA ≥ 192 ng/mL [17–19]. There are two types of neoplastic mucinous cysts that share common cytomorphological features but have distinct clinical and biological characteristics: *intraductal papillary mucinous neoplasm (IPMN)* and *mucinous cystic neoplasm (MCN)*. Both are stratified into low/intermediate-grade versus high-grade dysplasia with or without an invasive carcinoma component; invasive carcinoma is the most important negative prognostic factor. The distinction between IPMN and MCN is not always possible by cytology alone. However, it is important to distinguish MCN from IPMN, as surgical resection is recommended for all patients with MCN irrespective of grade, while most branch-duct IPMN can be managed conservatively without surgery.

Cyst fluid CEA levels have been shown to be the most accurate method for identifying a mucinous cyst, while cytology is the best modality for identifying high-risk cysts [17, 18, 20]. A cutoff of CEA $\geq$ 192 ng/mL has an overall accuracy of ~80% (sensitivity of 75% and specificity of 84%). Amylase levels are highly variable in mucinous cysts and do not reliably distinguish between cyst types.

Molecular studies have shown that in the setting of a pancreatic cyst, *KRAS* mutations are highly specific but only moderately sensitive for a mucinous etiology [6, 21]. A recent large prospective study performed NGS on 626 PCF specimens detected *KRAS* and/or *GNAS* mutations in 100% of IPMNs, with *GNAS* mutations being 100% specific for an IPMN; *KRAS* mutations were detected in 30% of MCNs. Overall, *KRAS/GNAS* mutations were found to have a sensitivity of 89% and specificity of 100% for the detection of a mucinous cyst [22]. *RNF43* mutations are also found in both IPMNs and MCNs [15, 23].

Intraductal papillary mucinous neoplasms (IPMNs) comprise 3–5% of pancreatic tumors and 20% of neoplastic pancreatic cysts; 70% arise in the head of the pancreas [24]. The prognosis for noninvasive IPMNs is excellent, and they can be managed conservatively by surveillance. High-risk features that may prompt surgical resection include main duct involvement, presence of a mural nodule, and the identification of high-grade dysplasia or invasive carcinoma [25]. Massively parallel sequencing of IPMN cyst fluid showed that *GNAS* mutations were present in 66% of cases and *KRAS* or *GNAS* mutations were present in 96% of cases [26]. *GNAS* mutations were not found in other types of pancreatic cystic neoplasms; thus, the detection of a *GNAS* mutation in PCF is diagnostic of an IPMN. *SMAD4/DPC4* and *p16/CDKN2A* mutations and/or loss of immunohistochemical expression can be seen in high-grade IPMNs (i.e., high-grade dysplasia or invasive carcinoma arising from IPMN) [27]. Recently, it was shown that preoperative detection of mutations/deletions in *TP53*, *PIK3CA*, *PTEN*, and/or *AKT1* was highly sensitive and specific for IPMNs with high-grade dysplasia/invasive adenocarcinoma [22]. Mutant allele frequencies >55% for *GNAS* mutations were also correlated with IPMNs with high-grade dysplasia. These findings show promise for predicting the presence of high-risk cysts and may become more relevant as molecular diagnostics become integrated into routine clinical practice.

Mucinous cystic neoplasms (MCNs) comprise 5–6% of pancreatic tumors and occur almost exclusively in women in the fourth to fifth decade; 90% arise in the body or tail of the pancreas. The presence of subepithelial ovarian-type stroma is the defining characteristic of MCN and can be evaluated if a biopsy specimen is available [28]. Immunohistochemistry for estrogen and progesterone receptors, which are expressed by the ovarian-type stromal cells, may be considered if morphologically ambiguous [29, 30]. There are no known genetic mutations specific to MCN [10, 31].

Solid Pancreatic Lesions

Tissue Management

FNA smears are typically made for solid pancreatic lesions and can then be air-dried for Romanowsky stain and/or alcohol-fixed for Papanicolaou stain. Liquid-based preparations (ThinPrep™ or SurePath™) can also be made. Importantly, allocation of material for cellblock preparation and/or having a concurrent core biopsy allows for immunohistochemical staining, which significantly aids in the diagnosis of certain neoplasms. Currently, molecular testing is not routinely performed for the purposes of diagnosis; instead, immunostains are routinely used as surrogate markers for their respective gene mutations. However, if molecular testing is warranted, FNA smear specimens have been shown to be a more optimal source of DNA than formalin-fixed paraffin-embedded tissue [32] (Table 15.2).

Solid Neoplasms

Pancreatic ductal adenocarcinoma (PDAC) accounts for 90% of all pancreatic neoplasms and carries a poor prognosis, with an overall 5-year survival rate of <10% [33]. The four key driver mutations in PDAC are *KRAS*, *TP53*, p16 (*CDKN2A*), and *SMAD4/DPC4*. Immunostains for p53 and SMAD4 are surrogate markers for their respective mutations [34] and can be helpful in challenging cases: most PDACs have mutated p53, which would show overexpression or complete absence of nuclear p53 (compared to scattered positivity in wild-type p53), and about half of cases (~55%) show loss of SMAD4 nuclear expression (Fig. 15.1). In contrast, CDX2 immunohistochemistry is not helpful in the diagnosis of PDAC, as studies have shown conflicting results regarding its expression in normal pancreatic tissue and PDAC, but may be performed in the context of an adenocarcinoma of unknown origin. CDX2 expression is downregulated during the transformation from pancreatic intraepithelial neoplasia to PDAC. Furthermore, tumors with some level of retained CDX2 expression (around one-third of cases) have been shown to have a shorter survival compared to those that were negative for CDX2 [35]. *KRAS* mutations are non-specific and are found in low-grade pancreatic intraepithelial neoplasia, as well as other pancreatic neoplasms. Thus, routine

TABLE 15.2 Practical analysis of solid pancreatic lesions

	Cytology	Immunoprofile	Molecular mutations
PDAC	Cellular/hypercellular specimen "Drunken honeycomb" pattern of unevenly spaced, crowded ductal cells Marked anisonucleosis (>4:1) Variable cytoplasmic mucin	CK7, CK19 CA19–9 SMAD4 loss p53 ++/or total loss	*KRAS* (>90%) *TP53* (50–75%) p16 (*CDKN2A*) (>95%) *SMAD4/DPC4* (55%)
PanNET	Discohesive, solid-cellular pattern Uniform, monotonous plasmacytoid cells "Salt-and-pepper" chromatin Dense, finely granular cytoplasm	Synaptophysin Chromogranin CD56 DAXX loss ATRX loss	11q loss (70%) *MEN1* (40%) *DAXX/ATRX* (40%)
PanNEC	Clusters of small-to-larger cells with high nuclear-to-cytoplasmic ratio, nuclear molding, crush artifact, mitoses, tumor necrosis	Synaptophysin Chromogranin CD56 DAXX + ATRX + p53 ++ Rb or p16 loss	*TP53* (95%) *Rb* (>50%) or *p16/CDKN2A*

(continued)

TABLE 15.2 (continued)

	Cytology	Immunoprofile	Molecular mutations
ACC	Solid-cellular pattern Non-cohesive irregular cell clusters Monomorphic bland cells Stripped naked nuclei with coarse chromatin Variably granular cytoplasm	Trypsin Chymotrypsin	11p loss (50%)
Pancreatoblastoma	Solid-cellular pattern Multilineage epithelial cells with predominantly acinar differentiation Squamous corpuscles Primitive stroma	Variable markers of acinar, ductal, endocrine differentiation	11p loss β-catenin/APC (50–80%)
SPN	Solid cellular pattern Fibrovascular myxoid stromal papillae Bland cells with nuclear grooves, fine chromatin, inconspicuous nucleoli Scant cytoplasm with perinuclear vacuoles	β-catenin (nuclear) CD10 CD56	β-catenin (95–100%)

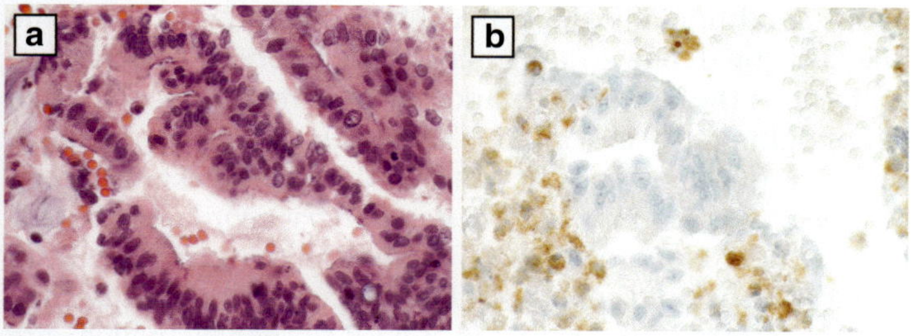

FIGURE 15.1 Well-differentiated pancreatic ductal adenocarcinoma on (**a**) hematoxylin and eosin stain (cellblock, 600×) with (**b**) loss of nuclear SMAD4 expression (cytoplasmic staining is non-specific) by immunohistochemistry (cellblock, 600×)

molecular testing is not helpful in distinguishing PDAC from premalignant lesions. A recent study evaluated the relationship between these four driver gene mutations and patient outcomes after tumor resection and found that *KRAS* mutants and tumors with p16 (*CDKN2A*) loss had worse disease-free and overall survival, while *TP53* mutants only predicted disease-free survival; *SMAD4* mutations were not predictive of survival [36].

Currently, there are clinical trials underway investigating the effectiveness of immune checkpoint inhibitors (targeting CTLA-4, PD-1, and PD-L1) in patients with PDAC. While some preliminary studies have shown promising results, these treatments have yet to be clinically implemented, and at present there is no role for the testing of PD-L1 by immunohistochemistry or other mutations by NGS in routine practice [37].

Pancreatic neuroendocrine tumors (PanNETs) represent 1–2% of all pancreatic neoplasms, most of which are nonfunctional [38]. On cytology, the most important role in grading is to distinguish well-differentiated PanNETs from *poorly differentiated pancreatic neuroendocrine carcinomas (PanNECs)*. Ki67 proliferation index is a requirement for grading and should be performed on cellblock preparations and core biopsies that are sufficiently cellular. PanNETs can undergo cystic degeneration and mimic a primary pancreatic cystic neoplasm. Immunohistochemical stains help to establish the diagnosis by demonstrating endocrine differentiation: synaptophysin is the preferred marker, as it is more sensitive than chromogranin A and relatively specific. CD56 is the most sensitive but least specific neuroendocrine marker and can also be expressed in *solid pseudopapillary neoplasms (SPN)*.

The most common PanNET mutations are in the death domain-associated protein (*DAXX*) and α-thalasesemia/mental retardation X-linked (*ATRX*) genes, which are detected in almost half of cases [10, 39]. Immunohistochemical stains are available as surrogate markers for the mutations. Loss of *DAXX* and *ATRX* are associated with increased risk of metastasis and shorter overall survival in PanNETs [40]. Up to 45% of sporadic PanNETs show somatic *MEN1* mutations, though these mutations are classically germline in multiple endocrine neoplasia type I (MEN1) syndrome. Other germline mutations associated with syndromes include neurofibromatosis type 1 (*NF1* gene), tuberous sclerosis (either *TSC1* or *TSC2* genes), and von Hippel Lindau (*VHL* gene) syndromes. In contrast, PanNECs are infrequently associated with MEN1 and retain *DAXX* and *ATRX* immunoreactivity; instead, they overexpress p53 (95%) and can lose pRb (60–90%) or p16 expression (10–40%), consistent with mutations in those respective genes [10, 41].

Acinar cell carcinoma (ACC) is a rare, aggressive tumor and accounts for <2% of all pancreatic neoplasms [24]. Immunohistochemical detection of specific enzymes produced by acinar cells (i.e., trypsin, chymotrypsin) supports the diagnosis [42]. Chromosomal analysis shows allelic loss on chromosome 11p [10, 43]. ACC harbors *APC* and *TP53* mutations, *RAF* gene fusions (*SND1-BRAF* fusions most common, up to 23% of cases) and inactivation of DNA repair genes (mutually exclusive with *RAF* rearrangements). APC/β-catenin mutations have been described; however, the common PDAC- and panNET-associated mutations are not seen in ACC.

Pancreatoblastoma is a rare multilineage malignant epithelial tumor that comprises <0.5% of all pancreatic neoplasms and is the most common pancreatic malignancy in children, typically seen in the first decade [44]. Immunohistochemical stains can be used to highlight the multiple lines of differentiation within the tumor: acinar (trypsin, chymotrypsin), ductal (cytokeratin), and neuroendocrine (synaptophysin, chromogranin). β-catenin stain can highlight the pathognomonic squamoid morules (nonreactive for cytokeratins), which are thought to be a manifestation of aberrant overexpression of β-catenin (nuclear and cytoplasmic) coupled with estrogen receptor-β [10], and can help distinguish pancreatoblastoma from ACC. Similar to ACC, the most common genetic abnormality is allelic loss on chromosome 11p [10]. Somatic mutations in the APC and β-catenin genes have also been described. The common PDAC-associated mutations are not seen in pancreatoblastoma.

Solid pseudopapillary neoplasms (SPNs) are tumors with low malignant potential and account for <2% of all pancreatic neoplasms. They harbor activating mutations of the β-catenin (*CTNNB1*) gene (95–100% of cases) without any other genetic alterations [10, 15]. These mutations result in nuclear (and cytoplasmic) accumulation of β-catenin, which can be routinely detected with β-catenin immunohistochemistry (Fig. 15.2).

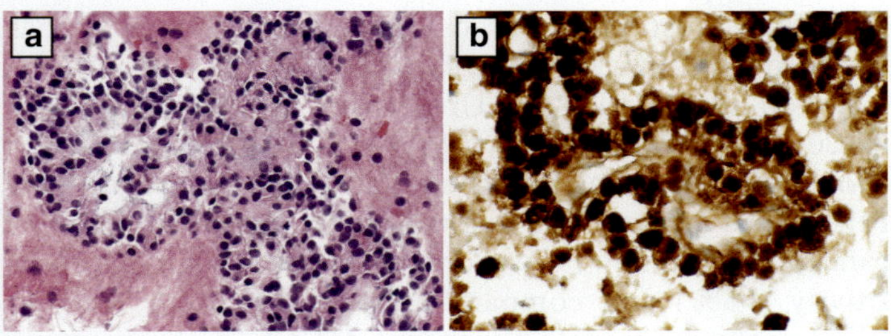

Figure 15.2 Solid pseudopapillary neoplasm on (**a**) hematoxylin and eosin stain (cellblock, 400×) with (**b**) nuclear β-catenin expression by immunohistochemistry (cellblock, 600×)

Biliary Duct Brushings

Tissue Management

The biliary tract is most frequently sampled using brush cytology obtained during endoscopic retrograde cholangiopancreatography, with the goal of distinguishing between reactive versus neoplastic processes to direct clinical management. Biliary brushing cytology has a high specificity for detecting malignancy but a low sensitivity (6–64%) [45]. EUS-FNA has also been used to sample biliary lesions, but is not routinely recommended due to concern for needle-track seeding. The material collected for biliary brush cytology can be used for FISH and molecular studies. A triple-modality approach using a combination of brush cytology, concurrent forceps biopsy, and FISH has demonstrated a significantly increased sensitivity of 82% and specificity of 100% [46].

Fluorescent In Situ Hybridization (FISH)

FISH is an established ancillary test for diagnosing bile duct carcinoma [46, 47]. Clinically, the multicolor FISH UroVysion probe set (Abbott Molecular Inc., Des Plaines, IL) is the most widely used and consists of four probes targeted against chromosomes 3, 7, 9p21, and 17. The reported sensitivities for UroVysion (35–60%) are only modestly improved over cytology [48–50]. More recently, a cholangiocarcinoma-/PDAC-specific FISH probe set (PB FISH) was created and reportedly increased the rate of cancer detection by 19% over UroVysion, with higher sensitivity (65%) and comparable specificity [51]. This PB FISH probe set targets oncogenes *MCL1* on chromosome 1q, *EGFR* on chromosome 7p, and *MYC* on chromosome 8q, all of which are often gained in cholangiocarcinomas and PDACs.

Next-Generation Sequencing

A recent study compared adjunctive molecular testing with targeted NGS versus FISH (UroVysion probe set) for the detection of high-risk neoplasia (i.e., main duct IPMN, high-grade dysplasia) or malignancy in 81 biliary duct brushings [52]. When added to cytology, NGS increased the sensitivity to 85%, while FISH only increased sensitivity to 76%. These results suggest that ancillary NGS may offer advantages over FISH in biliary duct brushings and warrant further validation in larger cohorts.

References

1. Genevay M, Mino-Kenudson M, Yaeger K, Konstantinidis IT, Ferrone CR, Thayer S, et al. Cytology adds value to imaging studies for risk assessment of malignancy in pancreatic mucinous cysts. Ann Surg. 2011;254(6):977–83.
2. Khashab MA, Kim K, Lennon AM, Shin EJ, Tignor AS, Amateau SK, et al. Should we do EUS/FNA on patients with pancreatic cysts? The incremental diagnostic yield of EUS over CT/MRI for prediction of cystic neoplasms. Pancreas. 2013;42(4):717–21.
3. Pitman MB, Deshpande V. Endoscopic ultrasound-guided fine needle aspiration cytology of the pancreas: a morphological and multimodal approach to the diagnosis of solid and cystic mass lesions. Cytopathology. 2007;18(6):331–47.
4. Tanaka M, Fernandez-Del Castillo C, Kamisawa T, Jang JY, Levy P, Ohtsuka T, et al. Revisions of international consensus Fukuoka guidelines for the management of IPMN of the pancreas. Pancreatology. 2017;17(5):738–53.
5. Pitman MB. Pancreatic cyst fluid triage: a critical component of the preoperative evaluation of pancreatic cysts. Cancer Cytopathol. 2013;121(2):57–60.
6. Jones M, Zheng Z, Wang J, Dudley J, Albanese E, Kadayifci A, et al. Impact of next-generation sequencing on the clinical diagnosis of pancreatic cysts. Gastrointest Endosc. 2016;83(1):140–8.
7. Kadayifci A, Atar M, Wang JL, Forcione DG, Casey BW, Pitman MB, et al. Value of adding GNAS testing to pancreatic cyst fluid

KRAS and carcinoembryonic antigen analysis for the diagnosis of intraductal papillary mucinous neoplasms. Dig Endosc. 2017;29(1):111–7.
8. Rosenbaum MW, Jones M, Dudley JC, Le LP, Iafrate AJ, Pitman MB. Next-generation sequencing adds value to the preoperative diagnosis of pancreatic cysts. Cancer Cytopathol. 2017;125(1):41–7.
9. Singhi AD, Nikiforova MN, Fasanella KE, McGrath KM, Pai RK, Ohori NP, et al. Preoperative GNAS and KRAS testing in the diagnosis of pancreatic mucinous cysts. Clin Cancer Res. 2014;20(16):4381–9.
10. Reid MD, Lewis MM, Willingham FF, Adsay NV. The evolving role of pathology in new developments, classification, terminology, and diagnosis of pancreatobiliary neoplasms. Arch Pathol Lab Med. 2017;141(3):366–80.
11. Chai SM, Herba K, Kumarasinghe MP, de Boer WB, Amanuel B, Grieu-Iacopetta F, et al. Optimizing the multimodal approach to pancreatic cyst fluid diagnosis: developing a volume-based triage protocol. Cancer Cytopathol. 2013;121(2):86–100.
12. Valsangkar NP, Morales-Oyarvide V, Thayer SP, Ferrone CR, Wargo JA, Warshaw AL, et al. 851 resected cystic tumors of the pancreas: a 33-year experience at the Massachusetts General Hospital. Surgery. 2012;152(3 Suppl 1):S4–12.
13. Singhi AD, Zeh HJ, Brand RE, Nikiforova MN, Chennat JS, Fasanella KE, et al. American Gastroenterological Association guidelines are inaccurate in detecting pancreatic cysts with advanced neoplasia: a clinicopathologic study of 225 patients with supporting molecular data. Gastrointest Endosc. 2016;83(6):1107–17.e2.
14. Lilo MT, VandenBussche CJ, Allison DB, Lennon AM, Younes BK, Hruban RH, et al. Serous cystadenoma of the pancreas: potentials and pitfalls of a preoperative cytopathologic diagnosis. Acta Cytol. 2017;61(1):27–33.
15. Springer S, Wang Y, Dal Molin M, Masica DL, Jiao Y, Kinde I, et al. A combination of molecular markers and clinical features improve the classification of pancreatic cysts. Gastroenterology. 2015;149(6):1501–10.
16. Reid MD, Choi H, Balci S, Akkas G, Adsay V. Serous cystic neoplasms of the pancreas: clinicopathologic and molecular characteristics. Semin Diagn Pathol. 2014;31(6):475–83.
17. Brugge WR, Lewandrowski K, Lee-Lewandrowski E, Centeno BA, Szydlo T, Regan S, et al. Diagnosis of pancreatic cystic

neoplasms: a report of the cooperative pancreatic cyst study. Gastroenterology. 2004;126(5):1330–6.
18. Cizginer S, Turner BG, Bilge AR, Karaca C, Pitman MB, Brugge WR. Cyst fluid carcinoembryonic antigen is an accurate diagnostic marker of pancreatic mucinous cysts. Pancreas. 2011;40(7):1024–8.
19. Pitman MB, Centeno BA, Ali SZ, Genevay M, Stelow E, Mino-Kenudson M, et al. Standardized terminology and nomenclature for pancreatobiliary cytology: the Papanicolaou Society of Cytopathology guidelines. Diagn Cytopathol. 2014;42(4):338–50.
20. Scourtas A, Dudley JC, Brugge WR, Kadayifci A, Mino-Kenudson M, Pitman MB. Preoperative characteristics and cytological features of 136 histologically confirmed pancreatic mucinous cystic neoplasms. Cancer Cytopathol. 2017;125(3):169–77.
21. Rockacy M, Khalid A. Update on pancreatic cyst fluid analysis. Ann Gastroenterol. 2013;26(2):122–7.
22. Singhi AD, McGrath K, Brand RE, Khalid A, Zeh HJ, Chennat JS, Fasanella KE, Papachristou GI, Slivka A, Bartlett DL, Dasyam AK, Hogg M, Lee KK, Marsh JW, Monaco SE, Ohori NP, Pingpank JF, Tsung A, Zureikat AH, Wald AI, Nikiforova MN. Preoperative next-generation sequencing of pancreatic cyst fluid is highly accurate in cyst classification and detection of advanced neoplasia. Gut. 2017. [Epub ahead of print].
23. Wu J, Jiao Y, Dal Molin M, Maitra A, de Wilde RF, Wood LD, et al. Whole-exome sequencing of neoplastic cysts of the pancreas reveals recurrent mutations in components of ubiquitin-dependent pathways. Proc Natl Acad Sci U S A. 2011;108(52):21188–93.
24. Hruban RH, Pitman MB, Klimstra DS. Tumors of the pancreas. Atlas of tumor pathology, Fourth series, Fascicle 6. Washington, DC: American Registry of Pathology; Armed Forces Institutes of Pathology; 2007.
25. Pitman MB, Centeno BA, Daglilar ES, Brugge WR, Mino-Kenudson M. Cytological criteria of high-grade epithelial atypia in the cyst fluid of pancreatic intraductal papillary mucinous neoplasms. Cancer Cytopathol. 2014;122(1):40–7.
26. Wu J, Matthaei H, Maitra A, Dal Molin M, Wood LD, Eshleman JR, et al. Recurrent GNAS mutations define an unexpected pathway for pancreatic cyst development. Sci Transl Med. 2011;3(92):92ra66.
27. Amato E, Molin MD, Mafficini A, Yu J, Malleo G, Rusev B, et al. Targeted next-generation sequencing of cancer genes dissects

the molecular profiles of intraductal papillary neoplasms of the pancreas. J Pathol. 2014;233(3):217–27.

28. Zhang ML, Arpin RN, Brugge WR, Forcione DG, Basar O, Pitman MB. Moray micro forceps biopsy improves the diagnosis of specific pancreatic cysts. Cancer Cytopathol. 2018;126(6):414–20.
29. Yamao K, Yanagisawa A, Takahashi K, Kimura W, Doi R, Fukushima N, et al. Clinicopathological features and prognosis of mucinous cystic neoplasm with ovarian-type stroma: a multi-institutional study of the Japan pancreas society. Pancreas. 2011;40(1):67–71.
30. Reddy RP, Smyrk TC, Zapiach M, Levy MJ, Pearson RK, Clain JE, et al. Pancreatic mucinous cystic neoplasm defined by ovarian stroma: demographics, clinical features, and prevalence of cancer. Clin Gastroenterol Hepatol. 2004;2(11):1026–31.
31. Pittman ME, Rao R, Hruban RH. Classification, morphology, molecular pathogenesis, and outcome of premalignant lesions of the pancreas. Arch Pathol Lab Med. 2017;141(12):1606–14.
32. Hartley CP, Mahajan AM, Selvaggi SM, Rehrauer WM. FNA smears of pancreatic ductal adenocarcinoma are superior to formalin-fixed paraffin-embedded tissue as a source of DNA: comparison of targeted KRAS amplification and genotyping in matched preresection and postresection samples. Cancer Cytopathol. 2017;125(11):838–47.
33. Siegel RL, Miller KD, Jemal A. Cancer Statistics, 2017. CA Cancer J Clin. 2017;67(1):7–30.
34. van Heek T, Rader AE, Offerhaus GJ, McCarthy DM, Goggins M, Hruban RH, et al. K-ras, p53, and DPC4 (MAD4) alterations in fine-needle aspirates of the pancreas: a molecular panel correlates with and supplements cytologic diagnosis. Am J Clin Pathol. 2002;117(5):755–65.
35. Xiao W, Hong H, Awadallah A, Zhou L, Xin W. Utilization of CDX2 expression in diagnosing pancreatic ductal adenocarcinoma and predicting prognosis. PLoS One. 2014;9(1):e86853.
36. Qian ZR, Rubinson DA, Nowak JA, Morales-Oyarvide V, Dunne RF, Kozak MM, et al. Association of alterations in main driver genes with outcomes of patients with resected pancreatic ductal adenocarcinoma. JAMA Oncol. 2018;4(3):e173420.
37. Johansson H, Andersson R, Bauden M, Hammes S, Holdenrieder S, Ansari D. Immune checkpoint therapy for pancreatic cancer. World J Gastroenterol. 2016;22(43):9457–76.
38. Lee DW, Kim MK, Kim HG. Diagnosis of pancreatic neuroendocrine tumors. Clin Endosc. 2017;50(6):537–45.

39. Jiao Y, Shi C, Edil BH, de Wilde RF, Klimstra DS, Maitra A, et al. DAXX/ATRX, MEN1, and mTOR pathway genes are frequently altered in pancreatic neuroendocrine tumors. Science. 2011;331(6021):1199–203.
40. Park JK, Paik WH, Lee K, Ryu JK, Lee SH, Kim YT. DAXX/ATRX and MEN1 genes are strong prognostic markers in pancreatic neuroendocrine tumors. Oncotarget. 2017;8(30):49796–806.
41. Shi C, Klimstra DS. Pancreatic neuroendocrine tumors: pathologic and molecular characteristics. Semin Diagn Pathol. 2014;31(6):498–511.
42. Sigel CS, Klimstra DS. Cytomorphologic and immunophenotypical features of acinar cell neoplasms of the pancreas. Cancer Cytopathol. 2013;121(8):459–70.
43. Abraham SC, TT W, Hruban RH, Lee JH, Yeo CJ, Conlon K, et al. Genetic and immunohistochemical analysis of pancreatic acinar cell carcinoma: frequent allelic loss on chromosome 11p and alterations in the APC/beta-catenin pathway. Am J Pathol. 2002;160(3):953–62.
44. Ogawa B, Okinaga K, Obana K, Nakamura K, Hattori T, Ito T, et al. Pancreatoblastoma treated by delayed operation after effective chemotherapy. J Pediatr Surg. 2000;35(11):1663–5.
45. Burnett AS, Calvert TJ, Chokshi RJ. Sensitivity of endoscopic retrograde cholangiopancreatography standard cytology: 10-y review of the literature. J Surg Res. 2013;184(1):304–11.
46. Nanda A, Brown JM, Berger SH, Lewis MM, Barr Fritcher EG, Gores GJ, et al. Triple modality testing by endoscopic retrograde cholangiopancreatography for the diagnosis of cholangiocarcinoma. Therap Adv Gastroenterol. 2015;8(2):56–65.
47. Boldorini R, Paganotti A, Sartori M, Allegrini S, Miglio U, Orsello M, et al. Fluorescence in situ hybridisation in the cytological diagnosis of pancreatobiliary tumours. Pathology. 2011;43(4):335–9.
48. Kipp BR, Fritcher EG, Clayton AC, Gores GJ, Roberts LR, Zhang J, et al. Comparison of KRAS mutation analysis and FISH for detecting pancreatobiliary tract cancer in cytology specimens collected during endoscopic retrograde cholangiopancreatography. J Mol Diagn. 2010;12(6):780–6.
49. Kipp BR, Stadheim LM, Halling SA, Pochron NL, Harmsen S, Nagorney DM, et al. A comparison of routine cytology and fluorescence in situ hybridization for the detection of malignant bile duct strictures. Am J Gastroenterol. 2004;99(9):1675–81.

50. Levy MJ, Baron TH, Clayton AC, Enders FB, Gostout CJ, Halling KC, et al. Prospective evaluation of advanced molecular markers and imaging techniques in patients with indeterminate bile duct strictures. Am J Gastroenterol. 2008;103(5):1263–73.
51. Barr Fritcher EG, Voss JS, Brankley SM, Campion MB, Jenkins SM, Keeney ME, et al. An optimized set of fluorescence in situ hybridization probes for detection of pancreatobiliary tract cancer in cytology brush samples. Gastroenterology. 2015;149(7):1813–24.e1.
52. Dudley JC, Zheng Z, McDonald T, Le LP, Dias-Santagata D, Borger D, et al. Next-generation sequencing and fluorescence in situ hybridization have comparable performance characteristics in the analysis of pancreaticobiliary brushings for malignancy. J Mol Diagn. 2016;18(1):124–30.

Chapter 16
Fluorescence *In Situ* Hybridization (FISH) Testing in Urinary Tract Cytology

Güliz A. Barkan and Stefan E. Pambuccian

Abbreviations

AMH	Asymptomatic microscopic hematuria
AUC	Atypical urothelial cells
CEP	Centromere enumeration probes
DAPI	4′6-Diamidino-2-phenylindole
FISH	Fluorescence *in situ* hybridization
H&E	Hematoxylin and eosin
HGUC	High-grade urothelial carcinoma
HPF	High-power field
LGUN	Low-grade urothelial neoplasia
LSI	Locus-specific identifier
NHGUC	Negative for high-grade urothelial carcinoma
QNS	Quantity not sufficient
RBC	Red blood cell

G. A. Barkan (✉) · S. E. Pambuccian
Department of Pathology and Laboratory Medicine,
Loyola University Medical Center, Maywood, IL, USA
e-mail: gbarkan@lumc.edu; spambuccian@lumc.edu

S. Roy-Chowdhuri et al. (eds.), *Molecular Diagnostics in Cytopathology*, https://doi.org/10.1007/978-3-319-97397-5_16

SHGUC	Suspicious for high-grade urothelial carcinoma
TPS	The Paris System for reporting urinary cytopathology

Key Terminology

Aneuploidy	Change in normal copy number of entire chromosomes, i.e., an abnormal number of chromosomes in a cell (e.g., monosomy, trisomy, tetrasomy, etc.)
Chromosome enumerating probe (CEP)	Specific probe designed to bind repetitive sequences of DNA. Enumeration of chromosome copies
DAPI (4′-6-Diamidino-2-phenylindole)	Fluorescent counterstain that binds to background double-stranded DNA
Denaturation	The process of separating two complementary strands of DNA, typically using heat
Fluorescence *in situ* hybridization (FISH)	A molecular detection technique that uses fluorescently labeled DNA to hybridize to complementary regions within the target DNA
Gene	A part of double-stranded DNA that codes for a protein
Heterozygous	Most diploid cells such as tumor cells contain two different alleles at any gene locus
Hybridization	Inducing a DNA probe sequence to bind to its complementary sequence on a chromosome
Locus-specific identifier	Probe designed to bind to the loci of a specific target region or gene to detect loss or gain of loci
Polysomy	The condition in which there may be three or more copies of the chromosome rather than the expected two copies

Key Points

Multi-target FISH remains an excellent molecular diagnostics tool to improve diagnosis in urinary cytopathology provided that the following points are considered:

- Understand the basic principles and limitations of the UroVysion® FISH test being used for appropriate molecular cytopathologic correlation
- Urinary FISH is better analyzed by morphologists (such as cytopathologists, cytotechnologists), since uncritical FISH analysis of activated, tetraploid umbrella cells can lead to false-positive results
- FISH results must be interpreted in the light of the clinical findings
- FISH adds no value in case of clearly positive (HGUC) or negative (NHGUC) cytology; analysis of equivocal cytology is the most reasonable application of urinary FISH
- Whatever the techniques used, there should be a clear communication between the cytopathologist and the urologist with regard to the meaning of urothelial atypias to avoid misinterpretation and unnecessary invasive procedures

Carcinoma of the urinary bladder is the second most common urological cancer and fifth most prevalent cancer overall with an estimated 79,030 new cases (60,490 in men and 18,540 in women) diagnosed and 16,870 deaths (12,240 men and 4630 women) occurring in the United States in 2017 [1]. Urothelial carcinoma is responsible for the majority of urinary bladder and upper urinary tract carcinomas, most of which are low-grade, superficial, non-muscle-invasive tumors with a good prognosis. Currently, the gold standard for detecting UCs and monitoring patients for recurrent UCs is cystoscopy with urinary cytology [2].

Urinary cytology is a simple, noninvasive, and relatively inexpensive method for detecting urothelial carcinoma. Although urinary cytology has relatively high specificity, and a relatively good sensitivity for detecting high-grade urothelial carcinoma (urothelial carcinoma *in situ* and high-grade papillary urothelial carcinoma), it has been plagued by low sensitivity for low-grade urothelial neoplasms (LGUN, including papilloma, papillary low-grade urothelial neoplasms of undetermined malignant potential, and low-grade urothelial carcinoma) [3]. These low-grade tumors are characterized by a high recurrence rate, but otherwise nonaggressive behavior [4]. The less common high-grade urothelial carcinoma (HGUC) also has a high recurrence rate but, more importantly, has a high risk of progression to muscle invasion and lymph node and systemic metastases. Therefore, while the detection of both LGUN and HGUC are important, the diagnosis of HGUC is of much higher clinical significance. This has been the guiding principle of The Paris System for reporting urinary cytopathology (TPS). The major accomplishments of TPS have been the shift in emphasis to the detection of HGUC and the standardization of cytologic reporting with a universally acceptable and globally applicable diagnostic terminology.

In addition, TPS offered strict definitions of the morphologic criteria necessary for the various categories in urinary tract cytopathology. The diagnostic categories included in TPS are:

1. Nondiagnostic
2. Negative for high-grade urothelial carcinoma (NHGUC)
3. Atypical urothelial cells (AUC)
4. Suspicious for high-grade urothelial carcinoma (SHGUC)
5. High-grade urothelial carcinoma (HGUC)
6. Low-grade urothelial neoplasm (LGUN)
7. Other malignancies

A number of ancillary tests have been proposed over the last decades to increase the sensitivity of urinary cytology.

These tests have included the use of markers like nuclear matrix protein (NMP22) and bladder tumor-associated antigen (BTA) and immunohistochemical stains (uCyt+/ImmunoCyt) using three fluorescent monoclonal antibodies (M344, LDQ10, and 19A211). However, the oldest and most widely used ancillary tests used in conjunction with urinary cytology to detect urothelial carcinoma were based on the fact that they may show complex genetic abnormalities, which render their cells aneuploid. This aneuploidy has been initially detected by flow and image cytometry [5], but these methods have been gradually replaced by more targeted detection of specific chromosome aneusomies, using *in situ* hybridization techniques like FISH [6, 7]. After various combinations of probes directed against chromosomes 1, 7, 8, 9, 12, 17, and Y had been used in the 1990s [8–10], the study by Sokolova et al. [11], using centromeric probes (CEP) against chromosomes 3, 7, 8, 9, 11, 17, and 18 and locus-specific identifier (LSI) probe for 9p21, showed that the combination of four probes (CEP3, CEP7, CEP17, and LSI 9p21) had the highest sensitivity for UC detection. The same group of researchers followed up with a study showing that the sensitivity of FISH using this probe set is superior to that of cytology, while the test's specificity was not significantly inferior [12]. Based on these results, the UroVysion® test was developed by Vysis, Downers Grove, IL (currently owned by Abbott Diagnostics, Abbott Park, IL) and gained FDA approval "for use in conjunction with and not in lieu of current standard diagnostic procedures" in 2001. Initially approved for "monitoring for tumor recurrence in patients previously diagnosed with bladder cancer," it was additionally approved by the FDA in 2005 "as an aid for initial diagnosis of bladder carcinoma in patients with hematuria." Both FDA approvals were for voided urine specimens only; other urinary tract specimens like washings/barbotage specimens and brushings were not included. After the FDA approval, the UroVysion® FISH test rapidly gained popularity and was used extensively in the United States and Europe. A recent SEER study showed that during 2004–2009, one of the FDA-approved ancillary tests (UroVysion® FISH, NMP22®, or BTA Stat®) was used, in addition to urine cytology, in almost a third of patients with bladder cancer [13]. However, following this peak use, the percentage of cases in which UroVysion® FISH test was employed has declined, most likely due to the lack of endorsement of the test by any of the numerous bladder cancer management guidelines, a perceived lack of benefit, uncertainly regarding its usefulness and the appropriate clinical scenario in which it should be used, and concerns about cost and reimbursement [13].

The theoretical underpinning of the use of UroVysion® is the presence of specific numerical changes (aneuploidy) in the chromosomes 3, 7, and 17, which occur most often in HGUC, and the loss of the *p16* gene located at 9p21, which is an early event in both LGUN and HGUC. It has been long known that urothelial carcinoma has two distinct pathogenetic pathways: a hyperplasia pathway leading to LGUN and a dysplasia pathway leading to HGUC. The hyperplasia pathway is more common, accounting for about 80% of cases, and starts with urothelial hyperplasia that progresses to low-grade papillary urothelial carcinoma (LGUC). One of the first molecular changes seen in the development of LGUC is the deletion of the gene *CDKN2A* (cyclin-dependent kinase inhibitor 2A), located on the short arm of chromosome 9 (9p21), which encodes the p16INK4A protein. This pathway is genetically stable and is characterized by *FGFR3* alterations, especially activating point mutations in *FGFR3*, which are detected in over 80% of LGUC.

The second pathway, the dysplasia pathway, is less frequent and leads to high-grade urothelial tumors. It starts with dysplasia, which progresses either to the formation of a high-grade papillary tumor or, in a smaller percentage of cases, to urothelial carcinoma *in situ*. This pathway is genetically unstable and is associated with a number of additional mutations; the most significant of them are inactivating mutations of *TP53*, which are seen in approximately 60% of these tumors [14].

Clinical Indications of FISH Testing

UroVysion® FISH testing has been used in four different clinical scenarios [15]:

1. Screening for urothelial carcinoma
2. Evaluation of patients with microscopic or gross hematuria
3. Surveillance of urothelial carcinoma recurrence
4. Atypical cytology or cystoscopic findings

Screening for Urothelial Carcinoma

Despite the theoretical appeal of identifying urothelial carcinomas at earlier stages and the ease of collection of a urine specimen, the US Preventive Services Task Force reviewed the published studies and deemed that there is insufficient evidence to support screening the general population of asymptomatic adults for urothelial carcinoma [16]. Since this is most likely due to the low prevalence of urothelial carcinoma in this population, more recent studies have used UroVysion® FISH testing and other urinary markers to screen high-risk populations (heavy smokers [17] and individuals with occupational exposure to known carcinogens [18]) for urothelial carcinoma. These studies have also concluded that screening for urothelial carcinoma with UroVysion® FISH testing and other urinary markers cannot be recommended, most likely because the prevalence of urothelial carcinoma is low even in these higher-risk populations. However, the use of UroVysion® FISH testing with or without concomitant urine cytology may be effective and cost-effective in certain populations at very high risk for urothelial carcinoma, based on individualized risk scores [19].

Evaluation of Patients with Microscopic or Gross Hematuria

Gross or microscopic hematuria is the main presentation symptom leading to the diagnosis of urothelial carcinoma and 20–25% of patients present with microscopic hematuria. However, while about 10% of adults with gross hematuria have underlying urothelial carcinoma, recent studies have shown that only a small minority of adult patients (less than 1% of women and up to 2% of men) with microscopic hematuria (defined as ≥3 RBCs/HPF) have underlying urothelial carcinoma, while the vast majority have no discernible underlying cause of hematuria. Therefore, despite the fact that the 2012 guideline developed by the American Urological Association (AUA) [20] recommends cystoscopy and upper urinary tract imaging for all adults over 35 with unexplained asymptomatic microscopic hematuria (AMH), the optimal management of these patients is still controversial [21]. Workup of AMH may have to be more nuanced, depending on the presence of other risk factors and the number of RBCs/HPF defining the presence of hematuria, especially in younger patients (35–50 years of age) and in women [22]. Currently, the guidelines developed in the United States, Canada, Europe, or Japan recommend cystoscopy and upper urinary tract evaluation for patients over 35, 40, or 50 years, but the use of cytology or UroVysion® FISH in the initial workup of AMH [23, 24] is either not mentioned or not recommended. These guidelines have not been prospectively validated and may change as new evidence accumulates. Recently, the Danish guideline performing urological investigation in all patients with AMH has been withdrawn [21], and an international panel of experts concluded that there is a need for better pre-cystoscopy risk assessment for patients with AMH. Because the "harms" may outweigh the benefits when working up patients with AMH with very low underlying risk of urothelial carcinoma, risk stratification of patients with AMH may reduce the need to perform cystoscopy on very low-risk patients [15]. In this context, urinary cytology and UroVysion® FISH testing may be used in conjunction with the patients' age, sex, and smoking history to better assess their risk for urothelial carcinoma.

Surveillance of Urothelial Carcinoma Recurrence

Low-grade and especially high-grade urothelial carcinomas have a strong tendency to recur after resection. Non-muscle-invasive tumors (Ta, T1), which represent about 70% of all urothelial carcinomas, have a 60–80% recurrence rate after local (transurethral) resection [25], while muscle-invasive tumors have a 2–6% upper urinary tract and 4–17% urethral post-cystectomy recurrence rate. These high recurrence rates stress the need for surveillance of patients with urothelial carcinoma to allow early detection of tumor recurrence. Surveillance recommendations vary but usually include cystoscopy and urinary cytology every 3–6 months for 2–3 years and at least yearly thereafter. UroVysion® FISH may be used in conjunction with urine cytology; negative results on both examinations may then be used to extend the interval between cystoscopies.

Bacillus Calmette-Guérin (BCG) is the recommended adjuvant intravesical therapy for intermediate- or high-risk non-muscle-invasive bladder cancer. UroVysion® FISH testing, which is not influenced by the prominent inflammatory reaction induced by BCG, can be used not only to detect recurrences but also to assess response to intravesical BCG therapy [26]. A positive FISH result at 3 months after the initiation of BCG therapy usually indicates lack of response to BCG and is associated with 4× greater risk of UC recurrence compared to patients with a negative FISH test [27]. Such patients may benefit from switching to another adjuvant intravesical therapy.

Atypical Cytology or Cystoscopic Findings

When UroVysion® FISH is used in conjunction with urinary cytology, it is important to assess the added value of using both tests over using urinary cytology alone. Of the seven diagnostic categories of The Paris System, the only

Table 16.1 The performance of UroVysion® FISH testing in cases with concomitant atypical urine cytology (atypical urothelial cells)

	Lowest	**Highest**
Sensitivity	44.6%	91.2%
Specificity	61.4%	100%
Positive predictive value	39.7%	100%
Negative predictive value	46.9%	95.9%
Accuracy	54.7%	85.7%
Positive likelihood ratio	1.22	8.00
Negative likelihood ratio	0.10	0.86

one that appears to possibly benefit from the addition of UroVysion® FISH is the AUC category, for the AUA guidelines suggest that UroVysion® FISH may be used to "adjudicate equivocal cytology" in certain clinical scenarios. Studies have shown that UroVysion® FISH testing does not offer additional benefits to the management of patients with "negative" (NHGUC), "suspicious," and "positive" cytologic diagnoses [28, 29].

The performance of UroVysion® FISH testing in the setting of AUC depends on the population's underlying prevalence of urothelial carcinoma, clinical scenario, type of urine specimen, and methodology of FISH testing ("target" FISH or FISH performed on the residual specimen). A review of the literature [30] demonstrating that the performance of UroVysion® FISH testing for AUC is presented in Table 16.1.

Based on these performance data, it seems that UroVysion® FISH testing cannot be used as a triage method, similar to cervical HPV testing for atypical squamous cells of undetermined significance (ASC-US), but rather as an additional tool for risk stratification of the patient, potentially determining the need for cystoscopy in patient with hematuria or modifying the interval between cystoscopies in patients under surveillance for urothelial carcinoma.

Technique

Fluorescence *in situ* hybridization (FISH) allows for visualization of specific DNA sequences and can, therefore, be used for quantitation of chromosomes and genes, including aneusomies, chromosomal deletions, or amplifications. The commercial assay UroVysion® (Vysis, Inc., Downers Grove, IL, USA) has made the FISH technique available for routine use in hospital cytology laboratories, but most UroVysion® tests are performed at large reference laboratories. The UroVysion® assay is composed of four single-stranded fluorescently labeled nucleic acid probes – three chromosome enumeration probes (CEP) for the chromosomes 3, 7, and 17 and the single locus-specific identifier (LSI) probe 9p21. The DNA probes are directly labeled with the four different fluorescent dyes SpectrumRed (CEP3), SpectrumGreen (CEP7), SpectrumAqua (CEP17), and SpectrumGold (LSI 9p21).

Methodology

A detailed description of the materials required for specimen preparation, hybridization, and scoring is provided in the package insert of the UroVysion® assay (Vysis, Inc./Abbott Laboratories). Several authors have suggested minor alterations to the preparation methodology as well [31]. The steps involve specimen pretreatment, denaturation and probe hybridization, post-hybridization washes, and counterstaining by 4′ 6-diamidino-2-phenylindol (DAPI), followed by scoring and interpretation using the red, green, aqua, and yellow filters at a magnification of 400X. The whole specimen is examined, including cell clusters. Nuclei are characterized as morphologically suspicious if they occur in clusters (overlapping nuclei are excluded from analysis) or are enlarged, irregular in shape, and/or are showing irregular/nonuniform (patchy) DAPI staining. A minimum number of 25 morphologically abnormal cells are initially examined. If the purpose of the UroVysion® test is the elucidation of the significance of AUC, then ideally the FISH test should be performed on the same slide as the cytological examination, which is destained and then subjected to FISH ("target FISH") with the results are read in the previously marked ("targeted") atypical cells [32]. However, this is technically demanding and is mostly done in cytology laboratories outside the United States, since the FDA-approved protocol involves the preparation of new slides, which are then subjected to FISH.

Interpretation of the Test

The UroVysion® FISH test is interpreted as "positive" if:

1. Four or more cells demonstrate polysomy (numeric gains) in two or more chromosomes (3, 7, and 17) in the same cell, i.e., four or more nuclei each show >2 red signals in any two of the centromeric probe (red and green and aqua) signals (2-4-3-2 or similar pattern).
2. At least 12 morphologically abnormal cells demonstrate homozygous loss of 9p21, i.e., show no locus-specific 9p21 (gold) signals.

If none of the above findings are present, the test is interpreted as "negative."

See Figs. 16.1a, b and 16.2a, b.

A scoring sheet can be used for recording the number of signals observed in each of the 25 most abnormal cells or the entire sample. Examples are shown in Fig. 16.3a–c. Incidentally, the evaluation and analysis of UroVysion® FISH may be automated using systems such as Bioview (Billerica, MA) (shown in Fig. 16.4), Applied Spectral Imaging (Carlsbad, CA), Ikonisys (New Haven, CT), or others. The reporting is based on the information provided by the score sheet, examples are shown in Fig. 16.5a, b.

Some alternative, modified positivity criteria and cutoff points have been proposed and may have better sensitivity and/or specificity to the manufacturer recommended FDA-approved criteria in instrumented urinary tract specimens.

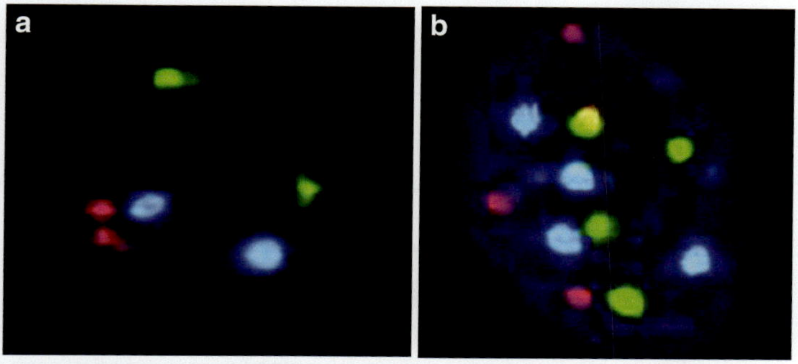

FIGURE 16.1 Negative (**a**) and positive (**b**) UroVysion® FISH test (1000×). (**a**) Note the presence of two of each red, green, and aqua signals corresponding to the centromeric probes for chromosomes 3, 7, and 17 in the cell depicted. (**b**) Nucleus showing aneuploidy, i.e., 3 red, 3 green, and 4 aqua signals in the cell depicted. Images courtesy of Ediz Cosar, MD, University of Massachusetts

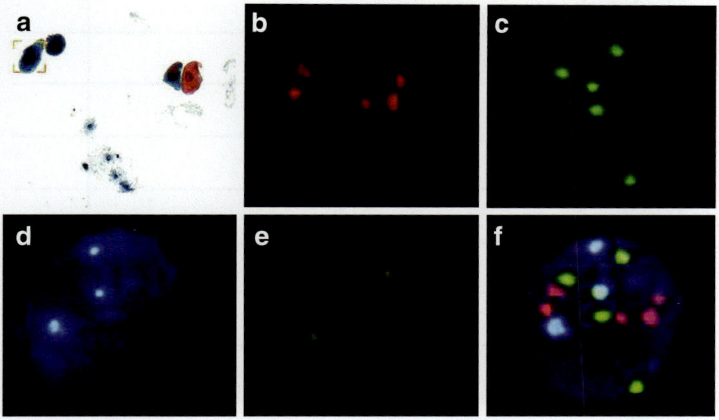

FIGURE 16.2 UroVysion® FISH test in a case of atypical urothelial cells (AUC) showing the Papanicolaou-stained cytologic preparation (**a**, 400×) and high-power (1000×) images of a nucleus with the red (**b**), green (**c**), aqua (**d**), and gold (**e**) filters and a summation image overlaying the images obtained with all four filters (**f**). The cell is aneuploid showing 5 chromosomes 3, 5 chromosomes 7, 3 chromosomes 17, and 4 9p21loci. (Images courtesy of Ediz Cosar, MD, University of Massachusetts)

a

Nucleus#	CEP 3 (RED)	CEP 7 (GREEN)	CEP 17 (AQUA)	LSI 9p21 (GOLD)	Aneu-ploidy	Homozygous deletion	Tetra-ploidy
Criterion					≥4	≥12	<10
Cell 1	2	2	1	2			
Cell 2	2	2	3	2			
Cell 3	3	2	2	2			
Cell 4	4	3	3	2	x		
Cell 5	4	4	3	0	x	x	
Cell 6	2	2	3	2			
Cell 7	3	3	2	2	x		
Cell 8	2	3	2	0		x	
Cell 9	2	4	5	2	x		
Cell 10	2	2	2	2			
Cell 11	2	2	2	2			
Cell 12	4	4	5	2	x		
Cell 13	2	2	2	2			
Cell 14	3	3	3	2	x		
Cell 15	2	2	2	2			
Cell 16	2	2	2	2			
Cell 17	5	2	3	2	x		
Cell 18	2	2	2	2			
Cell 19	2	2	2	2			
Cell 20	2	2	2	2			
Cell 21	2	2	2	2			
Cell 22	2	2	2	2			
Cell 23	2	2	2	2			
Cell 24	2	2	2	2			
Cell 25	2	2	2	2			
Cell 26							
Cell 27							
Cell 28							
Cell 29							
Cell 30							
Analysis					Present	Absent	Absent
Result						**POSITIVE**	

FIGURE 16.3 Scoring sheet of UroVysion® FISH. (**a**) Scoring lead to a "positive" test due to aneuploidy. (**b**) Scoring lead to a "positive" test due to deletion of 9p21 in more than 12 cells. (**c**) This score shows that there are nine aneuploid cells (that are tetraploid). While this would be considered positive under the FDA-approved interpretation criteria, it would be negative applying modified positivity criteria

b

Nucleus#	CEP 3 (RED)	CEP 7 (GREEN)	CEP 17 (AQUA)	LSI 9p21 (GOLD)	Aneu-ploidy	Homozygous deletion	Tetra-ploidy
Cell 1	2	2	2	2	≥4	≥12	<10
Cell 2	2	2	2	0		x	
Cell 3	2	4	2	0		x	
Cell 4	2	2	2	2			
Cell 5	2	2	2	2			
Cell 6	2	2	4	0		x	
Cell 7	2	2	2	2		x	
Cell 8	2	2	2	0		x	
Cell 9	2	2	2	2			
Cell 10	3	2	2	0		x	
Cell 11	2	2	2	2			
Cell 12	2	2	2	0		x	
Cell 13	2	3	2	0		x	
Cell 14	2	2	2	1			
Cell 15	2	2	2	0		x	
Cell 16	2	3	2	0		x	
Cell 17	2	2	2	2			
Cell 18	2	2	2	0		x	
Cell 19	2	2	2	0		x	
Cell 20	2	2	3	2		x	
Cell 21	2	2	2	2			
Cell 22	2	2	2	0		x	
Cell 23	3	2	2	0		x	
Cell 24	2	2	2	2			
Cell 25	2	2	2	2			
Cell 26							
Cell 27							
Cell 28							
Cell 29							
Cell 30							
Analysis					Absent	Present	Absent
Result						**POSITIVE**	

FIGURE 16.3 (continued)

c

Nucleus#	CEP 3 (RED)	CEP 7 (GREEN)	CEP 17 (AQUA)	LSI 9p21 (GOLD)	Aneu-ploidy	Homozygous deletion	Tetra-ploidy
Criterion					≥4	≥12	<10
Cell 1	4	4	4	4	x		x
Cell 2	8	8	8	8	x		x
Cell 3	2	4	2	0			
Cell 4	2	2	2	2			
Cell 5	4	4	4	4	x		x
Cell 6	4	4	4	4	x		x
Cell 7	2	2	2	2			
Cell 8	8	8	8	8	x		x
Cell 9	4	4	4	4	x		x
Cell 10	3	2	2	0			
Cell 11	2	2	2	2			
Cell 12	2	2	2	0			
Cell 13	4	3	4	4	x		x
Cell 14	2	2	2	2			
Cell 15	4	4	4	4	x		x
Cell 16	4	4	4	4	x		x
Cell 17	2	2	2	2			
Cell 18	2	4	2	2			
Cell 19	2	2	2	2			
Cell 20	2	2	3	0			
Cell 21	2	2	2	2			
Cell 22	2	2	2	2			
Cell 23	3	2	2	2			
Cell 24	2	2	2	2			
Cell 25	2	2	2	2			
Cell 26							
Cell 27							
Cell 28							
Cell 29							
Cell 30							
Analysis					Present	Absent	Present
Result						**POSITIVE-**	

Figure 16.3 (continued)

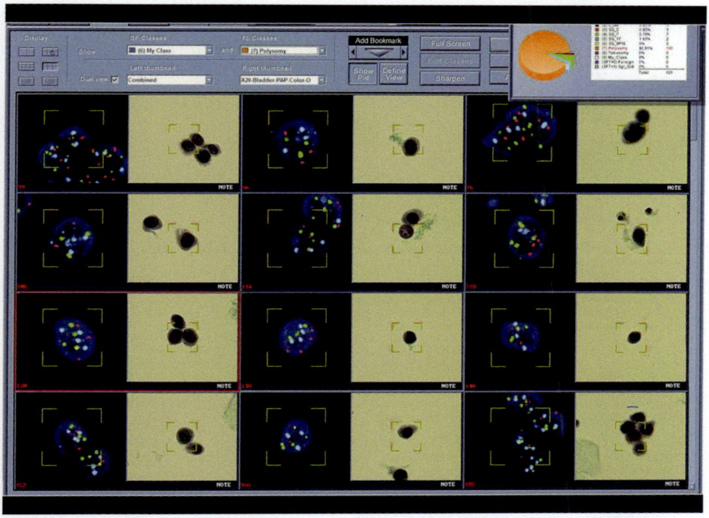

FIGURE 16.4 Automated cell imaging and analysis of UroVysion® FISH using the Bioview system. (Images courtesy of Ediz Cosar, MD, University of Massachusetts)

One of these modifications is the exclusion of 10 or fewer cells with a balanced polyploidy [33], i.e., when the number of FISH positive cells (polysomic in two or more chromosomes in the same cell), was ≥4 after subtracting the tetraploid cells. Balanced polyploidy is present when the nucleus shows 4 or 8 complete sets of chromosomes (4N or 8N) resulting in or 4 or 8 signals of each probe (a 4-4-4-4 or 8-8-8-8 pattern). In practice, such "uniform tetraploid cells" also include cases in which one of the 4 signals is absent, i.e., showing a 4-4-4-3 pattern [34, 35]. Abnormal DNA ploidy, especially tetraploidy is common in umbrella cells in normal urinary tract cytology specimens and has been well-described in bladder washes evaluated by image analysis [36]. This was particularly true when the largest and most atypical cells were selected by a cytologically inexperienced operator, who tended to

a

Addendum Diagnosis
Fluorescence In situ Hybridization (FISH) Report

Bladder Cancer Detection by Vysis (R) UroVysion*

Result:	Negative
Specimen Site/Type:	Bladder Washings
Indication for Study:	UROVYSION

Interpretation:
nuc ish (D3Z1, (D7Z1, p16, (D17Z1)x2[450]

Fluorescence in situ hybridization(FISH) analysis was performed using the Vysis UroVysion Kit on analyzable cells from urine specimens to detect aneuploidy of chromosomes 3, 7, and 17, and loss of 9p21 locus.

A total of 450 cells were examined and a negative UroVysion FISH profile was observed.

A positive UroVysion result is defined as 4 or more cells with gains of multiple chromosomes (3, 7, and/or 17) or 12 or more cells with homozygous loss of 9p21.

These results should be interpreted with caution. The criteria for positive UroVysion findings have not been established in bladder/ureteral/renal pelvis wash, instrumented, or catheterized specimens. These types of specimens often yield abundant superficial or "umbrella" cells, particularly when they are in a reactive state, are often tetraploid and, therefore, can give rise to abnormal UroVysion findings in the absence of neoplasia.

b

Addendum Diagnosis
Fluorescence In situ Hybridization (FISH) Report

Bladder Cancer Detection by Vysis (R) UroVysion*

Result:	Positive
Specimen Site/Type:	Urinary Bladder Washing
Indication for Study:	UroVysion

Interpretation:
nuc ish (D3Z1x3~6),(D7Z1x3~5),(p16x2~6),(D17Z1x2~4)[4/250]

Fluorescence in situ hybridization(FISH) analysis was performed using the Vysis UroVysion Kit on analyzable cells from bladder washing specimens to detect aneuploidy of chromosomes 3, 7, and 17, and loss of 9p21 locus.

A total of 250 cells were examined and 4 cells showed aneuploidy of at least two chromosomes (3, 7, or 17), indicating positive UroVysion FISH profile.

A positive UroVysion result is defined as 4 or more cells with gains of multiple chromosomes (3, 7, and/or 17) or 12 or more cells with homozygous loss of 9p21.

These results should be interpreted with caution. The criteria for positive UroVysion findings have not been established in bladder/ureteral/renal pelvis wash, instrumented, or catheterized specimens. These types of specimens often yield abundant superficial or "umbrella" cells, particularly when they are in a reactive state, are often tetraploid and, therefoer, can give rise to abnormal UroVysion findings in the absence of neoplasia.

FIGURE 16.5 Sample FISH reports issued as addenda to the urine cytology reports. (**a**) Sample "negative" UroVysion® FISH report. (**b**) Sample "positive" UroVysion® FISH report

predominantly score umbrella cells. Tetraploidy was also commonly seen with UroVysion® FISH in a variety of reactive conditions [32], especially in instrumented urine specimens in which umbrella cells are more numerous.

In general, if cutoff points for UroVysion® test positivity other than those recommended by the manufacturer and approved by the FDA can be used, different cutoff points could be used in different settings, since a high sensitivity and NPV of the test are preferable for patients under surveillance, whereas a high specificity and PPV are better in the primary diagnostic setting [37].

Interpretation of the UroVysion® Test Results in Clinical Context

Table 16.2 shows the overall sensitivity, specificity, and likelihood ratios of UroVysion® FISH testing, compared to cytology [38] as calculated in a meta-analysis. This meta-analysis shows that FISH testing is more sensitive and less specific than urinary cytology. FISH testing results in both false-negative and false-positive cases (Table 16.2). In addition, a variable percentage of cases (2.7–16.8%) may be not yield valid FISH results due to insufficient volume or numbers of cells or delay in testing.

False-Negative Results

These can be due to several factors, including technical factors, sample-related factors (insufficient cellularity of the sample, degenerated cells, presence of blood, inflammation/instrumentation), and tumor-related factors, including diploid tumors without *p16* deletion. However, compared to other ancillary tests, the performance of FISH testing is less impacted by the presence of blood, inflammation, prior intravesical therapy, and age of the patient [39]. A serious limitation of the current practice of reflex testing urinary cytology specimens initially diagnosed as equivocal (AUC or SHGUC) is the fact that the atypical/suspicious cells may not be present at all in the residual sample submitted for FISH testing.

Therefore a negative UroVysion® test does not rule out low-grade or high-grade urothelial carcinoma. This is especially true in urinary cytology specimens initially diagnosed as equivocal (AUC or SHGUC) (Table 16.3).

False-Positive Results

Certain circumstances can lead to problems in the FISH test resulting in a false-positive interpretation. It is well known

TABLE 16.2 The overall sensitivity, specificity, and likelihood ratios of UroVysion® FISH testing compared to cytology

	UroVysion® FISH			**Cytology**		
	Pooled	**95% CI low**	**95% CI high**	**Pooled**	**95% CI low**	**95% CI high**
Sensitivity	72%	69%	75%	42%	38%	45%
Specificity	83%	82%	85%	96%	95%	97%
Positive likelihood ratio	4.8	3.5	6.5	8.5	5.1	14.2
Negative likelihood ratio	0.3	0.2	0.4	0.6	0.6	0.7

TABLE 16.3 Reasons for false-negative and false-positive interpretation of UroVysion® FISH testing

Interpretation	Cause	Comment
False negative: Cytologically positive but FISH negative	Technical factors Sample-related factors (e.g., insufficient cellularity, degenerated cells, presence of blood, inflammation/ instrumentation) Tumor-related factors (e.g., diploid tumors without *p16* deletion)	Compared to other ancillary tests, the performance of FISH testing is less impacted by the presence of blood, inflammation, prior intravesical therapy, and age of the patient
False positive: Cytologically negative but FISH positive	Umbrella cell Polyomavirus Seminal vesicle cells	Due to polyploidy seen in these cells
False false positive	"Anticipatory positive" FISH	FISH results would be false positives, if only histologic results obtained within a 3–12-month follow-up period have been considered and have been termed "anticipatory positive" results

that umbrella cells, cells showing polyomavirus cytopathic changes, and seminal vesicle cells can be aneuploid and have an abnormal FISH pattern. A positive urinary FISH test after radiation therapy (in the pelvic field for prostate or endometrial cancer) and/or chemotherapy (local or systemic) must also be interpreted with caution, as both can lead to persistent chromosomal aberrations. It is therefore important to interpret FISH findings in the context of the morphologic findings of the urine cytology as well as the clinical setting.

Due to the occurrence of such false-positive results, a positive UroVysion® test result does not indicate a more aggressive workup of patients with an equivocal cytology result and a negative cystoscopic evaluation [30].

"False False-Positive" Results or Anticipatory Positive FISH Results

In the study by Yoder et al. [40], some of the patients with positive FISH results with concomitant negative or atypical urine cytology and negative initial cystoscopic examination developed recurrent UC beyond the study follow-up period but within 29 months of the FISH test results. These FISH results would be false positives, if only histologic results obtained within a 3–12-month follow-up period had been considered, and have been termed "anticipatory positive" results. According to this study, for 56 cases with a positive FISH result, there was a 65% chance (95% CI, 50%–80%) of developing recurrent UC within 29 months of having a the positive FISH test. However, this has not been confirmed in other studies [30]. For example, the largest study regarding the use of UroVysion® FISH in the setting of AUC found a high false-positive rate (28/53, 53%) that remained high even after extended follow-up (up to 36 months), arguing against a significant contribution of "anticipatory positive" results, and supporting the interpretation that instrumented urine specimens, which made up the majority of cases in the study, can give false-positive results due to the presence of high numbers of reactive umbrella cells.

Utilization Guidelines

As previously mentioned, the FDA has approved the UroVysion® FISH test to be used in conjunction with current standard diagnostic procedures for the following:

- Initial diagnosis of bladder carcinoma in patients with hematuria
- Subsequent monitoring for tumor recurrence in patients previously diagnosed with bladder cancer

According to the Center for Medicare Services (CMS), only one bladder cancer test per single date of service is considered reasonable and necessary. For high-risk patients with persistent hematuria and an initial negative FISH test result, one repeat FISH test within 1 year of the original attempted diagnosis, in conjunction with cystoscopy, is considered reasonable and necessary.

Billing Codes for UroVysion® Testing

The CPT codes for UroVysion® FISH are 88120 and 88121, but not codes 88271, 88274, or 88291, as outlined in Table 16.4.

In conclusion, the judicious use of this test in select clinical circumstances requires cost considerations, in addition to having a clear understanding of the limitations of the test and issues related to its interpretation.

Table 16.4 Billing codes (CPT codes) for UroVysion® FISH testing

CPT code	Description
88120	Cytopathology, *in situ* hybridization (e.g., FISH), urinary tract specimen with morphometric analysis, 3–5 molecular probes, each specimen; manual
88121	Cytopathology, *in situ* hybridization (e.g., FISH), urinary tract specimen with morphometric analysis, 3–5 molecular probes, each specimen; using computer-assisted technology
88271	Molecular cytogenetic, DNA probe, each
88274	Interphase *in situ* hybridization, analyze 25–99 cells, each
88291	Molecular cytogenetic, interpretation and report

References

1. Siegel RL, Miller KD, Jemal A. Cancer statistics, 2017. CA Cancer J Clin. 2017;67(1):7–30.
2. Power NE, Izawa J. Comparison of guidelines on non-muscle invasive bladder Cancer (EAU, CUA, AUA, NCCN, NICE). Bladder Cancer. 2016;2(1):27–36.
3. Yafi FA, Brimo F, Auger M, Aprikian A, Tanguay S, Kassouf W. Is the performance of urinary cytology as high as reported historically? A contemporary analysis in the detection and surveillance of bladder cancer. Urol Oncol. 2014;32(1):27.e21–6.
4. Amin MB, Smith SC, Reuter VE, et al. Update for the practicing pathologist: the international consultation on urologic disease-European association of urology consultation on bladder cancer. Mod Pathol. 2015;28(5):612–30.
5. Wojcik EM. Urine cytology, DNA ploidy and morphometry. In: Lokeshwar VB, editor. Bladder tumors: molecular aspects and clinical management, cancer drug discovery and development. New York: Springer Science+Business Media; 2011. p. 79–90.
6. Cajulis RS, Haines GK 3rd, Frias-Hidvegi D, McVary K, Bacus JW. Cytology, flow cytometry, image analysis, and interphase cytogenetics by fluorescence in situ hybridization in the diagnosis of transitional cell carcinoma in bladder washes: a comparative study. Diagn Cytopathol. 1995;13(3):214–23; discussion 224
7. Meloni AM, Peier AM, Haddad FS, et al. A new approach in the diagnosis and follow-up of bladder cancer. FISH analysis of urine, bladder washings, and tumors. Cancer Genet Cytogenet. 1993;71(2):105–18.
8. Cajulis RS, Haines GK 3rd, Frias-Hidvegi D, McVary K. Interphase cytogenetics as an adjunct in the cytodiagnosis of urinary bladder carcinoma. A comparative study of cytology, flow cytometry and interphase cytogenetics in bladder washes. Anal Quant Cytol Histol. 1994;16(1):1–10.
9. Pycha A, Mian C, Haitel A, Hofbauer J, Wiener H, Marberger M. Fluorescence in situ hybridization identifies more aggressive types of primarily noninvasive (stage pTa) bladder cancer. J Urol. 1997;157(6):2116–9.
10. Zhang FF, Arber DA, Wilson TG, Kawachi MH, Slovak ML. Toward the validation of aneusomy detection by fluorescence in situ hybridization in bladder cancer: comparative analysis with cytology, cytogenetics, and clinical features predicts

recurrence and defines clinical testing limitations. Clin Cancer Res. 1997;3(12 Pt 1):2317–28.
11. Sokolova IA, Halling KC, Jenkins RB, et al. The development of a multitarget, multicolor fluorescence in situ hybridization assay for the detection of urothelial carcinoma in urine. J Mol Diagn. 2000;2(3):116–23.
12. Halling KC, King W, Sokolova IA, et al. A comparison of cytology and fluorescence in situ hybridization for the detection of urothelial carcinoma. J Urol. 2000;164(5):1768–75.
13. Narayan VM, Adejoro O, Schwartz I, Ziegelmann M, Elliott S, Konety BR. The prevalence and impact of urinary marker testing in patients with bladder Cancer. J Urol. 2018;199(1):74–80.
14. Sanli O, Dobruch J, Knowles MA, et al. Bladder cancer. Nat Rev Dis Primers. 2017;3:17022.
15. Clinton T, Lotan Y. Review of the clinical approaches to the use of urine-based tumor markers in bladder cancer. Rambam Maimonides Med J. 2017;8(4):1–10. https://www.ncbi.nlm.nih.gov/pmc/articles/PMC5652931/pdf/rmmj-8-4-e0040.pdf.
16. Moyer VA, Force USPST. Screening for bladder cancer: U.S. Preventive Services Task Force recommendation statement. Ann Intern Med. 2011;155(4):246–51.
17. Steiner H, Bergmeister M, Verdorfer I, et al. Early results of bladder-cancer screening in a high-risk population of heavy smokers. BJU Int. 2008;102(3):291–6.
18. Pesch B, Taeger D, Johnen G, et al. Screening for bladder cancer with urinary tumor markers in chemical workers with exposure to aromatic amines. Int Arch Occup Environ Health. 2014;87(7):715–24.
19. Vickers AJ, Bennette C, Kibel AS, et al. Who should be included in a clinical trial of screening for bladder cancer?: a decision analysis of data from the prostate, lung, colorectal and ovarian Cancer screening trial. Cancer. 2013;119(1):143–9.
20. Davis R, Jones JS, Barocas DA, et al. Diagnosis, evaluation and follow-up of asymptomatic microhematuria (AMH) in adults: AUA guideline. J Urol. 2012;188(6 Suppl):2473–81.
21. Ordell Sundelin M, Jensen JB. Asymptomatic microscopic hematuria as a predictor of neoplasia in the urinary tract. Scand J Urol. 2017;51(5):373–5.
22. Committee on Gynecologic Practice AUS. Committee opinion No.703: asymptomatic microscopic hematuria in women. Obstet Gynecol. 2017;129(6):e168–72.

23. Linder BJ, Bass EJ, Mostafid H, Boorjian SA. Guideline of guidelines: asymptomatic microscopic haematuria. BJU Int. 2018;121(2):176–83.
24. Schmitz-Drager BJ, Kuckuck EC, Zuiverloon TC, et al. Microhematuria assessment an IBCN consensus-based upon a critical review of current guidelines. Urol Oncol. 2016;34(10):437–51.
25. Nepple KG, O'Donnell MA. The optimal management of T1 high-grade bladder cancer. Can Urol Ass J. 2009;3(6 Suppl 4):S188–92.
26. Chang SS, Boorjian SA, Chou R, et al. Diagnosis and treatment of non-muscle invasive bladder Cancer: AUA/SUO guideline. J Urol. 2016;196(4):1021–9.
27. Liem E, Baard J, Cauberg ECC, et al. Fluorescence in situ hybridization as prognostic predictor of tumor recurrence during treatment with Bacillus Calmette-Guerin therapy for intermediate- and high-risk non-muscle-invasive bladder cancer. Medical Oncol (Northwood, London, England). 2017;34(10):172.
28. Bubendorf L, Piaton E. UroVysion(R) multiprobe FISH in the triage of equivocal urinary cytology cases. Ann Pathol. 2012;32(6):e52–6, 438–43
29. Youssef RF, Schlomer BJ, Ho R, Sagalowsky AI, Ashfaq R, Lotan Y. Role of fluorescence in situ hybridization in bladder cancer surveillance of patients with negative cytology. Urol Oncol. 2012;30(3):273–7.
30. Virk RK, Abro S, de Ubago JMM, et al. The value of the UroVysion(R) FISH assay in the risk-stratification of patients with "atypical urothelial cells" in urinary cytology specimens. Diagn Cytopathol. 2017;45(6):481–500.
31. Bubendorf L, Grilli B. UroVysion multiprobe FISH in urinary cytology. Methods Mol Med. 2004;97:117–31.
32. Savic S, Bubendorf L. Common fluorescence in situ hybridization applications in cytology. Arch Pathol Lab Med. 2016;140(12):1323–30.
33. Zellweger T, Benz G, Cathomas G, et al. Multi-target fluorescence in situ hybridization in bladder washings for prediction of recurrent bladder cancer. Int J Cancer. 2006;119(7):1660–5.
34. Moatamed NA, Apple SK, Bennett CJ, et al. Exclusion of the uniform tetraploid cells significantly improves specificity of the urine FISH assay. Diagn Cytopathol. 2013;41(3):218–25.
35. Zhou AG, Liu Y, Cyr MS, et al. Role of Tetrasomy for the diagnosis of urothelial carcinoma using UroVysion fluorescent in situ hybridization. Arch Pathol Lab Med. 2016;140(6):552–9.

36. Wojcik EM, Brownlie RJ, Bassler TJ, Miller MC. Superficial urothelial (umbrella) cells. A potential cause of abnormal DNA ploidy results in urine specimens. Anal Quant Cytol Histol. 2000;22(5):411–5.
37. Mischinger J, Guttenberg LP, Hennenlotter J, et al. Comparison of different concepts for interpretation of chromosomal aberrations in urothelial cells detected by fluorescence in situ hybridization. J Cancer Res Clin Oncol. 2017;143(4):677–85.
38. Hajdinjak T. UroVysion FISH test for detecting urothelial cancers: meta-analysis of diagnostic accuracy and comparison with urinary cytology testing. Urol Oncol. 2008;26(6):646–51.
39. Horstmann M, Todenhofer T, Hennenlotter J, et al. Influence of age on false positive rates of urine-based tumor markers. World J Urol. 2013;31(4):935–40.
40. Yoder BJ, Skacel M, Hedgepeth R, et al. Reflex UroVysion testing of bladder cancer surveillance patients with equivocal or negative urine cytology: a prospective study with focus on the natural history of anticipatory positive findings. Am J Clin Pathol. 2007;127(2):295–301.

Chapter 17
Molecular Diagnostics in Hematologic Malignancies

Rashmi Kanagal-Shamanna

Abbreviations

ABL1	ABL proto-oncogene 1
ALCL	Anaplastic large-cell lymphoma
ALK	Anaplastic lymphoma kinase or ALK receptor tyrosine kinase
ASXL1	Additional sex combs like 1
ATRA	All-trans-retinoic acid
BCL2/BCL6/BCL10	B-cell CLL/lymphoma 2/6/10
BCR	Breakpoint cluster region
BIRC3	Baculoviral IAP repeat-containing protein 3
BRAF	V-raf murine sarcoma viral oncogene homolog B
BTK	Bruton tyrosine kinase

R. Kanagal-Shamanna
Department of Hematopathology and Molecular Diagnostics, The University of Texas MD Anderson Cancer Center, Houston, TX, USA
e-mail: rkanagal@mdanderson.org

S. Roy-Chowdhuri et al. (eds.), *Molecular Diagnostics in Cytopathology*, https://doi.org/10.1007/978-3-319-97397-5_17

CEBPA	CCAAT-enhancer-binding protein alpha
CHOP	Cyclophosphamide, hydroxydaunorubicin (doxorubicin or Adriamycin), Oncovin (vincristine), and prednisone
CNS	Central nervous system
COO	Cell of origin
CXCR4	C-X-C motif chemokine receptor 4
DNA	Deoxyribonucleic acid
DNMT3A	DNA methyltransferase 3 alpha
DUSP22	Dual specificity phosphatase 22
EBV	Epstein-Barr virus
FDA	Food and Drug Administration
FFPE	Formalin-fixed paraffin-embedded
FISH	Fluorescence *in situ* hybridization
FL	Follicular lymphoma
FLT3	Fms-related tyrosine kinase 3
FNA	Fine-needle aspiration
FOXP1	Forkhead box P1
GEP	Gene expression profile
IDH	Isocitrate dehydrogenase
IGH	Immunoglobulin heavy chain locus
IGHV	Immunoglobulin heavy chain variable region
KIT	KIT proto-oncogene receptor tyrosine kinase
KRAS	Kirsten rat sarcoma viral oncogene homolog
MALT1	Mucosa-associated lymphoid tissue lymphoma translocation gene 1
MAP2K1	Mitogen-activated protein kinase 1
MYC	V-myc avian myelocytomatosis viral oncogene homolog
MYD88	Myeloid differentiation primary response 88
NK	Natural killer
NGS	Next-generation sequencing
NOTCH1	Notch (*Drosophila*) homolog 1 (translocation-associated)
NPM1	Nucleophosmin 1
PAX-5	Paired box 5
PDGFRA	Platelet-derived growth factor receptor alpha
PLCG2	Phospholipase C gamma 2

qPCR	Quantitative polymerase chain reaction
RUNX1	Runt-related transcription factor 1
SF3B1	Splicing factor 3b subunit 1
TCL1A	T-cell leukemia/lymphoma 1A
TCR	T-cell receptor
TET2	Tet methylcytosine dioxygenase 2
TP53/63	Tumor protein p53/p63

Key Points

- In hematologic malignancies, molecular testing of cytology specimens can be extremely useful in the context of tissue-based malignancies such as lymphomas and myeloid sarcomas when the source of nucleic acids can be limited
- Assessment of VDJ rearrangements in immunoglobulin heavy chain (IgH) and T-cell receptor (TCR) beta or gamma genes by PCR-based assays is a valuable adjunct for differentiating neoplastic and reactive B-cell and T-cell lymphoproliferative disorders
- Small B-cell lymphomas:
  - Assessment of characteristic translocations by either FISH or RT-PCR is useful for diagnosis, subclassification, and monitoring
  - Lymphoplasmacytic lymphoma is frequently associated with *MYD88* mutation; *CXCR4* mutation status is helpful to predict prognosis
  - Unmutated *IGHV* is associated with decreased survival in CLL/SLL independent of disease stage and high-risk genomic abnormalities
- Large B-cell lymphomas:
  - *MYC* rearrangement is prognostic in diffuse large B-cell lymphomas; in addition to *MYC*, testing for rearrangements in *BCL2* and *BCL6* genes is

  essential for the recognition of double-hit and triple-hit high-grade B-cell lymphomas
  - To determine the cell-of-origin classification, immunohistochemistry is often used as a surrogate for gene expression analysis
- *BRAF* mutations in hairy cell leukemia and Langerhans cell histiocytosis, as well as *MAP2K1* mutations in hairy cell leukemia variant, are useful for targeted therapeutics with vemurafenib and MEK inhibitors, respectively
- Currently, FDA has approved drugs for targeted therapies in AML with mutations in *IDH1*/2 and *FLT3* gene mutations
- Screening for drug resistance mutations is an important monitoring tool in CML treated with TKIs for *BCR/ABL1* kinase domain mutations, and CLL treated with B-cell signaling pathway inhibitors for mutations in *BTK* and *PLCG2* genes
- *In situ* hybridization for EBV-encoded mRNA (EBER) and PCR for viral DNA is used for the diagnosis of classical Hodgkin lymphomas, B-cell and T-cell/NK non-Hodgkin lymphomas, as well as monitoring lymphoproliferative disorders arising in the setting of immunodeficiency such as post-stem cell transplantation
- In post-allogeneic stem cell transplant patients, microsatellite-based chimerism assays are performed at regular intervals to monitor donor engraftment and determine the donor versus recipient origin of tumor

Precision medicine is currently the standard of care in most hematologic malignancies. Clinical trials targeting molecular biomarkers are ongoing for many others [1]. Since molecular testing is integral for personalized therapy, it has become a critical aspect of patient management. Within the setting of a broader multidisciplinary team, pathologists are at the forefront to process diagnostic specimens and facilitate appropriate triaging for various ancillary testing [2]. Blood-based hematologic malignancies such as leukemia(s) generally have abundant and easy access to diagnostic material for molecular work-up such as bone marrow aspirates and peripheral blood specimens. The role of FNA cytology aspirates and small biopsies comes into play in the diagnostics of tissue-based hematologic malignancies and in specific contexts of blood-based malignancies as detailed below:

1. Diagnostic work-up of tissue-based hematologic malignancies:
   (a) Myeloid sarcoma
   (b) Extramedullary B-cell lymphoblastic lymphoma(s)
   (c) B-cell and T-cell lymphoma(s)
   (d) Histiocytic neoplasms such as follicular dendritic cell sarcomas, Langerhans cell histiocytosis
   (e) Rosai-Dorfman disease
2. Involvement of CSF and serous effusions
3. Testing precluded on bone marrow aspirates due to limited neoplastic cells due to (a) marrow fibrosis such as hairy cell leukemia, (b) underestimation of plasmacytic component by flow cytometry as in lymphoplasmacytic lymphoma, and (c) technically poor BM.

With the increasing use of minimally invasive procedures, judicious use of the specimen for morphology, immunohistochemistry, flow cytometry, cytogenetic, and molecular genetic work-up is needed. Specifically, for molecular testing of hematologic malignancies, the need for simultaneous assessment of gene mutations, copy number assessment, translocations, gene expression, etc. warrants an adequate amount of high-quality nucleic acids. However, since the diagnosis of malignancy is often not anticipated, these cases lack fresh or frozen tissue for genomic testing. It is difficult to obtain high-quality DNA from FFPE samples. In these instances, molecular testing on FNA specimens offers distinct advantages compared to FFPE specimens. FNA provides unprocessed high-molecular-weight nucleic acids; the quantitative tumor burden information based on the concurrent multi-parametric flow cytometry analysis is readily available for use in downstream interpretation [3].

A wide variety of molecular aberrations are present in hematological malignancies. Often times, these malignancies have to be screened for multiple types of genetic aberrations, thus requiring DNA- and RNA-based testing. Hence, a multimodal approach for molecular biomarker assessment, when feasible, is preferred. Further, judicious utilization of these limited FNA specimens and FFPE blocks is essential, thereby underscoring the important role of the cytopathologist in triaging samples for effective integration of molecular ancillary testing.

Lymphoid Malignancies

Molecular testing is a critical adjunct for personalized therapy in lymphoid malignancies and provides valuable information for diagnosis, prognostication, and treatment selection.

Translocations

In lymphoid malignancies, identification of characteristic translocations can facilitate diagnosis, subtyping, and prognostication. Detection of t(11;14) is diagnostic for mantle cell lymphoma [4–7]. Both FISH and PCR-based testing have been well established in cytology specimens. FISH offers a distinct advantage of higher detection yield in most cases due to significant breakpoint heterogeneity that limits the proportion of translocations that can be interrogated by PCR, such as in mantle cell lymphoma. However, qPCR, if positive, can be used for the evaluation of minimal residual disease [8–10]. In the right clinical and morphologic context, molecular studies for characteristic translocations can help in subtyping specific types of small B-cell lymphomas. FISH studies can be easily performed on fine-needle aspirates from follicular lymphoma (FL) for t(14;18)(q32;q21) [4, 11–13], which is seen in more than 90% of low-grade FL. Marginal zone lymphomas have a variety of translocations, such as t(11;18)(q21;q21) *BIRC3-MALT1* in gastric and pulmonary locations, t(14;18)(q32;q21) *IGH@-MALT1* in ocular adnexa, t(3;14)(p14.1;q32) *FOXP1-IGH@* in thyroid, and t(1;14)(p22;q32) *IGH@-BCL10* in lung [4]. In these occasions, molecular results serve as valuable adjuncts to support a suspected diagnosis. In addition, translocations are important in prognostication of large B-cell lymphomas. Burkitt lymphoma is characterized by the presence of t(8;14)(q24;q32) involving *MYC* and *IGH@* or, rarely, kappa or lambda light chains. In diffuse large B-cell lymphoma (DLBCL), *MYC* rearrangement is associated with poor prognosis. For high-grade B-cell lymphomas, testing for translocations in *MYC*, *BCL2,* and *BCL6* is a part of routine standard of care for appropriate management due to poor outcome seen in these patients. These are designated as double-hit and triple-hit lymphomas in the new 2016 WHO classification system. Similarly, in T-cell lymphomas, *ALK* rearrangement, most frequent being t(2;5)(p23;q35), is seen in ALK-positive anaplastic large-cell lymphoma (ALCL) cases, although ALK positivity by immunohistochemistry is an easy surrogate marker for FISH [14]. Among *ALK*-negative ALCL, predictive biomarkers include *DUSP22* rearrangement, which has a favorable outcome, and *TP63* rearrangement, which may portend a poor outcome [15]. T-prolymphocytic leukemia often presents with cutaneous involvement and is associated with *TCL1* rearrangement or inversion in majority of cases [16].

In addition to translocations, characteristic chromosomal alterations have a significant role in prognostic evaluation of chronic lymphocytic leukemia (CLL)/small lymphocytic lymphoma (SLL). While translocations are rare in CLL/SLL, standard gene copy number assessment for del(13q), del(11q), del(17p), and trisomy 12, routinely performed by either FISH or array-based comparative genomic hybridization, is prognostic beyond other clinical factors [17, 18]. Although not of similar significance, abnormalities such as trisomy of chromosomes 3, 7, and 18 and loss of chromosome 7q are frequent in marginal zone B-cell and splenic marginal zone B-cell lymphomas, respectively.

Gene Mutation Analysis

Multi-gene mutation profiling can be readily performed using next-generation sequencing or other techniques on FNA specimens from suspected lymphoma [19–21]. Testing for *MYD88* L265P and *CXCR4* mutations is a routine practice for lymphoplasmacytic lymphoma (LPL). LPL can involve lymph nodes and extranodal sites affected by marginal zone B-cell lymphoma, and the differential diagnosis between the two entities is extremely difficult. *MYD88* mutations are seen in over 90% of patients with LPL [22]. Identification of *MYD88* mutation favors the diagnosis of LPL. In addition to diagnosis, the knowledge of *MYD88* and *CXCR4* mutation status is useful for prognostication of LPL. Further, *CXCR4* mutations are associated with inferior response to ibrutinib therapy [23, 24]. Similarly, gene mutation analysis is integral to the work-up of CLL/SLL due to prognostic value. Rossi et al. have proposed an integrated prognostic model combining gene mutations in *NOTCH1*, *SF3B1,* and *BIRC3* and standard FISH abnormalities [25]. However, other than *TP53* aberrations, most other mutations do not influence the choice of treatment at this time [17]. Hairy cell leukemia and variant can rarely present in extramedullary sites [26]. Hairy cell leukemia is characterized by a high frequency of *BRAF* mutations [27] and has shown good response with vemurafenib, which is a potent inhibitor of kinase domain [28]. A subset of variant hairy cell leukemia cases with certain *MAP2K1* mutations may respond to MEK inhibitors [29]. Potentially targetable clonal genetic aberrations have also been identified in the histiocytic disorders, such as *BRAF* V600E mutations in Langerhans cell histiocytosis [30] and *KRAS* and *MAP2K1* mutations in Rosai-Dorfman disease [31].

Gene Expression Profiling

Gene expression profiling (GEP) has identified two distinct biological subtypes of DLBCL based on cell of origin (COO) – germinal center versus activated B-cell phenotype [32]. Determination of the COO subtype is important for clinical trials for prognosis and may warrant modification to the standard R-CHOP regimens [33]. While determination of COO subtype by GEP is not a standard of practice due to the need for fresh tissue, adjunct low-density gene expression assays applicable for FFPE specimens are potentially available [34–36]. FNA specimens have been shown to be feasible alternates for transcription profiling of lymphomas [37].

Myeloid Malignancies

In myeloid malignancies, the role of molecular biomarkers cannot be overemphasized for the purposes of (1) diagnosis, (2) prognostication, (3) selection of therapy, and (4) monitoring of minimal residual disease. Cytopathology plays a major role in molecular profiling of leukemias presenting as soft tissue masses (myeloid sarcomas), effusions, or CNS-based disease. Each of the hematologic malignancies has a characteristic chromosomal genomic profile, including copy number changes and copy-neutral heterozygosity, which can be assessed using microarray platforms in addition to gene translocations and mutation analysis [38]. However, for the purpose of this chapter, we will only focus on gene translocations and gene mutations.

Gene Translocations

Similar to their medullary counterparts, detection of specific genetic alterations is critical for diagnosis and subclassification within the broader diagnostic categories. Generally, selected translocations are tested using FISH or PCR-based assays depending on the morphologic suspicion. These include abnormal eosinophils in AML with inv(16), B-cell markers such as PAX-5 expression in blasts of AML with t(8;21), and bilobed "apple-core" morphology of blasts with strong myeloperoxidase expression in acute promyelocytic leukemia with t(15;17). These specific translocations are important to identify due to distinct prognostic outcome that may warrant a specific therapy, such as ATRA therapy for acute promyelocytic leukemia, a subtype of AML, defined by t(15;17). Similarly, chronic myeloid leukemia patients and a subset of B-lymphoblastic leukemia/ lymphoma with *BCR/ABL1* rearrangement, myeloid/lymphoid neoplasms with rearrangements involving *PDGFRA*, and advanced systemic mastocytosis without *KIT* D816V mutation respond to treatment with tyrosine kinase inhibitors [39–42]. Advances in nanofluidic technology have permitted simultaneous screening for many of these translocations with limited amounts of RNA. PCR-based assays for the translocations permit evaluation of residual disease; however, these are feasible in peripheral blood or bone marrow.

Gene Mutations

Advances in NGS-based technology have shed extensive light on the spectrum of gene mutations in AML and other myeloid neoplasms. The 2016 WHO classification of AML has formally incorporated the entities of AML with mutated *NPM1* and AML with bi-allelic *CEBPA* mutations and the provisional entity of AML with mutated *RUNX1* [43]. In addition, several gene mutations such as *FLT3, TET2, ASXL1, DNMT3A, IDH1, IDH2,* and *TP53* are of prognostic significance. Some of the gene mutations have been incorporated into the NCCN guidelines and 2017 ELN risk stratification of AML [44, 45]; ELN includes, in addition to cytogenetic abnormalities and translocations, mutations in *NPM1, FLT3, CEBPA, RUNX1, ASXL1,* and *TP53*. The feasible mode of interrogating these mutations would be by a multi-gene NGS panel almost routinely done in most laboratories. Non-formalin-fixed FNA specimens provide high-molecular-weight DNA that permits testing for a broader spectrum of mutations than might be possible from FFPE cell blocks; hence, procuring adequate material up front for molecular testing is important. A recent significant development included FDA approval of two drugs for targeted treatment of AML with mutated *FLT3* or mutated *IDH* [46, 47]. Testing for these gene mutations, at a minimum, is warranted to identify targets of therapy in addition to several gene mutations in clinical trials. And with the rapid evolution in the field of molecular biomarkers, this list is likely to increase in the future.

Resistance Mutations

With the availability and use of drugs that target specific pathways, tumors can develop mutations leading to drug resistance. Examples include mutations in the *BCR/ABL1* kinase domain for tyrosine kinase inhibitors in CML [48] and, more recently, mutations in *BTK* and *PLCG2* genes in CLL patients treated with ibrutinib [49]. Consequentially, testing for resistance mutations while on treatment is an important aspect of monitoring and is emerging as standard of care testing. Often, due to the need for early detection of these drug resistance mutations, testing requires the use of a highly sensitive technique with a much lower limit of detection than that used at the time of initiation of treatment.

Malignancy-Associated Viruses

Molecular testing for malignancy-associated viruses, specifically Epstein-Barr virus, plays an important role in the diagnosis and monitoring of a variety of hematologic conditions including classical Hodgkin lymphomas, B-cell and T-cell/NK non-Hodgkin lymphomas, as well as lymphoproliferative disorders arising in the setting of immunodeficiency such as post-stem cell transplantation [50–53]. Molecular techniques such as *in situ* hybridization for EBV-encoded mRNA (EBER) and PCR for viral DNA are standard clinical practices for diagnosis and monitoring. In certain conditions, such as post-stem cell transplant, EBV status guides disease management; hence sensitive PCR-based techniques are vital.

Other Molecular Assays Unique to Hematologic Malignancies

In addition to translocations, copy number assessments, and mutation analysis, certain tests are unique to hematologic malignancies.

Differentiation of low-grade lymphomas and reactive lymphoid proliferations can be very challenging despite the use of standard immunohistochemical ancillary techniques [54]. In addition to genetic translocations and mutations, the identification of monoclonal gene rearrangements, e.g., VDJ rearrangements in immunoglobulin heavy chain (IgH) and T-cell receptor (TCR) beta or gamma genes, is a useful adjunct in diagnostically challenging cases, and often essential for interpreting skin biopsies [3, 4, 9, 54–58]. Clinical testing for monoclonal gene rearrangements plays a vital role in identifying the neoplastic nature of lymphoid proliferations. In order to achieve consensus across institutions with respect to primers and procedures and hence avoid false-negatives and false-positives, EuroClonality/BIOMED-2 consortium was established to standardize testing methods across the institutions [59–63]. Once a monoclonal rearrangement has been identified, it can be used as a biomarker for serial follow-up to monitor residual disease. This is especially feasible in the context of the development of NGS-based clonality testing that can provide patient-specific sequence at sufficient sensitivity. *IGHV* mutational status (aka somatic hypermutation) is a standard of care test in CLL/SLL. Unmutated *IGHV* (defined as greater than or equal to 98% sequence homology with germline) is associated with decreased survival independent of disease stage and high-risk genomic abnormalities [64, 65]. Use of VH3-21 is associated with poor survival irrespective of the mutation status [66]. In hairy cell leukemia, a minor subset of cases showing unmutated *IGHV* is associated with refractoriness to single-agent cladribine [67]. Further, hairy cell leukemia and variant with VH4-34 usage is associated with poor prognosis and absent *BRAF* mutations [68, 69]. Currently NGS-based techniques using high-molecular-weight DNA are often employed to accurately determine the degree of somatic hypermutation and the sequence and, hence, could be potentially assessed on FNA specimens [70]. In post-allogeneic stem cell transplant patients, microsatellite-based chimerism assays are performed at regular intervals to monitor donor engraftment and determine the donor versus recipient origin of tumor.

In summary, molecular testing is a crucial component of evaluation and management of hematologic malignancies. FNA cytology specimens are especially well suited for testing in hematologic malignancies as they provide adequate amounts of high-molecular-weight DNA; the interpretation of the results can be done in the context of the estimated tumor burden by simultaneous flow cytometry analysis. The importance of integrating molecular testing along with other diagnostic modalities including histopathologic evaluation, flow cytometry immunophenotypic analysis, and cytogenetic studies cannot be overemphasized.

References

1. Kanagal-Shamanna R, Singh RR, Routbort MJ, Patel KP, Medeiros LJ, Luthra R. Principles of analytical validation of next-generation sequencing based mutational analysis for hematologic neoplasms in a CLIA-certified laboratory. Expert Rev Mol Diagn. 2016;16(4):461–72.
2. Dietel M. Molecular pathology: a requirement for precision medicine in cancer. Oncol Res Treat. 2016;39(12):804–10.

3. Peluso AL, Ieni A, Mignogna C, Zeppa P. Lymph node fine-needle cytology: beyond flow cytometry. Acta Cytol. 2016;60(4):372–84.
4. Ochs RC, Bagg A. Molecular genetic characterization of lymphoma: application to cytology diagnosis. Diagn Cytopathol. 2012;40(6):542–55.
5. da Cunha Santos G, Ko HM, Geddie WR, Boerner SL, Lai SW, Have C, et al. Targeted use of fluorescence in situ hybridization (FISH) in cytospin preparations: results of 298 fine needle aspirates of B-cell non-Hodgkin lymphoma. Cancer Cytopathol. 2010;118(5):250–8.
6. Bentz JS, Rowe LR, Anderson SR, Gupta PK, McGrath CM. Rapid detection of the t(11;14) translocation in mantle cell lymphoma by interphase fluorescence in situ hybridization on archival cytopathologic material. Cancer. 2004;102(2):124–31.
7. Caraway NP, Gu J, Lin P, Romaguera JE, Glassman A, Katz R. The utility of interphase fluorescence in situ hybridization for the detection of the translocation t(11;14)(q13;q32) in the diagnosis of mantle cell lymphoma on fine-needle aspiration specimens. Cancer. 2005;105(2):110–8.
8. Baró C, Espinet B, Salido M, García M, Sánchez B, Florensa L, et al. Cryptic IGH/BCL2 rearrangements with variant FISH patterns in follicular lymphoma. Leuk Res. 2011;35(2):256–9.
9. Grosso LE, Collins BT. DNA polymerase chain reaction using fine needle aspiration biopsy smears to evaluate non-Hodgkin's lymphoma. Acta Cytol. 1999;43(5):837–41.
10. Rambaldi A, Carlotti E, Oldani E, Della Starza I, Baccarani M, Cortelazzo S, et al. Quantitative PCR of bone marrow BCL2/IgH(+) cells at diagnosis predicts treatment response and long-term outcome in follicular non-Hodgkin lymphoma. Blood. 2005;105(9):3428–33.
11. Richmond J, Bryant R, Trotman W, Beatty B, Lunde J. FISH detection of t(14;18) in follicular lymphoma on Papanicolaou-stained archival cytology slides. Cancer. 2006;108(3):198–204.
12. Safley AM, Buckley PJ, Creager AJ, Dash RC, Dodd LG, Goodman BK, et al. The value of fluorescence in situ hybridization and polymerase chain reaction in the diagnosis of B-cell non-Hodgkin lymphoma by fine-needle aspiration. Arch Pathol Lab Med. 2004;128(12):1395–403.
13. Gong Y, Caraway N, Gu J, Zaidi T, Fernandez R, Sun X, et al. Evaluation of interphase fluorescence in situ hybridization for the t(14;18)(q32;q21) translocation in the diagnosis of follicular

lymphoma on fine-needle aspirates: a comparison with flow cytometry immunophenotyping. Cancer. 2003;99(6):385–93.
14. Shin HJ1, Thorson P, Gu J, Katz RL. Detection of a subset of CD30+ anaplastic large cell lymphoma by interphase fluorescence in situ hybridization. Diagn Cytopathol. 2003;29(2):61–6.
15. Xing X, Feldman AL. Anaplastic large cell lymphomas: ALK positive, ALK negative, and primary cutaneous. Adv Anat Pathol. 2015;22(1):29–49.
16. Hsi AC, Robirds DH, Luo J, Kreisel FH, Frater JL, Nguyen TT. T-cell prolymphocytic leukemia frequently shows cutaneous involvement and is associated with gains of MYC, loss of ATM, and TCL1A rearrangement. Am J Surg Pathol. 2014;38(11):1468–83.
17. Wierda WG, Zelenetz AD, Gordon LI, Abramson JS, Advani RH, Andreadis CB, et al. NCCN guidelines insights: chronic lymphocytic leukemia/small lymphocytic leukemia, version 1.2017. J Natl Compr Cancer Netw. 2017;15(3):293–311.
18. Malcikova J, Tausch E, Rossi D, Sutton LA, Soussi T, Zenz T, et al., European Research Initiative on Chronic Lymphocytic Leukemia (ERIC) — TP53 network. ERIC recommendations for TP53 mutation analysis in chronic lymphocytic leukemia-update on methodological approaches and results interpretation. Leukemia. 2018;32(5):1070–80.
19. Kanagal-Shamanna R, Portier BP, Singh RR, Routbort MJ, Aldape KD, Handal BA, et al. Next-generation sequencing-based multi-gene mutation profiling of solid tumors using fine needle aspiration samples: promises and challenges for routine clinical diagnostics. Mod Pathol. 2014;27(2):314–27.
20. Santos Gda C, Saieg MA, Ko HM, Geddie WR, Boerner SL, Craddock KJ, et al. Multiplex sequencing for EZH2, CD79B, and MYD88 mutations using archival cytospin preparations from B-cell non-Hodgkin lymphoma aspirates previously tested for MYC rearrangement and IGH/BCL2 translocation. Cancer Cytopathol. 2015;123(7):413–20.
21. Saieg MA, Geddie WR, Boerner SL, Bailey D, Crump M, da Cunha Santos G. EZH2 and CD79B mutational status over time in B-cell non-Hodgkin lymphomas detected by high-throughput sequencing using minimal samples. Cancer Cytopathol. 2013;121(7):377–86.
22. Treon SP, Xu L, Yang G, Zhou Y, Liu X, Cao Y, Sheehy P, et al. MYD88 L265P somatic mutation in Waldenström's macroglobulinemia. N Engl J Med. 2012;367:826–33.

23. Treon SP, Cao Y, Xu L, Yang G, Liu X, Hunter ZR. Somatic mutations in MYD88 and CXCR4 are determinants of clinical presentation and overall survival in Waldenström macroglobulinemia. Blood. 2014;123(18):2791–6.
24. Hunter ZR, Xu L, Yang G, Zhou Y, Liu X, Cao Y, et al. The genomic landscape of Waldenström macroglobulinemia is characterized by highly recurring MYD88 and WHIM-like CXCR4 mutations, and small somatic deletions associated with B-cell lymphomagenesis. Blood. 2014;123(11):1637–46.
25. Rossi D, Rasi S, Spina V, Bruscaggin A, Monti S, Ciardullo C, et al. Integrated mutational and cytogenetic analysis identifies new prognostic subgroups in chronic lymphocytic leukemia. Blood. 2013;121(8):1403–12.
26. Liu H, Wang W, Tang G, Yin CC, Muzzafar T, Medeiros LJ, Hu S. Lymphomatous variant of hairy cell leukaemia: a distinctive presentation mimicking low-grade B-cell lymphoma. Histopathology. 2015;67(5):740–5.
27. Tiacci E, Trifonov V, Schiavoni G, Holmes A, Kern W, Martelli MP, et al. BRAF mutations in hairy-cell leukemia. N Engl J Med. 2011;364(24):2305–15.
28. Tiacci E, Park JH, De Carolis L, Chung SS, Broccoli A, Scott S, et al. Targeting mutant BRAF in relapsed or refractory hairy-cell leukemia. N Engl J Med. 2015;373(18):1733–47.
29. Angelova E, et al. Clinicopathologic and molecular features in hairy cell leukemia variant: single institutional experience. Mod Pathol. 2018. https://doi.org/10.1038/s41379-018-0093-8.
30. Badalian-Very G, Vergilio JA, Degar BA, MacConaill LE, Brandner B, Calicchio ML, et al. Recurrent BRAF mutations in Langerhans cell histiocytosis. Blood. 2010;116(11):1919–23.
31. Garces S, Medeiros LJ, Patel KP, Li S, Pina-Oviedo S, Li J, et al. Mutually exclusive recurrent KRAS and MAP 2K1 mutations in Rosai-Dorfman disease. Mod Pathol. 2017;30(10):1367–77.
32. Alizadeh AA, Eisen MB, Davis RE, Ma C, Lossos IS, Rosenwald A, et al. Distinct types of diffuse large B-cell lymphoma identified by gene expression profiling. Nature. 2000;403(6769):503–11.
33. Leonard JP, Kolibaba KS, Reeves JA, Tulpule A, Flinn IW, Kolevska T, et al. Randomized phase II study of R-CHOP with or without Bortezomib in previously untreated patients with non-germinal center B-cell-like diffuse large B-cell lymphoma. J Clin Oncol. 2017;35(31):3538–46.
34. Scott DW, Mottok A, Ennishi D, Wright GW, Farinha P, Ben-Neriah S, et al. Prognostic significance of diffuse large B-cell

lymphoma cell of origin determined by digital gene expression in formalin-fixed paraffin-embedded tissue biopsies. J Clin Oncol. 2015;33(26):2848–56.
35. Scott DW, Wright GW, Williams PM, Lih CJ, Walsh W, Jaffe ES, et al. Determining cell-of-origin subtypes of diffuse large B-cell lymphoma using gene expression in formalin-fixed paraffin-embedded tissue. Blood. 2014;123(8):1214–7.
36. Rimsza LM, Wright G, Schwartz M, Chan WC, Jaffe ES, Gascoyne RD, et al. Accurate classification of diffuse large B-cell lymphoma into germinal center and activated B-cell subtypes using a nuclease protection assay on formalin-fixed, paraffin-embedded tissues. Clin Cancer Res. 2011;17(11):3727–32.
37. Goy A1, Stewart J, Barkoh BA, Remache YK, Katz R, Sneige N, Gilles F. The feasibility of gene expression profiling generated in fine-needle aspiration specimens from patients with follicular lymphoma and diffuse large B-cell lymphoma. Cancer. 2006;108(1):10–20.
38. Campo E. Whole genome profiling and other high throughput technologies in lymphoid neoplasms—current contributions and future hopes. Mod Pathol. 2013;26(S1):S97.
39. Baccarani M, Cilloni D, Rondoni M, Ottaviani E, Messa F, Merante S, et al. The efficacy of imatinib mesylate in patients with FIP1L1-PDGFRalpha-positive hypereosinophilic syndrome. Results of a multicenter prospective study. Haematologica. 2007;92(9):1173–9.
40. Cools J, DeAngelo DJ, Gotlib J, Stover EH, Legare RD, Cortes J, et al. A tyrosine kinase created by fusion of the PDGFRA and FIP1L1 genes as a therapeutic target of imatinib in idiopathic hypereosinophilic syndrome. N Engl J Med. 2003;348(13):1201–14.
41. Legrand F, Renneville A, MacIntyre E, Mastrilli S, Ackermann F, Cayuela JM, et al., French Eosinophil Network. The spectrum of FIP1L1-PDGFRA-associated chronic eosinophilic leukemia: new insights based on a survey of 44 cases. Medicine (Baltimore) 2013;92(5):e1–9.
42. Vega-Ruiz A, Cortes JE, Sever M, Manshouri T, Quintás-Cardama A, Luthra R, et al. Phase II study of imatinib mesylate as therapy for patients with systemic mastocytosis. Leuk Res. 2009;33(11):1481–4.
43. Arber DA, Orazi A, Hasserjian R, Thiele J, Borowitz MJ, Le Beau MM, et al. The 2016 revision to the World Health Organization (WHO) classification of myeloid neoplasms and acute leukemia. Blood. 2016;127(20):2391–405.

44. O'Donnell MR, Tallman MS, Abboud CN, Altman JK, Appelbaum FR, Arber DA, et al. Acute myeloid leukemia, version 3.2017, NCCN clinical practice guidelines in oncology. J Natl Compr Cancer Netw. 2017;15(7):926–57.
45. Döhner H, Estey E, Grimwade D, Amadori S, Appelbaum FR, Büchner T, et al. Diagnosis and management of AML in adults: 2017 ELN recommendations from an international expert panel. Blood. 2017;129(4):424–47.
46. Stein EM, DiNardo CD, Pollyea DA, Fathi AT, Roboz GJ, Altman JK, et al. Enasidenib in mutant IDH2 relapsed or refractory acute myeloid leukemia. Blood. 2017;130(6):722–31.
47. Levis M. Midostaurin approved for FLT3-mutated AML. Blood. 2017;129(26):3403–6.
48. Baer C, Kern W, Koch S, Nadarajah N, Schindela S, Meggendorfer M, et al. Ultra-deep sequencing leads to earlier and more sensitive detection of the tyrosine kinase inhibitor resistance mutation T315I in chronic myeloid leukemia. Haematologica. 2016;101(7):830–8.
49. Woyach JA, Ruppert AS, Guinn D, Lehman A, Blachly JS, Lozanski A. BTK C481S-mediated resistance to ibrutinib in chronic lymphocytic leukemia. J Clin Oncol. 2017;35(13):1437–43.
50. Gulley ML, Tang W. Laboratory assays for Epstein-Barr virus-related disease. J Mol Diagn. 2008;10(4):279–92.
51. Engelmann I, Alidjinou EK, Lazrek M, Pouillaude JM, Ogiez J, Rose F, et al. Comparison of two commercial quantitative PCR assays for EBV DNA detection and their correlation with the first WHO International Standard for EBV. J Med Microbiol. 2018;67(4):529–36.
52. Semenova T, Lupo J, Alain S, Perrin-Confort G, Grossi L, Dimier J, et al. Multicenter evaluation of whole-blood Epstein-Barr viral load standardization using the WHO international standard. J Clin Microbiol. 2016;54(7):1746–50.
53. Gulley ML. Molecular diagnosis of Epstein-Barr virus-related diseases. J Mol Diagn. 2001;3(1):1–10.
54. Venkatraman L, Catherwood MA, Patterson A, Lioe TF, McCluggage WG, Anderson NH. Role of polymerase chain reaction and immunocytochemistry in the cytological assessment of lymphoid proliferations. J Clin Pathol. 2006;59(11):1160–5.
55. Bagg A. Immunoglobulin and T-cell receptor gene rearrangements: minding your B's and T's in assessing lineage and clonality in neoplastic lymphoproliferative disorders. J Mol Diagn. 2006;8(4):426–9. quiz 526-7

56. Zhang S, Abreo F, Lowery-Nordberg M, Veillon DM, Cotelingam JD. The role of fluorescence in situ hybridization and polymerase chain reaction in the diagnosis and classification of lymphoproliferative disorders on fine-needle aspiration. Cancer Cytopathol. 2010;118(2):105–12.
57. Maroto A, Martinez M, Martinez MA, de Agustin P, Rodriguez-Peralto JL. Comparative analysis of immunoglobulin polymerase chain reaction and flow cytometry in fine needle aspiration biopsy differential diagnosis of non-Hodgkin B-cell lymphoid malignancies. Diagn Cytopathol. 2009;37(9):647–53.
58. Peluso AL, Cozzolino I, Bottiglieri A, Lucchese L, Di Crescenzo RM, Langella M, et al. Immunoglobulin heavy and light chains and T-cell receptor beta and gamma chains PCR assessment on cytological samples. A study comparing FTA cards and cryopreserved lymph node fine-needle cytology. Cytopathology. 2017;28(3):203–15.
59. Langerak AW, Groenen PJ, Brüggemann M, Beldjord K, Bellan C, Bonello L, et al. EuroClonality/BIOMED-2 guidelines for interpretation and reporting of Ig/TCR clonality testing in suspected lymphoproliferations. Leukemia. 2012;26(10):2159.
60. van Dongen JJ, Langerak AW, Brüggemann M, Evans PA, Hummel M, Lavender FL, et al. Design and standardization of PCR primers and protocols for detection of clonal immunoglobulin and T-cell receptor gene recombinations in suspect lymphoproliferations: report of the BIOMED-2 concerted action BMH4-CT98-3936. Leukemia. 2003;17(12):2257–317.
61. Patel KP, Pan Q, Wang Y, Maitta RW, Du J, Xue X, Lin J, Ratech H. Comparison of BIOMED-2 versus laboratory-developed polymerase chain reaction assays for detecting T-cell receptor-γ gene rearrangements. J Mol Diagn. 2010;12(2):226–37.
62. Evans PA, Pott C, Groenen PJ, Salles G, Davi F, Berger F, et al. Significantly improved PCR-based clonality testing in B-cell malignancies by use of multiple immunoglobulin gene targets. Report of the BIOMED-2 concerted action BHM4-CT98-3936. Leukemia. 2007;21(2):207–14.
63. McClure RF, Kaur P, Pagel E, Ouillette PD, Holtegaard CE, Treptow CL, Kurtin PJ. Validation of immunoglobulin gene rearrangement detection by PCR using commercially available BIOMED-2 primers. Leukemia. 2006;20(1):176–9.
64. Damle RN, Wasil T, Fais F, Ghiotto F, Valetto A, Allen SL, et al. Ig V gene mutation status and CD38 expression as novel

prognostic indicators in chronic lymphocytic leukemia. Blood. 1999;94(6):1840–7.
65. Oscier D, Wade R, Davis Z, Morilla A, Best G, Richards S, et al., Chronic Lymphocytic Leukaemia Working Group, UK National Cancer Research Institute. Prognostic factors identified three risk groups in the LRF CLL4 trial, independent of treatment allocation. Haematologica. 2010;95(10):1705–12.
66. Tobin G, Thunberg U, Johnson A, Thörn I, Söderberg O, Hultdin M, et al. Somatically mutated Ig V(H)3-21 genes characterize a new subset of chronic lymphocytic leukemia. Blood. 2002;99(6):2262–4.
67. Forconi F, Sozzi E, Cencini E, Zaja F, Intermesoli T, Stelitano C, et al. Hairy cell leukemias with unmutated IGHV genes define the minor subset refractory to single-agent cladribine and with more aggressive behavior. Blood. 2009;114(21):4696–702.
68. Arons E, Suntum T, Stetler-Stevenson M, Kreitman RJ. VH4-34+ hairy cell leukemia, a new variant with poor prognosis despite standard therapy. Blood. 2009;114(21):4687–95.
69. Xi L, Arons E, Navarro W, Calvo KR, Stetler-Stevenson M, Raffeld M, Kreitman RJ. Both variant and IGHV4-34-expressing hairy cell leukemia lack the BRAF V600E mutation. Blood. 2012;119(14):3330–2.
70. McClure R, Mai M, McClure S. High-throughput sequencing using the Ion Torrent personal genome machine for clinical evaluation of somatic hypermutation status in chronic lymphocytic leukemia. J Mol Diagn. 2015;17(2):145–54.

Chapter 18
Molecular Diagnostics in Bone and Soft Tissue Tumors

Vickie Y. Jo and Xiaohua Qian

Abbreviations

ABC	Aneurysmal bone cyst
ALK	Anaplastic lymphoma kinase or ALK receptor tyrosine kinase
ALT	Atypical lipomatous tumor
APC	Adenomatous polyposis coli
ASPS	Alveolar soft part sarcoma
ASPSCR1	Alveolar soft part sarcoma critical region 1
ATF1	Activating transcription factor 1
BCOR	BCL6 corepressor
BNCT	Benign notochordal cell tumor

V. Y. Jo (✉) · X. Qian
Harvard Medical School, Department of Pathology, Brigham and Women's Hospital, Boston, MA, USA
e-mail: vjo@bwh.harvard.edu; xqian@bwh.harvard.edu

S. Roy-Chowdhuri et al. (eds.), *Molecular Diagnostics in Cytopathology*, https://doi.org/10.1007/978-3-319-97397-5_18

BRAF	V-raf murine sarcoma viral oncogene homolog B
CAMTA1	Calmodulin-binding transcription activator 1
CCLTGT	Clear cell sarcoma-like tumor of the gastrointestinal tract
CCNB3	Cyclin B3
CDH11	Cadherin 11
CDK4	Cyclin-dependent kinase 4
CIC	Capicua transcriptional repressor
CLTC	Clathrin heavy chain
COL1A1/COL2A1	Collagen type I/type II alpha 1 chain
COL6A3	Collagen type VI alpha 3 chain
CREB1	cAMP-responsive element-binding protein 1
CREB3L1/CREB3L2	cAMP responsive element binding protein 3-like 1/protein 3-like 2
CSF1	Colony-stimulating factor 1
CTNNB1	Catenin beta 1
DDIT3	DNA damage-inducible transcript 3
DDLPS	Dedifferentiated liposarcoma
DFSP	Dermatofibrosarcoma protuberans
DNA	Deoxyribonucleic acid
DOG1	Discovered on GIST-1
DSRCT	Desmoplastic round cell tumor
DUX4	Double homeobox 4
EHE	Epithelioid hemangioendothelioma
EMA	Epithelial membrane antigen
EMC	Extraskeletal myxoid chondrosarcoma
ERG	V-ets erythroblastosis virus E26 oncogene like
ETS	Erythroblast transformation-specific; ETS proto-oncogene 1
ETV1/ETV4	ETS variant 1/ETS variant 4
EWSR1	Ewing sarcoma breakpoint region 1
FET (TET) family	FUS/EWS/TLS (TAF15/EWS/TLS)

FEV	Fifth Ewing variant
FGFR1-4	Fibroblast growth factor receptor 1-4
FLI1	Friend leukemia integration 1
FISH	Fluorescence *in situ* hybridization
FFPE	Formalin-fixed, paraffin-embedded
FOXO1	Forkhead box O1
FNA	Fine-needle aspiration
FUS	Fused in sarcoma
GCT	Giant cell tumor
GFAP	Glial fibrillary acidic protein
GIST	Gastrointestinal stromal tumor
GNAS1	GNAS complex locus (guanine nucleotide-binding protein (G protein), alpha-stimulating activity polypeptide 1)
H&E	Hematoxylin and eosin
H3.3	H3 histone family
H3F3A/H3F3B	H3 histone family member 3A/3B
H3K27me3	Histone 3 lysine 27 trimethylation
HEY1	Hes-related family bHLH transcription factor with YRPW motif 1
HMB-45	Human melanoma black
HMGA2	High-mobility group AT-hook 2
IAF	E1A enhanced-binding protein, E1AF
IDH1/IDH2	Isocitrate dehydrogenase 1/2
IHC	Immunohistochemistry
IMT	Inflammatory fibroblastic tumor
INI1	Integrase interactor 1
LCH	Langerhans cell histiocytosis
LGFMS	Low-grade fibromyxoid tumor
MAPK	Mitogen-activated protein kinase
Mart-1	Melanoma antigen recognized by T-cell 1
MDM2	Protein 53 E3 ubiquitin protein ligase homolog (mouse)
MiTF	Microphthalmia-associated transcription factor
MPNST	Malignant peripheral nerve sheath tumor

MUC4	Mucin 4
Myf-4	Myogenic factor 4
MYH9	Myosin heavy chain 9
MyoD1	Myogenic differentiation 1
NAB2	NGFI-A-binding protein 2
NCOA2	Nuclear receptor coactivator 2
NKX2.2	NK2 homeobox *2*
NR4A3	Nuclear receptor subfamily 4 group A member 3
NSE	Neuron-specific enolase
PAX3/PAX7	Paired box 3/Paired box 7
PBX1	PBX homeobox 1 (pre-B-cell leukemia homeobox 1)
PCR	Polymerase chain reaction
PDGFRA/PDGFRB	Platelet-derived growth factor receptor alpha/beta
POU5F1	POU class 5 homeobox 1 (POU domain class 5, transcription factor 1)
PRC2	Polycomb repressor complex 2
PRKAR1A	Protein kinase cAMP-dependent type I regulatory subunit alpha
RANBP2	RAN-binding protein 2
RAS	RAS type GTPase family
Rb	Retinoblastoma
RMS	Rhabdomyosarcoma
RNA	Ribonucleic acid
ROSE	Rapid on-site evaluation
RPMI	Roswell Park Memorial Institute
RT-PCR	Reverse transcription-polymerase chain reaction
SDH	Succinate dehydrogenase
SFT	Solitary fibrous tumor
SMA	Smooth muscle actin
SMARCB1	SWI/SNF-related matrix-associated actin-dependent regulator of chromatin subfamily B member 1
SOX10	Sry-related HMG-box gene 10

SS18	Synovial sarcoma translocation, chromosome 18
SSX1/SSX2/SSX4	SSX family member 1; synovial sarcoma, X breakpoint 1/ breakpoint 2/ breakpoint 4
STAT6	Signal transducer and activator of transcription 6
TAF15	TATA-box binding protein-associated factor 15
TFE3	Transcription factor binding to immunoglobulin heavy constant
TKI	Tyrosine kinase inhibitor
TLE1	Transducin-like enhancer of split 1
TPM3/TPM4	Tropomyosin 3/Tropomyosin 4
USP6	Ubiquitin-specific peptidase 6
VGLL2	Vestigial-like family member 2
WDL	Well-differentiated liposarcoma
WHO	World Health Organization
WT1	Wilms' tumor suppressor protein
WWTR1	WW domain containing transcription regulator 1
YAP1	Yes-associated protein 1
ZNF444	Zinc finger protein 444

Key Terminologies

Actionable alteration	A genomic event that has diagnostic, prognostic, or therapeutic disease-specific significance
Chromosomal karyotype	Evaluation of the number and structure of chromosomes from metaphase-arrested tumor cell nuclei to detect gross chromosomal abnormalities
Chromosomal translocation	Chromosomal rearrangement secondary to exchange of

	material between nonhomologous chromosomes
Fluorescence *in situ*	A molecular detection hybridization technique that uses fluorescently labeled DNA to hybridize to complementary regions within the target DNA
Fusion gene	A hybrid gene that is formed from a translocation that joins two otherwise-separated genes by mechanisms such as translocation or interstitial deletion
Fusion type	The specific exon combination between two genes for a given fusion variant of a tumor type
Fusion variant	Specific combination of partnered fusion gene to a commonly rearranged gene within a tumor type
IHC	A laboratory technique that allows the visualization of specific antigens in tissue by conjugating them to complementary antibodies with a reporter molecule. Common reporters are enzymes such as horseradish peroxidase. Enzymatic activation of the reporter leads to the production of a colored product that can be visualized with light microscopy
Immunophenotype	Tumor type-specific expression patterns of antigens detected by IHC

Mutation	Change in the nucleotide sequence of a gene or a chromosome. It may be classified into various ways. One of these classifications involves classifying mutations based on the effect on structure: (1) small-scale mutations and (2) large-scale mutations
NGS	A high-throughput approach using massively parallel sequencing (either targeted sequencing or transcriptome sequencing) to detect genetic alterations
RT-PCR	PCR-based assay that detects and quantifies in "real time" the amplification of a given target using specific fluorescent probes
Targeted sequencing (DNA-seq)	NGS approach to detect single nucleotide variants using DNA probes for a panel of selected genes from a tumor sample
Transcriptome sequencing (RNA-seq)	NGS approach to extract and sequence RNA molecules from a tumor sample
Wild-type	A phenotype/genotype/gene that predominates in a natural population. Wild-type allele is the one that is the most common one in the natural population

Key Points

- Definitive cytologic diagnosis is now possible for many soft tissue and bone tumors given the numerous advances in ancillary test development
- The diagnosis of soft tissue and bone neoplasms requires integration of morphologic, clinical, and radiographic features with relevant immunohistochemical and molecular tests
- Although immunohistochemistry, FISH, and sequencing assays can be performed on all cytology samples, rapid on-site evaluation is helpful to ensure specimen adequacy and to triage material for cell block preparation, which is frequently the preferred substrate for ancillary testing
- Most soft tissue and bone tumors that harbor recurrent molecular alterations have chromosomal translocations, gene amplifications, or point mutations, which can be detected by FISH and sequencing-based methods (such as RT-PCR)
- In order to optimize work-up of small cytologic biopsies, immunohistochemistry should be performed first, using panels selected based on clinical and morphologic features to address the differential diagnosis, and those results should then guide further molecular testing
- Immunohistochemistry can be used to identify line of differentiation and confirm characteristic immunophenotypes for many entities, including protein correlates of underlying molecular alterations
- The cytopathologist should be aware that many tumor types share immunohistochemical and genetic features, which may pose numerous diagnostic pitfalls
- Sarcomas with pleomorphic morphology can have complex karyotypes/genomic profiles and often lack distinctive immunophenotypes

- FISH has high utility in cytology specimens, and break-apart probes are most commonly employed to identify gene rearrangements; however, FISH cannot detect specific fusion type
- For some entities, identification of the fusion type (i.e., partner gene), such as by RT-PCR, may be required for definitive diagnosis given that many entities can share gene rearrangements
- While the rapidly growing NGS technologies have no current diagnostic role for soft tissue and bone neoplasms, NGS has had a significant role in tumor discovery and has many exciting potential applications in the future
- Because decalcification with harsh acid solutions (e.g., nitric acid, hydrochloric acid) damages nucleic acids and compromises most molecular tests including sequencing and FISH, FNA material (non-decalcified) and/or bone biopsy cores treated with EDTA-based decalcification are preferred for molecular testing of bone tumor biopsy samples

Introduction

Molecular genetics has an important role in the characterization, classification, and diagnosis of soft tissue and bone neoplasms. The identification of defining molecular alterations for numerous soft tissue and bone neoplasms has facilitated the recognition of novel entities, refinements in tumor classification, and development of many useful diagnostic immunohistochemical and molecular tests. These ancillary tools can be performed on cytologic preparations, and it is increasingly feasible to render accurate diagnoses on these limited volume samples. Soft tissue and bone neoplasms are rare but present frequent diagnostic challenges in cytopathology practice. Soft tissue and bone tumors are organized by the WHO classification [1] based on common histogenesis as determined by clinical, morphologic, immunohistochemical, and

TABLE 18.1 Classification of soft tissue and bone tumors based on the 2013 (4th edition) WHO [1]

Tumors of soft tissue	Tumors of bone
Adipocytic tumors	Chondrogenic tumors
Fibroblastic/myofibroblastic tumors	Osteogenic tumors
So-called fibrohistiocytic tumors	Fibrogenic tumors
Smooth muscle tumors	Fibrohistiocytic tumors
Pericytic tumors	Ewing sarcoma
Skeletal muscle tumors	Osteoclastic giant cell-rich tumors
Vascular tumors	Notochordal tumors
Chondro-osseous tumors	Vascular tumors
Gastrointestinal stromal tumors	Myogenic, lipogenic, and epithelial tumors
Nerve sheath tumors	Tumors of undefined neoplastic potential
Tumors of uncertain differentiation	Undifferentiated high-grade pleomorphic sarcoma
Undifferentiated/unclassified sarcomas	

molecular genetic features (see Table 18.1); it should be noted that there remain categories of "uncertain differentiation" for soft tissue and bone tumors. These neoplasms encompass a large number and wide diversity of tumor types, and there is considerable morphologic overlap between entities, and ancillary testing is often necessary for diagnosis.

The diagnostic approach to any soft tissue and bone tumor on small biopsy begins with the evaluation of the cytomorphologic features and correlation with clinical and imaging data to guide the differential diagnosis and ancillary testing. Many tumors are sampled by fine-needle aspiration (FNA) either by palpation or image guidance. Rapid on-site evaluation (ROSE) has an additional advantage for specimen triage to ensure allocation of material for ancillary studies. Direct smears are best for visualization of cytomorphologic features, and formalin-fixed, paraffin-embedded (FFPE) cell blocks are the favored substrate for immunohistochemistry (IHC) and most molecular testing methods as most IHC and molecular tests are validated for clinical applications on FFPE material only. However it should be noted that ancillary studies are feasible on all types of cytologic preparations including liquid-based preparations and smears (for details see Chap. 2). ROSE also has the added benefit of providing guidance for adequate core biopsies, which are often obtained concurrently with FNA in many practice settings [2]. In addition to enabling precise classification to guide appropriate clinical management, molecular tests can also provide prognostic and therapeutic information for several tumor types.

Molecular testing has particularly helpful applications in soft tissue and bone pathology and can often allow for more efficient work-up of small cytology samples. Molecular tests can provide diagnostic confirmation for tumor types presenting in the setting of unexpected clinical features, such as unusual patient age or sex or tumor site, or when a tumor shows uncharacteristic morphologic features or discordant immunohistochemical features. Clinical trials may require diagnostic molecular confirmation for patient enrollment. Many tumor types are associated with important therapeutic or prognostic features; for example, patients with GISTs may benefit from molecular testing given the correlation between response to tyrosine-kinase inhibitor (TKI) therapy and *KIT* mutation type.

Methods

Many soft tissue and bone neoplasms harbor recurrent genetic/molecular alterations, which can be detected by numerous methodologies including conventional karyotype analysis, fluorescence *in situ* hybridization (FISH), and sequencing-based assays. Generally, soft tissue and bone neoplasms with recurrent alterations have simple cytogenetic features that can be targeted for diagnosis and are predominantly balanced translocations or single-gene mutations. There are also sarcomas that harbor complex karyotypes and bear no specific immunohistochemical profiles; most of these tumor types have pleomorphic morphology and include myxofibrosarcoma, pleomorphic liposarcoma, leiomyosarcoma, and osteosarcoma. The diagnostic utility of conventional karyotype analysis and FISH has been well-established for the evaluation of mesenchymal neoplasms [2].

Conventional chromosome analysis by karyotype has long been utilized in soft tissue and bone pathology and facilitated many of the original discoveries of defining chromosomal translocations. Chromosomal karyotype requires allocation of fresh material (often needle rinses washed in RPMI); tumor cells are grown in culture, arrested in metaphase, treated with trypsin, and finally Giemsa-stained for G-banding pattern analysis. All chromosomal material is thus evaluated, which can identify gross chromosomal abnormalities, but lacks resolution for cryptic events. Karyotyping is not available in all practice settings, as this methodology is timely and costly and requires high-level technical skills and expertise interpretation.

FISH has high efficacy in cytology samples and can be performed on fresh material, cytospins, touch preparations, smears, and cell blocks. FISH is employed to detect chromosomal translocations and amplifications using targeted DNA probes. Break-apart probes for a targeted locus to confirm gene rearrangement are most commonly used, although a positive result does not provide specific information about the fusion variant or type present. Fusion variants can be detected using combination probes that target two separate gene loci; however results depend on the assay design as probe sets are required for each potential fusion partner. Break-apart FISH is useful in the diagnosis of tumor types that have numerous fusion variants but may present diagnostic pitfalls given the "promiscuity" of certain gene fusions, such as *EWSR1* rearrangements being present in a wide spectrum of tumor types.

Numerous sequencing-based methods have relevant applications in the cytologic diagnosis of soft tissue and bone tumors and can be performed on fresh or FFPE material, as well as on direct smears. Single-gene sequencing analysis can be useful in the diagnosis and prognostication of certain tumor types, such as *KIT* mutations in GIST. Reverse transcription-PCR (RT-PCR) detects specific fusion variants and types and is advantageous for small samples as it does not require tumor DNA enrichment; however, RT-PCR results are dependent on probe design. Next-generation sequencing (NGS) (e.g., massively parallel sequencing) is gaining widespread use and has been established to have utility for detecting actionable mutations for some diseases, such as lung adenocarcinoma. Most routinely used NGS panels are whole exome (RNA-seq) or targeted panel (DNA-seq). RNA-seq provides information about present structural rearrangements and expression levels and has enabled the discovery of novel fusion genes in many mesenchymal neoplasms. Targeted panel NGS detects single nucleotide variants, and computational approaches allow for the estimation of copy number alterations and identification for structural rearrangements (albeit with low sensitivity). While NGS may have replaced "low-throughput" sequencing tests in some practice settings, no standardized diagnostic role for NGS currently exists for soft tissue and bone pathology.

Immunohistochemistry: Differentiation Markers and Surrogates for Molecular Alterations

IHC has been well-established in diagnostic soft tissue and bone pathology for its utility for determining the line of differentiation and identifying characteristic immunophenotypes (including protein correlates of molecular alterations) for soft tissue and bone neoplasms. While traditional markers to identify intermediate filament proteins are still commonly used, such as keratin for epithelial differentiation and desmin for muscle differentiation, numerous lineage-specific markers are also available, such as CD31, CD34, and ERG for endothelial; S-100, SOX10, and GFAP for neural crest; and myogenin (myf-4) for skeletal muscle differentiation. Table 18.2 summarizes commonly used differentiation-specific immunohistochemical markers. It should be noted that these markers only support the line of differentiation, but do not necessarily distinguish normal tissue counterparts from neoplastic cells or benign from malignant neoplasms. Furthermore, many mesenchymal tumors show overlapping patterns of protein expression that are not necessarily lineage-specific. Numerous soft tissue tumors can show expression of epithelial markers

Table 18.2 Immunohistochemical markers of differentiation in soft tissue and bone tumors

Line of differentiation	Immunohistochemical markers
Epithelial	Keratin, EMA
Smooth muscle	SMA, desmin, caldesmon
Skeletal muscle	Desmin, muscle-specific actin, myogenin
Endothelial	CD34, CD31, ERG
Fibroblastic/ myofibroblastic	CD34±, SMA±, desmin±
Myoepithelial	Keratin, EMA, S-100, GFAP, p63 (40%), SOX10
Nerve sheath	S-100, GFAP, SOX10
Perineurial	EMA, CD34, claudin-1
Melanocytic	S-100, Mart-1, HMB-45, SOX10
Histiocytic	CD163, PU.1
Osteoblastic	SATB2
Chondroid	S-100

(keratin or EMA), including epithelioid sarcoma, synovial sarcoma, and desmoplastic small round cell tumor.

Several diagnostic immunohistochemical markers have been developed after identification by gene expression profiling, including MUC4 for low-grade fibromyxoid sarcoma (and a subset of genetically related sclerosing epithelioid fibrosarcoma) [3, 4], DOG1 for gastrointestinal stromal tumor (GIST) [5], and TLE1 for synovial sarcoma [6].

Molecular genetic insights have also facilitated the development of antibodies against protein correlates of specific molecular alterations for many tumor types; IHC can detect protein products of genetic alterations (such as mutations or fusion genes) and is less costly to perform than routine molecular testing. Examples include β-catenin expression in desmoid fibromatosis secondary to *CTNNB1* [7] or *APC* mutations [8], MDM2 for chromosome 12q13-15 amplification in atypical lipomatous tumor/well-differentiated liposarcoma and dedifferentiation liposarcoma, STAT6 overexpression secondary to *NAB2-STAT6* fusion for solitary fibrous tumor [9, 10], and loss of retinoblastoma (Rb) expression secondary to 13q rearrangements in spindle cell/pleomorphic lipomas, mammary-type myofibroblastoma, and cellular angiofibroma (three tumors that share morphologic and genetic features) [11]. Numerous diagnostic markers that identify protein surrogates of underlying genetic alterations are available, which are included in Table 18.3 and discussed below.

Understanding the expected immunophenotypes, expression patterns, sensitivity, and specificity for diagnostic markers is important for accurate interpretation and avoiding diagnostic pitfalls. For instance, ERG, a highly sensitive and specific marker for endothelial differentiation, can be positive in up to 40% of epithelioid sarcoma which can be mistaken for epithelioid hemangioendothelioma [12]. CD99 (identified by the monoclonal antibody O13) is often used to identify Ewing sarcoma for which a diffuse membranous staining pattern is expected. However, many other tumor types (including morphologic mimics) show CD99 expression, often in a cytoplasmic and/or weaker pattern. While

TABLE 18.3 Immunohistochemical and molecular features of selected soft tissue tumors

Tumor	Immunohistochemistry	Molecular features
Adipocytic tumors		
Atypical lipomatous tumor/well-differentiated liposarcoma	MDM2, CDK4, HMGA2	12q13–15 amplification
Dedifferentiated liposarcoma	MDM2, CDK4, HMGA2	12q13–15 amplification
Spindle cell lipoma	CD34, RB-loss	Monosomy or partial loss 13q or 16q
Myxoid liposarcoma	–	*FUS-DDIT3*
Fibroblastic/myofibroblastic tumors		
Nodular fasciitis	SMA multifocal	*MYH9-USP6*
Desmoid fibromatosis	β-Catenin, SMA±	*CTNNB1* or *APC* mutations
Mammary-type myofibroblastoma	CD34, desmin, RB1-loss	Monosomy or partial loss 13q or 16q
Cellular angiofibroma	CD34, desmin±, RB1-loss	Monosomy or partial loss 13q or 16q
Low-grade fibromyxoid sarcoma	MUC4	*FUS-CREB3L2*, *FUS-CREB3L1*; variant *EWSR1* in lieu of *FUS*

Myxoinflammatory fibroblastic sarcoma	–	*TGFBR3-MGEA5*, *TML1L2-BRAF*
Inflammatory myofibroblastic tumor	SMA±, ALK (50%)	*ALK* rearrangement with multiple partners (*TPM3*, *TPM4*, *CLTC*, *RANBP2*)
Solitary fibrous tumor	CD34, STAT6	*NAB2-STAT6*
Dermatofibrosarcoma protuberans	CD34	*COL1A1-PDGFB*
So-called fibrohistocytic tumors		
Tenosynovial giant cell tumor (localized and diffuse)	–	*CSF1* rearrangement (most commonly with *COL6A3* partner)
Pericytic tumors		
Glomus tumor	SMA, h-caldesmon	Heterogeneous: *BRAF* (V600E) and *KRAS* (G12A) mutations [16]; *NOTCH2/3* mutations [17]; association with NF1 [18]
Skeletal muscle tumors		
Alveolar rhabdomyosarcoma	Desmin and myogenin (diffuse)	*PAX3-FOXO1*; *rare PAX7-FOXO1*, *PAX3-NCOA1*, *PAX3-NCOA2*

(continued)

Table 18.3 (continued)

Tumor	Immunohistochemistry	Molecular features
Spindle cell rhabdomyosarcoma	Desmin, myogenin, MyoD1	*MyoD1* mutations
Vascular tumors		
Epithelioid hemangioendothelioma	CAMTA1, ERG, CD31, CD34, keratin (30%)	*CAMTA1-WWTR1*; subset with *YAP1-TFE3*
Angiosarcoma	ERG, CD31, CD34, keratin (30%)	Heterogeneous: *KDR* mutations [19], *CIC* rearrangement [20], MYC amplification [21]
Pseudomyogenic hemangioendothelioma	ERG, CD31, AE1/AE3, FOSB N.B.: CD34 negative	*SERPINE1-FOSB* [22]
Gastrointestinal stromal tumors		
Gastrointestinal stromal tumor	KIT, DOG1	*KIT* mutations (~80%); subset with *PDGFRA* mutations
SDH-deficient GIST	KIT, DOG1, SDHB loss, SDHA loss if *SDHA*-mutant	Mutations in *SDHA*, *B*, *C*, *D*; SDHC promoter hypermethylation
Nerve sheath tumors		
Malignant peripheral nerve sheath tumor	Limited S100, SOX10, GFAP; H3K27me3 loss (50%)	*NF1, CDKN2A, SUZ12, EED1* mutations

Tumors of uncertain differentiation		
Intramuscular myxoma	–	*GNAS1* mutation
Synovial sarcoma	EMA, keratin, TLE1	*SS18-SSX1, SS18-SSX2, SS18-SSX4*
Desmoplastic small round cell tumor	EMA, NSE, desmin, WT1 (C-terminus)	*EWSR1-WT1*
Myoepithelial neoplasms of soft tissue	Keratin, EMA, S100, SOX10, p63, INI1-loss	*EWSR1* rearrangement (various partners include *PBX1*, *PBX3*, *POU5F1*, *ZNF44*)
Epithelioid sarcoma	*EMA, keratin, CD34 (50%), INI1-loss*	*SMARCB1 alterations*
Clear cell sarcoma of soft tissue	S-100, HMB-45	*EWSR1-ATF1* or *EWSR1-CREB1*
Clear cell sarcoma-like tumor of the gastrointestinal tract	S-100	*EWSR1-ATF1* or *EWSR1-CREB1*
Angiomatoid fibrous histiocytoma	Desmin, EMA, CD99	*EWSR1-ATF1* or *EWSR1-CREB1*
Alveolar soft part sarcoma	TFE3	*ASPSCR1-TFE3*
Extraskeletal myxoid chondrosarcoma	Rare S100	*NR4A3* rearrangement (most commonly partnered with *EWSR1*)

(continued)

Table 18.3 (continued)

Tumor	Immunohistochemistry	Molecular features
Ossifying fibromyxoid tumor	S100, desmin	*PHF1* rearrangement [23]
Miscellaneous and unclassified sarcomas		
Ewing sarcoma	CD99, FLI1, NKX2.2	*EWSR1-FLI1* in majority
CIC-rearranged sarcoma	CD99±, WT1, ETV4	*CIC-DUX4;* rare *CIC-FOXO4*
BCOR-CCNB3 sarcoma	CD99±, CCNB3, BCOR, TLE1, SATB2, CyclinD1	*BCOR-CCNB3;* Rare: *BCOR-MAML3*, *ZC3H7B-BCOR* [24]

myogenin identifies skeletal muscle differentiation in all subtypes of rhabdomyosarcoma, diffusely strong nuclear staining is characteristic of alveolar rhabdomyosarcoma and distinguishes alveolar rhabdomyosarcoma from all other subtypes.

Application of Ancillary Tests for Common Soft Tissue Cytologic Differential Diagnoses

While soft tissue tumors are classified based on the line of differentiation, in routine cytopathologic practice, application of a pattern-based approach is often helpful in guiding differential diagnosis and application of appropriate ancillary testing. Most soft tissue neoplasms fall into one of the following morphologic patterns: adipocytic, myxoid, spindle, round cell, epithelioid, and pleomorphic [13]. Examples of application of ancillary testing for specific pattern-based differential diagnostic situations are briefly outlined below.

ALT/WDL may need to be distinguished from benign lipoma, fat necrosis, or hibernoma. MDM2, CDK4, and HMGA2 IHC identify most cases of ALT/WDL. Challenging cases can be resolved by MDM2 FISH, and molecular testing should be performed before any diagnosis of lipoma is assigned to an adipocytic neoplasm located in visceral sites (e.g., retroperitoneum or mediastinum) or sized greater than 10.0 cm in any location.

For hypocellular low-grade myxoid neoplasms with relatively bland spindle cells, the main diagnostic considerations are myxoma, perineurioma, and LGFMS. Perineurioma is usually positive for CD34, EMA, and claudin-1, but these markers are not entirely specific, especially in limited biopsy samples [4]. LGFMS also shows CD34 expression, but MUC4 is almost universally positive, and *FUS* FISH can also confirm the diagnosis. For cases with increased cytologic atypia, the diagnosis of myxofibrosarcoma (or other sarcoma) must be considered. For low-grade myxoid tumors showing an adipocytic component, *DDIT3* FISH can identify myxoid liposarcoma, and immunohistochemical Rb loss is helpful for spindle cell lipoma.

Spindle cell neoplasms may be particularly problematic to classify on cytology, and diagnostic efforts should focus on correct assignment of biologic grade. For low-grade spindle cell neoplasms in or near the gastrointestinal tract, most cases can be distinguished by IHC using KIT and DOG1 for gastrointestinal tumor, S100 for schwannoma, SMA and desmin for leiomyoma, and β-catenin for desmoid fibromatosis. Across a broader anatomic spectrum, diagnostic considerations for a low-grade spindle cell neoplasm include nodular fasciitis (*UPS6* fusion), desmoid fibromatosis (SMA and β-catenin), IMT (SMA and ALK), and SFT (CD34 and STAT6). For high-grade spindle cell sarcomas, an immunohistochemical panel should be applied first and should typically address synovial sarcoma (EMA, TLE1), leiomyosarcoma (SMA, desmin), MPNST (S-100, SOX10, GFAP, H3K27me3), and DDLPS (MDM2, CDK4, HMGA2); relevant molecular testing should then be selected based on immunohistochemical results.

Round cell sarcomas should always first undergo immunohistochemical testing using a panel to address a broad differential diagnosis, including Ewing sarcoma (CD99) and alveolar RMS (desmin), and exclusion of melanoma (S-100), carcinoma (keratin), and lymphoma (LCA or TdT). Additional immunohistochemical studies should be selected based on preliminary results and may either confirm a diagnosis (e.g., NKX2.2 and *EWSR1* FISH for Ewing sarcoma) or pursue additional diagnostic considerations, such as TLE1 and *SS18* FISH for poorly differentiated synovial sarcoma and *DDIT3* for high-grade myxoid liposarcoma. *EWSR1* rearrangements are also characteristic of DSRCT and myoepithelial neoplasms, and sequencing may be helpful in identifying the fusion partners in distinguishing from Ewing sarcoma. The pattern of CD99 staining should always be carefully examined, and alternative diagnoses to Ewing sarcoma should be considered for any tumor showing variable staining CD99 (including *CIC*-rearranged sarcoma and *BCOR-CCNB3* sarcoma).

Epithelioid tumors may be challenging as carcinoma and melanoma are often considered in the differential diagnosis. Keratin and S-100 should always be performed, but many sarcomas in the differential diagnosis show expression of keratin (e.g., epithelioid sarcoma and EHE) and S-100 (e.g., clear cell sarcoma of soft tissue). Using a SOX10/keratin double stain has been shown to be a focused approach for the work-up of an epithelioid neoplasm with a broad differential diagnosis including carcinoma, melanoma, and sarcoma with an epithelioid pattern [14]. Additional useful immunohistochemical studies include endothelial markers (ERG, CD34, CD31) and CAMTA1 for EHE, CD34 and INI1 for epithelioid sarcoma, FOSB for pseudomyogenic hemangioendothelioma [15], HMB-45 and *EWSR1* FISH for clear cell sarcoma of soft tissue, and TFE3 for ASPS (with confirmatory *TFE3* FISH).

The differential diagnosis for aspirates of pleomorphic sarcomas, namely, includes tumors having complex cytogenetic profiles, such as myxofibrosarcoma, pleomorphic liposarcoma, pleomorphic rhabdomyosarcoma, and unclassified pleomorphic sarcoma. However, MDM2 and CDK4 IHC (and potentially *MDM2* FISH) should be performed to identify DDLPS, which comprise a significant proportion of sarcomas showing pleomorphic morphology.

Specific Applications of Molecular Diagnostics for Soft Tissue Tumors

The application of ancillary testing for the diagnosis of the more commonly encountered soft tissue neoplasms in cytopathologic practice is briefly discussed below; Table 18.3 provides a more comprehensive reference list of soft tissue tumors that may be sampled by FNA and their respective immunohistochemical and molecular features.

MDM2 *Amplification*

Atypical lipomatous tumor/well-differentiated liposarcoma (ALT/WDL) and dedifferentiated liposarcoma (DDLPS) types are characterized by amplification of chromosome 12q13-15 via giant marker or ring chromosomes; this region includes *MDM2*, *CDK4*, and *HMGA2* [25–28]. Amplification of 12q13-15 can be visualized by conventional karyotype, but FISH for the *MDM2* locus is the most commonly employed method to detect amplification**.** IHC can detect resultant nuclear overexpression of MDM2, CDK4, and HGMA2, and positivity is sufficiently diagnostic in many scenarios, although challenging cases or equivocal staining should be confirmed by *MDM2* FISH which is considered the most reliable method [29–31]. MDM2, CDK4, and HMGA2 IHC are especially useful in distinguishing ALT/WDL from benign lipoma, especially because some ALT/WDL appear lipoma-like. ALT/WDL must be completely resected with clear margins given its risk for recurrence and dedifferentiation. One major pitfall is that histiocytes may express MDM2 [32], which can be problematic such as in the setting of extensive fat necrosis which can mimic ALT. A diagnosis of lipoma for an adipocytic tumor sized greater than 10.0 cm and/or located in the body cavities (mediastinum, retroperitoneum) requires molecular testing to exclude the more likely diagnosis of ALT/WDL. IHC for MDM2, CDK4, and HMGA2 is also useful for the diagnosis of DDLPS, which can show a wide range of non-lipogenic and lipogenic morphologies [28, 33–35]; DDLPS can show low-grade spindle morphology or mimic other tumor types (such as myxofibrosarcoma), as well as appear completely morphologically indistinct, such as a high-grade pleomorphic sarcoma (Fig. 18.1a–c). DDLPS should always be excluded using MDM2 and CDK4 IHC for any pleomorphic sarcoma before considering other diagnoses, such as myxofibrosarcoma, pleomorphic liposarcoma, and unclassified/undifferentiated sarcoma (all of which are characterized by complex karyotypes), especially in the retroperitoneum. It should be noted that weak MDM2 expression may be seen in other sarcoma types such as malignant peripheral nerve sheath tumor (MPNST)

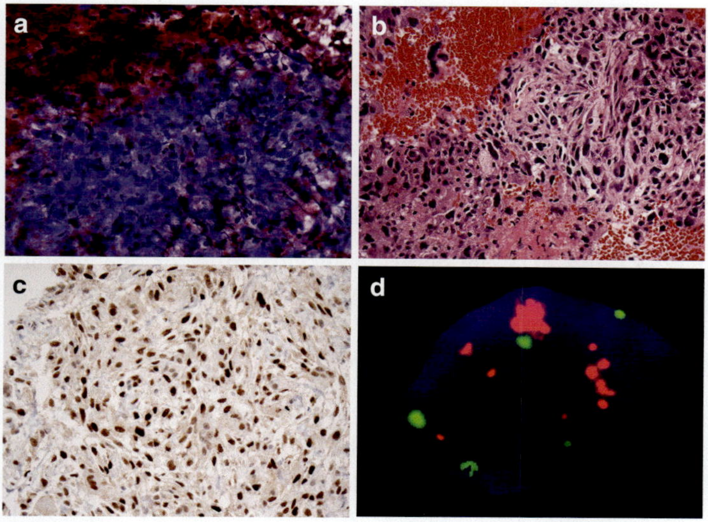

FIGURE 18.1 Dedifferentiated liposarcoma (DDLPS) frequently appears as a non-lipogenic pleomorphic sarcoma (**a**, Diff-Quik stained smear; **b**, H&E cell block section). Immunohistochemistry can detect nuclear overexpression of MDM2 (**c**), and MDM2 FISH confirms amplification of chromosome 12q13-15 (**d**; red MDM2 probe, green centromeric probe CEP12). (**d** Courtesy of Paola dal Cin, PhD, Brigham and Women's Hospital, Boston, MA)

[36]; thus, FISH to confirm *MDM2* amplification may be necessary (Fig. 18.1d).

MDM2 gene amplification is also characteristic of intimal sarcoma [37–39], parosteal osteosarcoma [40], and central low-grade osteosarcoma [41–43]. Association with a vessel wall supports intimal sarcoma, and correlation with radiologic data is required when considering a primary osseous tumor.

Tumors with EWSR1 *Rearrangement*

Rearrangements of *EWSR1*, a member of the FET (TET) family of RNA-binding proteins, are characteristic of numerous soft tissue tumors representing a broad range of morphologies, immunophenotypes, and biologic behavior and underscore the importance of judicious application of ancillary testing and appropriate interpretation of molecular test results. *EWSR1* FISH is a commonly used diagnostic approach, but a positive result is not necessarily diagnostic of one specific entity. Sequencing-based methods (such as RT-PCR) to identify the specific fusion partners may be required in some contexts. Furthermore, *FUS* is also a FET (TET) family member, and *EWSR1* and *FUS* can occasionally substitute for one another [44], and *FUS* testing should be considered if *EWSR1* is negative in this group of tumors.

EWSR1 rearrangements were first recognized in Ewing sarcoma, the vast majority of cases harboring the balanced translocation t(11;22)(q24;q12), resulting in *EWSR1-FLI1* [45, 46]. FLI1 is a member of the *ETS* family of transcription factors, and fusions involving other *ETS* family members, including *ERG*, *ETV1*, *ETV4* (*EIAF*), and *FEV* [47–50], occur in a small subset of Ewing sarcomas. Ewing sarcoma appears as a round cell sarcoma, and the diagnosis typically requires molecular confirmation, although IHC is employed to support the diagnosis and direct molecular testing. Ewing sarcoma shows a characteristic strong diffuse membranous staining pattern for CD99 (Fig. 18.2a, b); non-specific CD99 staining is seen in a broad range of morphologic mimics, including many other round cell sarcomas and non-mesenchymal mimics such as lymphoblastic lymphoma and carcinoid tumors, and should be interpreted with caution. Additional helpful immunohistochemical are FLI1 (positive in up to 70% of cases) and NKX2.2, which have high sensitivity (93%) but more modest specificity for Ewing sarcoma [51] (Fig. 18.2c). ERG is positive in the small subset (~5%) of cases that have *EWSR1-ERG* fusion, which are second most common in Ewing sarcoma [47, 52]. FISH for *EWSR1* rearrangement is a common diagnostic approach (Fig. 18.2d). Rare variant fusions with *FUS* in lieu of *EWSR1* also occur [53, 54].

Desmoplastic small round cell tumor (DSRCT) is characterized *EWSR1-WT1* [55, 56] and may also morphologically

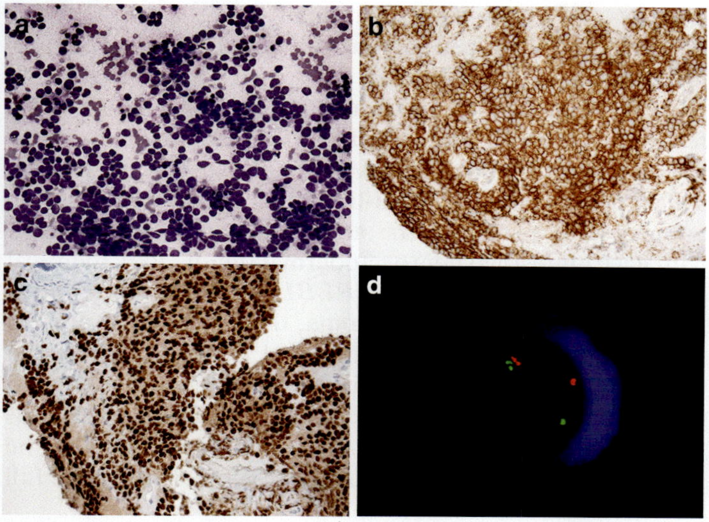

FIGURE 18.2 Ewing sarcoma is a round cell sarcoma (**a**, Diff-Quik stained smear) that requires ancillary testing for accurate classification. Strong diffuse membranous staining for CD99 is characteristic of Ewing sarcoma (**b**). Nuclear expression of NKX2.2 is highly sensitive, but only modestly specific, for Ewing sarcoma (**c**). FISH analysis detects *EWSR1* rearrangement, with separate green, telomeric *EWSR1* and red, centromeric *EWSR1* signals (**d**). (**d**, Courtesy of Sheng Xiao, PhD, Brigham and Women's Hospital, Boston, MA)

mimic Ewing sarcoma. The clinical presentation of most cases arising as an intraabdominal mass in young men is helpful. Apart from the identification of the specific fusion gene by RT-PCR, identifying the appropriate immunophenotype is crucial for interpreting positive FISH results for *EWSR1* rearrangement. DSRCT expresses keratin, EMA, NSE, desmin (frequently dot-like), and WT1 when using polyclonal antibodies to the C-terminus.

Specific *EWSR1* fusion variants are shared by some tumor types. Clear cell sarcoma of soft tissue is an epithelioid neoplasm showing melanocytic differentiation and is positive for S-100, HMB-45, and MiTF. Most tumors have

EWSR1-ATF1 fusions, and a small subset have *EWSR1-CREB1* [57]. Clear cell sarcoma-like tumor of the gastrointestinal tract (CCLTGT) also harbors *EWSR1-CREB1* and *EWSR1-ATF1* fusions and is also positive for S-100 but differs from clear cell sarcoma of soft tissue by being negative for melanocytic markers (HMB-45, MelanA) and showing solid growth and osteoclast-like giant cells [58, 59]; some authors have proposed the alternate terminology "malignant gastrointestinal neuroectodermal tumor" [60]. Identical *EWSR1-ATF1* and *EWSR1-CREB1* fusions are present in angiomatoid fibrous histiocytoma, the latter being present in >90% of cases [61]. Angiomatoid fibrous histiocytoma shows varying spindle cell histiocytic and small cell morphology and is positive for desmin and EMA as well as CD99; some cases with small cell morphology may thus be mistaken for Ewing sarcoma in small samples without a full immunohistochemical panel [62].

Other rare tumors with *EWSR1* rearrangements include extraskeletal myxoid chondrosarcoma (EMCS) and myoepithelial neoplasms of soft tissue and bone. EMCS (which notably does not show convincing cartilaginous differentiation) has either *EWSR1-NR4A3* or *TAF15-NR4A3* fusions [63, 64], and FISH probes for *NR4A3* are available and more specific for EMCS [65]. EMCS lacks a specific immunophenotype other than S-100 positivity in 20% of cases but shares morphologic features with myoepithelial neoplasms of soft tissue which also harbors *EWSR1* rearrangement. Soft tissue myoepithelioma and myoepithelial carcinoma (the latter defined by cytologic atypia) show varying positivity for pan-keratin, EMA, S-100, GFAP, and p63 [66]. A subset of myoepithelial neoplasms show an undifferentiated round cell morphology, most frequently in children [67], and *EWSR1* FISH results alone may be misleading for Ewing sarcoma. A heterogeneous group of fusion partners have been identified, including *POU5F1*, *PBX1*, and *ZNF444*, as well as variant fusion genes with *FUS* [68–75].

Tumors with FUS *Rearrangement*

Similarly to *EWSR1* rearrangements, *FUS* rearrangements characterize several diverse soft tissue neoplasms. Furthermore, as described earlier, variant fusions involving *EWSR1* in lieu of *FUS* may occur, and *EWSR1* testing may be helpful in the absence of *FUS* rearrangement.

Myxoid liposarcoma is characterized by *FUS-DDIT3* [76]; this tumor has several characteristic morphologic features (Fig. 18.3a) but otherwise has no specific immunophenotype, and many cases require molecular confirmation for diagnosis, especially for high-grade tumors which are hypercellular and may appear as round cell sarcomas. While *FUS* FISH is available, many laboratories employ *DDIT3* FISH, which is more specific for myxoid liposarcoma, which also detects the small subset having alternate *EWSR1-DDIT3* fusions [77, 78] (Fig. 18.3b).

LGFMS harbors translocations of *FUS*, most commonly with fusion partners *CREB3L2* or *CREB3L1* [79–81]. As mentioned previously, cytoplasmic staining for MUC4 is a

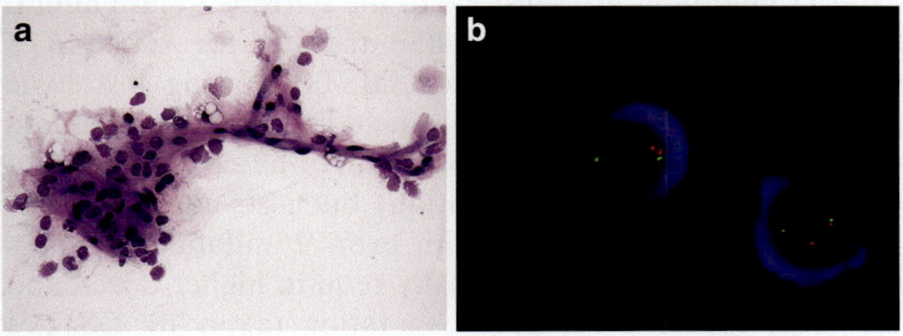

Figure 18.3 Myxoid liposarcoma showing the characteristic features of abundant myxoid stroma with uniform ovoid-to-round tumor cells, delicate branching capillaries, and small lipoblasts (**a**, Diff-Quik stained smear). Tumors harbor *FUS-DDIT3* fusions, which can be detected by FISH for *DDIT3* (**b**; green telomeric *DDIT3*, red centromeric *DDIT3*). (**b**, Courtesy of Adrian Dubuc, PhD, Brigham and Women's Hospital, Boston, MA)

highly sensitive and specific marker for LGFMS [3], which can be especially useful in cytology samples as LGFMS may be challenging to distinguish from other low-grade myxoid lesions, such as myxoma and soft tissue perineurioma [4].

A subset of sclerosing epithelioid fibrosarcoma shares the same *FUS-CREB3L1* translocation as LGFMS [3, 81, 82], and subset of tumors with hybrid features of LGFMS and sclerosing epithelioid fibrosarcoma are known to occur. Not surprisingly given the shared morphologic and genetic features, MUC4 is also positive in up to 70% of cases [3].

Gastrointestinal Stromal Tumors (Including SDH-Deficient Tumors)

Gastrointestinal stromal tumor (GIST) harbors *KIT* mutations in 80% of cases; exon 11 mutations are most common (80%), followed by exon 9 (11%); *PDGFRA* mutations occur in 10–15% [83]. Most GISTs appear as low-grade spindle cell neoplasms, though 30% show mixed spindle and epithelioid or epithelioid-predominant morphology. GISTs with *KIT* exon 11 mutations are sensitive to the tyrosine kinase inhibitor (TKI) imatinib, the first-line therapy for GIST. *KIT* sequencing may be helpful for GISTs showing histologic responses to imatinib treatment (including shift to epithelioid morphology, increased pleomorphism, or heterologous rhabdomyosarcomatous differentiation) but also may be therapeutically relevant. Tumors with exon 9 mutations are less sensitive to imatinib and typically require higher doses, and the most common *PDGFRA* mutation (exon 18; D842V) renders tumors unresponsive to imatinib. Other rare alterations among *KIT* "wild-type" GISTs are *BRAF* V600E and association with neurofibromatosis type 1. Mutational testing is also helpful diagnostically for the rare GISTs (~2%) that are negative for both KIT and DOG1 IHC [84].

Most GISTs (95%) show KIT immunoreactivity in a diffuse cytoplasmic or occasionally membranous and dot-like (Golgi) patterns, regardless of *KIT* mutation status. Most

KIT-negative GISTS are *PDGFRA*-mutant tumors that arise in the stomach and show epithelioid morphology and myxoid stroma [85]. DOG1 is a highly sensitive and specific marker for GIST and is positive in up to 30% of KIT-negative GISTs [86, 87]. DOG1 also shows more robust staining than KIT in cytology samples of GIST fixed in methanol-based solutions, such as CytoLyt [5].

Succinate dehydrogenase (SDH)-deficient GIST is an important clinicopathologic variant and comprises nearly half of all "wild-type" GISTs including pediatric GISTs, sporadic adult "wild-type" GISTs, and GISTs associated with Carney triad or Carney-Stratakis syndrome [88–90]. These tumors arise nearly exclusive in the stomach and show predominantly epithelioid morphology and a distinctive multinodular growth pattern through the gastric wall. Despite lacking *KIT* mutations, SDH-deficient GISTs strongly express both KIT and DOG1. The tetrameric SDH complex is comprised of four subunits SDHA, SDHB, SDHC, or SDHD, and mutation of any of the coding genes for the four subunits (or other mechanisms such as epigenetic events) causes dysfunction of the entire SDH complex. SDH deficiency can be identified by IHC for SDHB, which is ubiquitously expressed in normal tissue [91, 92]. The loss of SDHB expression in tumor cells indicates SDH deficiency but is not specific for the mechanism of SDH dysfunction. SDHA IHC should be performed if SDHB expression is lost, and the loss of SDHA expression correlates with *SDHA* mutations (accounting for 30% of SDH-deficient GISTs) [93, 94]. SDH-deficient GISTs differ from conventional *KIT*-mutant GISTs by showing frequent vascular invasion and nodal and distant metastases; their biologic behavior cannot be predicted using conventional NCCN risk stratification, and tumors follow an overall indolent course despite the propensity for metastases [95]. SDH-deficient GISTs are not responsive to imatinib and typically require second- and third-generation TKI therapy (sunitinib, sorafenib, dasatinib). Patients diagnosed with SDH-deficient GIST are referred for genetic counseling and often undergo germline mutational testing given several syndromic associations. GIST may arise in the setting of the autosomal dominant Carney-Stratakis syndrome; these patients have germline *SDH* mutations and also develop paragangliomas [96]. Carney triad syndrome (GIST, paraganglioma, pulmonary chondroma) is nonhereditary; most affected patients are female and are associated with *SDHC* promoter hypermethylation [97]. SDHB IHC should be used to screen for SDH deficiency in gastric GISTs with epithelioid morphology, as well as metastatic GISTs in young patients.

Molecular Alterations in Selected Other Soft Tissue Tumor Types

Synovial sarcoma appears as a spindle cell sarcoma, either as monophasic (exclusively spindle cell morphology) or biphasic with epithelial differentiation (Fig. 18.4a); there is no prognostic significance between these two subtypes. Both spindle cell and epithelial components express EMA and keratin. Tumors show diffuse nuclear staining for TLE1,

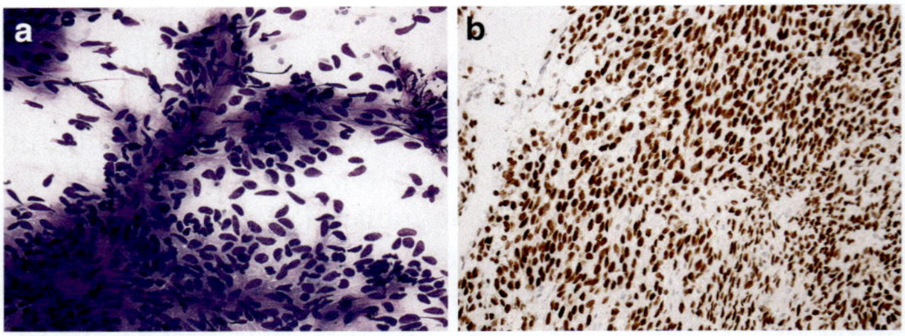

FIGURE 18.4 Synovial sarcoma yields cellular smears of uniform spindle cells that are singly dispersed and arranged in clusters with thin branching capillaries (**a**, Diff-Quik stained smear). TLE1 immunohistochemistry is a useful diagnostic marker, and most cases of synovial sarcoma show diffuse nuclear staining (**b**); however, specificity is more modest and *SS18* FISH may be necessary in challenging cases

which is highly sensitive but more modestly specific (Fig. 18.4b) but is helpful in the differential diagnosis of spindle cell sarcomas. Synovial sarcoma harbors *SS18-SSX* fusions, with fusion of *SS18* to *SSX1* or *SSX2* (and rarely, *SSX4*). *SS18* FISH or sequencing can identify *SS18* rearrangement or present fusion variants, respectively. Of note, 10% of synovial sarcomas are poorly differentiated and appear as either a round cell or epithelioid sarcoma, for which molecular testing may be necessary for diagnosis [98].

Rhabdomyosarcoma (RMS) encompasses embryonal, alveolar, spindle cell/sclerosing, and pleomorphic subtypes. Accurate classification is important for appropriate clinical management as patients are treated with subtype-specific regiments. All RMS subtypes show desmin and myogenin (myogenic factor 4, myf4) expression; however, alveolar RMS (a round cell sarcoma) characteristically shows diffuse nuclear staining for myogenin that allows distinction from other subtypes. Alveolar RMS harbors *PAX3-FOXO1* and *PAX7-FOXO1* fusions [99, 100], which can be identified by RT-PCR; *FOXO1* FISH is also commonly employed. Spindle cell/sclerosing RMS are characterized by *MyoD1* L122R mutations, and tumors show diffuse nuclear staining for MyoD1 IHC which is helpful in distinguishing spindle cell RMS from other spindle cell sarcomas [101–103]. A rare subset of congenital/infantile spindle cell RMS has recurrent *NCOA2* and *VGLL2* rearrangements [104, 105]. There are no specific diagnostic features for embryonal and pleomorphic RMS subtypes. Pleomorphic RMS shows a complex karytyope; embryonal RMS has *FGFR4* and *RAS* mutations and non-specific features of loss of heterozygosity of 11p15 and trisomies of chromosomes 2, 8, and 20 [106, 107].

Solitary fibrous tumor (SFT) is characterized by *NAB2-STAT6* fusion resulting from an intrachromosomal rearrangement on 12q13 [108, 109]. The two involved genes are located in close proximity such that the rearrangement cannot be detected by conventional karyotype analysis or FISH and require sequencing for detection. Resultant nuclear STAT6 overexpression can be detected by IHC, and STAT6 is highly sensitive and specific for SFT [9, 10, 110] and is often used in combination with CD34, which is positive in most SFTs but not specific.

Dermatofibrosarcoma protuberan (DFSP) may be a cytomorphologic mimic of SFT and shows CD34 expression but is negative for STAT6. DFSP harbors *COL1A1-PDGFB* fusion [111–113], and *PDGFRB* FISH can be helpful for challenging cases or for cases showing fibrosarcomatous differentiation, which appear as an indistinct spindle cell sarcoma.

ALK rearrangements are present in up to half of all cases of inflammatory fibroblastic tumor (IMT); these fusions involve a heterogeneous group of partners (including *TPM3*, *TPM4*, *CLTC*, and *RANBP2*), and localization of the ALK immunohistochemical expression appears to reflect the function of the involved fusion partner and is most commonly cytoplasmic (for instance, TPM3 and TPM4 are cytoplasmic proteins) [114, 115]. The epithelioid variant of IMT harbors *ALK-RANBP2* and shows a nuclear membranous staining pattern for ALK as RANBP2 is a nuclear pore protein [116, 117]. Epithelioid IMT also expresses CD30 and desmin which may pose diagnostic pitfalls; accurate classification is important as epithelioid IMT represents an aggressive subtype.

Epithelioid sarcoma (classified as either conventional distal and proximal subtypes) has *SMARCB1* alterations [118–120]. Secondary loss of INI1 expression can be detected by IHC; furthermore, epithelioid sarcoma expresses EMA and keratin, and CD34 is positive in half of all cases. There are numerous diagnostic pitfalls. Tumors may be mistaken for carcinoma if only EMA and keratin are performed [118, 121], and a subset express ERG which may be confused for an epithelioid vascular neoplasm. Loss of INI1 expression also occurs in many other tumor types, including malignant rhabdoid tumor, renal medullary carcinoma, and many tumors with *EWSR1* rearrangement due to function loss of material on chromosome 22q (such as myoepithelial neoplasms of soft tissue) [122]; thus, clinical correlation and an inclusive immunohistochemical panel are often required for accurate diagnosis.

Epithelioid hemangioendothelioma (EHE) harbors *CAMTA1-WWTR1* [123]. Endothelial differentiation can be identified using IHC for ERG, CD31, and CD34. Nuclear CAMTA1 expression is highly sensitive and specific for EHE and distinguishes EHE from other vascular tumors and other mimics, including epithelioid sarcoma (which may be ERG-positive) [124] (Fig. 18.5). CAMTA1 is especially helpful as 30% of EHE are positive for keratin or EMA, which are also positive in mimics such as epithelioid sarcoma and epithelioid angiosarcoma.

Several tumor types have *TFE3* fusions that can be detected by *TFE3* FISH or IHC for resultant nuclear TFE3 overexpression. *YAP1-TFE3* fusions characterize a subset of EHE showing vasoformative features [125]. Alveolar soft part sarcoma (ASPS) harbors *ASPSCR1-TFE3*, and TFE3 IHC and *TFE3* FISH are helpful diagnostic adjuncts as ASPS shows indistinct epithelioid morphology in cytology samples. TFE3 expression is also seen in the benign neoplasm granular cell tumor, a cytomorphologic mimic of ASPS; however granular cell tumor lacks *TFE3* rearrangements [126, 127]. Granular cell tumors express S-100 and SOX10, which are negative in ASPS. *TFE3* fusions are also present in a subset of PEComas, and IHC can demonstrate myoid and melanocytic

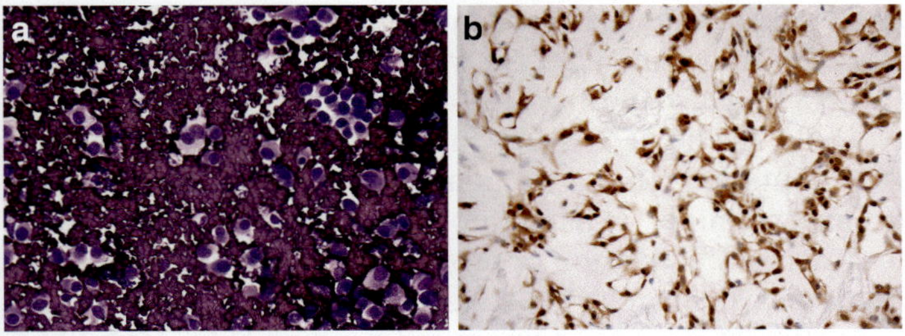

Figure 18.5 Epithelioid hemangioendothelioma (EHE) is comprised of singly dispersed epithelioid and polygonal cells with large nuclei (often eccentrically placed or binucleated) and abundant cytoplasm (**a**, Diff-Quik stained smear). Immunohistochemistry for CAMTA1 is highly sensitive and specific for EHE (**b**)

differentiation in these tumors in addition to nuclear TFE3 expression [128, 129].

Among undifferentiated/unclassified sarcomas, rare molecular "subsets" of round cell sarcomas (often previously classified as "atypical" or "variant" Ewing sarcoma) have been recognized, including *CIC*-rearranged sarcoma [130–133] and *BCOR-CCNB3* sarcoma [134–137]. *CIC*-rearranged sarcoma and *BCOR-CCNB3* sarcoma show variable (often negative) CD99 expression and more readily show increased cytologic atypia, distinctive nucleoli, increased cytoplasm, spindle cell morphology, myxoid stroma, and necrosis (which are features uncharacteristic of Ewing sarcoma) [138]. These sarcomas are more readily diagnosed by sequencing-based methods or FISH and should be considered after exclusion of Ewing sarcoma and other round cell sarcomas. The most common fusion in *CIC*-rearranged sarcoma is *CIC-DUX4*, which can be detected by *CIC* FISH. IHC is often helpful in selecting cases for molecular testing. *CIC*-rearranged sarcoma shows frequent nuclear positivity for WT1 and ETV4 [139–141]. *BCOR-CCNB3* sarcoma shows nuclear BCOR and CCNB3 expression, and frequent positivity for SATB2, TLE1, and cyclinD1 [142, 143], though owing to its rarity most cases undergo confirmation by molecular testing.

Some tumors are characterized by single-gene mutations that can be detected by both sequencing-based methods and immunohistochemical correlates, including desmoid fibromatosis and malignant peripheral nerve sheath tumor (MPNST). Desmoid fibromatosis includes sporadic tumors typically having *CTNNB1* mutations [7] or tumors with *APC* mutations that arise in association with Gardner syndrome (familial adenomatous polyposis) [8]. Nuclear β-catenin accumulation occurs secondary to either of these mutations and can be detected by IHC (Fig. 18.6), although only 80% of desmoid tumors are positive [144, 145]. SMA expression is variable; if β-catenin is negative, the diagnosis can be supported by appropriate clinical and morphologic features, and molecular testing may be performed in certain circumstances.

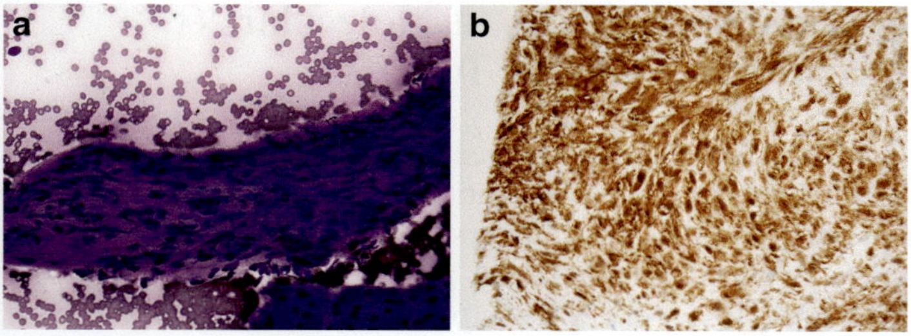

FIGURE 18.6 Desmoid fibromatosis comprised of fascicles of bland-appearing spindle cells within a dense collagenous stroma (**a**, Diff-Quik stained smear). Nuclear overexpression of β-catenin is a useful diagnostic feature (**b**)

MPNST, which may be sporadic or arise in association with radiation or neurofibromatosis I, is notoriously challenging to diagnose as most cases show limited (if any) expression of neural markers S100, SOX10, and GFAP. A subset of MPNST have mutations in *SUZ12* and *EED1*, which encode components of the polycomb repressor complex 2 (PRC2) [146, 147]; these alterations seem to be a marker of progression and are most commonly present in morphologically high-grade tumors. Dysregulation of PRC2 leads to the loss of trimethylation of the histone H3 at lysine 27, which can be detected by IHC using H3K27me3 [148–152]. However, there are some limitations to the diagnostic utility of H3K27me3, as loss is not seen in all MPNSTs and its specificity is modest, with H3K27me3 loss being observed in other tumor types including synovial sarcoma and DDLPS [151, 152].

It should be noted that many soft tissue tumors have straightforward diagnostic features and do not require molecular testing but may be subject to incidental identification with the increasing use of NGS. Examples include detection of *USP6-MYH9* fusion in nodular fasciitis [153], *GNAS1* mutations in myxoma [154, 155], *PRKAR1A* mutations in superficial angiomyxoma of Carney complex [156, 157], and *CSF1-COL6A3* fusion in tenosynovial giant cell tumor [158, 159].

Specific Applications of Molecular Diagnostics for Bone Tumors

In recent years, there has been remarkable progress in the discovery of molecular alterations in bone tumors, which has not only broadened our understanding of the pathogenesis of many bone tumors but also provided us novel diagnostic tools [160, 161]. An FNA sample with intact genetic material is particularly advantageous for bone tumors as it does not require decalcification, a routine tissue process for FFPE bone sections. Decalcification with harsh acid solutions damages DNA or RNA and compromises most molecular tests including sequencing, and FISH [162], although decalcification using chelating agents such as EDTA has shown better success for molecular testing. From a genetic perspective, bone tumors, like soft tissue tumors, can be divided into three categories: (a) tumors with point mutations or amplifications, (b) tumors with recurrent translocations or fusion genes, and (c) sarcomas with complex genomic profiles. Aggressive sarcomas such as conventional osteosarcoma and angiosarcoma are examples of the last category, where current molecular genetic testing is not diagnostically helpful due to the presence of inconsistent, non-specific molecular alterations [163]. Therefore, the entities in the first two categories are discussed below with an emphasis on clinical relevance.

Molecular alterations and related diagnostic immunohistochemical markers of selected bone tumors are summarized in Table 18.4.

Bone Tumors with Point Mutations or Amplifications

H3.3 Mutations in Chondroblastoma and Giant Cell Tumor of Bone

The differential diagnosis of many giant cell-rich tumors, especially in needle biopsy samples, can be very challenging

TABLE 18.4 Molecular alterations and associated immunohistochemistry of selected bone tumors

Tumor	Molecular alteration	Immunohistochemistry
Tumors with point mutations or amplifications		
Giant cell tumor of bone	*H3F3A* G34W/V/R/L mutations	Mutation-specific IHC G34W
Chondroblastoma	*H3F3B* K36M mutations	Mutation-specific IHC K36M
Enchondroma Chondrosarcomas	Somatic *IDH1* and *IDH2* mutations	N/A
Langerhans cell histiocytosis	*BRAF V600E*	BRAF V600E, CyclinD1
Low-grade osteosarcomas Parosteal osteosarcoma Low-grade central osteosarcoma	12q13–15 amplification	MDM2, CDK4
Chordoma	Germline duplication/somatic amplification of *T*	Brachyury
Poorly differentiated/pediatric variant	Deletions at *SMARCB1/INI-1* locus	Loss of INI1 expression
Tumors with recurrent translocations		
Aneurysmal bone cyst	*CDH11-USP6*	N/A
Mesenchymal chondrosarcoma	*HEY1-NCOA2*	N/A

due to significant morphologic and radiologic overlap [164–166]. Traditionally, correlation of morphology with clinical, radiologic, and laboratory findings is the only way to establish a correct diagnosis [167]. Now molecular testing and even better surrogate IHC can aid in difficult differential diagnosis, especially in settings where tumors arise in unusual anatomic sites and/or show atypical morphologic features [168].

Recently, highly recurrent somatic driver mutations in two genes, *H3F3A* (located at 1q42.12) and *H3F3B* (located at 17q25.1), have been identified in 92% of giant cell tumor (GCT) of the bone and in 95% of chondroblastomas, respectively [169]. Both *H3F3A* and *H3F3B* encode replication-independent histone H3.3 proteins with an identical amino acid sequence. In GCT of bone, *H3F3A* G34W mutations are most common (85% to 95%), but alternate G34V, G34R, and G34L mutations have been reported in a subset of cases [169–172]. Chondroblastomas harbor K36M mutations in >90% of cases, resulting from *H3F3B* mutations and rarely from *H3F3A* mutations [169, 172]. These mutations are not present in many other giant cell-containing bone tumors that frequently enter the morphologic differential diagnosis of GCT of bone and/or chondroblastoma, which includes solid aneurysmal bone cysts, non-ossifying fibromas, chondromyxoid fibromas, giant cell reparative granulomas, brown tumor of hyperparathyroidism, GCT of Paget disease, and giant cell-rich osteosarcomas [172, 173].

Using monoclonal antibodies directed against the mutant H3.3 G34W and H3.3 K36M proteins, mutation-specific IHC has been shown to be highly specific and sensitive for the diagnosis of GCT of bone and chondroblastoma, respectively, on both surgical resections and FNA/core biopsy samples [173–175]. *H3F3A* and *H3F3B* mutations as well as the resulting mutant H3.3 G34W and H3.3 K36M proteins are restricted to the mononuclear stromal cell population [174–176] (Fig. 18.7). Because of the admixed large population of non-neoplastic multinucleated giant cells and their mononuclear precursors in GCT of bone and chondroblastoma, the sensitivity of detecting these mutations depends on the

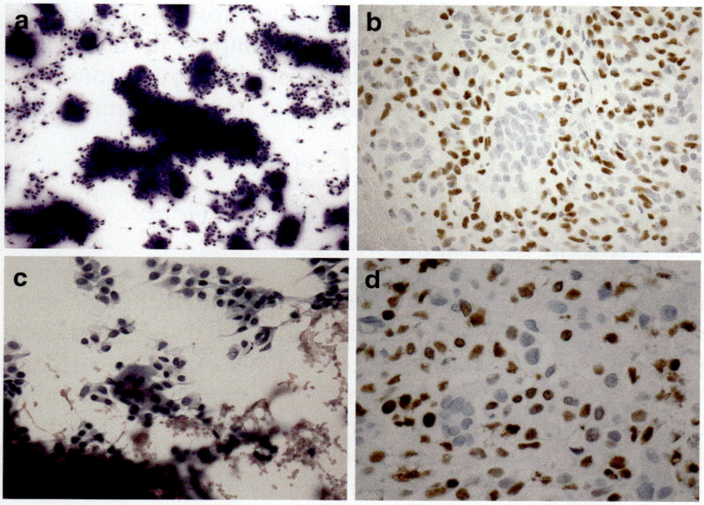

FIGURE 18.7 Giant cell tumor of bone on an aspirate (**a**, Diff-Quik stain) showing a cellular smear with cohesive clusters of spindled to oval cells admixed with many multinucleate giant cells. Immunohistochemistry for H3G34W (**b**) on cell block highlights the nuclei of the neoplastic mononucleate stromal cells. The multinucleate giant cells and their precursor cells are negative. Chondroblastoma on an aspirate (**c**, Papanicolaou stain) showing clusters and single chondroblasts with nuclear grooves. Scattered multinucleate giant cells are also present. Immunohistochemistry for H3K36M (**d**) on cell block highlights the nuclei of chondroblasts only

sequencing methods and ranges from 69% for Sanger sequencing to 96% for targeted highly parallel sequencing [170, 171, 177, 178]. However, mutation-specific IHC can detect just a few clusters of neoplastic cells on cell block sections, and on even otherwise nondiagnostic samples [174]. Undetected by G34W IHC, alternate *H3F3A* mutations, namely, H3.3 G34V, G34R, or G34L, account for H3 G34W IHC negativity in a subset of GCT of bone cases [173]. In such settings, mutation analysis as well as other mutation-specific markers such as antibodies against H3 G34R or G34V would be helpful [173]. The specificity of these mutation-specific antibodies has been proven high, so it is extremely helpful in small biopsy samples to distinguish chondroblastoma from rare cases of chondroblastoma-like osteosarcoma and GCT of bone from its benign and malignant mimics [173–176].

Isocitrate Dehydrogenenase (IDH1/2) Gene Mutations in Cartilage-Forming Tumors

Cartilage-forming tumors form a clinical and histologic spectrum ranging from benign (enchondroma, osteochondroma, periosteal chondroma) to intermediate (atypical cartilaginous tumor/chondrosarcoma grade 1) to malignant (chondrosarcoma, grades 2 and 3, dedifferentiated chondrosarcoma) [1]. A multidisciplinary approach with close histo-radiologic correlation is of paramount importance for a correct diagnosis. It is well known now that there is a variable prevalence of point mutations in *isocitrate dehydrogenenase* (*IDH1/2*) genes in a variant of benign and malignant cartilage-forming tumors, including enchondroma (about 40% in solitary lesions, 87% in syndromic multiple lesions), conventional central chondrosarcomas, grades 1–3 (38–70%), periosteal chondrosarcoma (variable), and dedifferentiated chondrosarcoma (50–60%). Hot-spot mutations are found at the *IDH1* R132 and the *IDH2* R172 positions [179, 180]. Additional genetic alterations in chondrosarcomas identified by NGS include mutations in *COL2A1* gene and aberrations in the p53 and Rb pathways [181].

Because of the low frequency and vast diversity in the variants of *IDH1/2* mutations, mutation-specific IHC is less useful in cartilage-forming tumors. Direct sequencing is the test of choice to increase diagnostic accuracy in addition to traditional histo-radiologic correlation [179]. Despite being incapable of distinguishing conventional low-grade chondrosarcomas from benign chondroid neoplasms, detection of *IDH1/2* mutations has proven value in separating chondrosarcomas from chondroblastic osteosarcomas and dedifferentiated chondrosarcomas from undifferentiated pleomorphic sarcomas of bone [182, 183].

BRAF V600E Mutation in Langerhans Cell Histiocytosis

Langerhans cell histiocytosis (LCH) is a clonal proliferation of Langerhans cells which can form mass lesions in the bone, skin, and lung. LCH may need to be distinguished from Rosai-Dorfman disease, reactive lymphoid hyperplasia, and Hodgkin lymphoma in bone [164]. It has been shown that the lesional Langerhans cells contain *BRAF* V600E mutation in about 57% of cases, which can be detected by mutation-specific IHC and molecular testing [184]. *BRAF* V600E mutations result in the activation of the mitogen-activated protein kinase (MAPK) pathway. Most recently, overexpression of cyclin D1, a downstream target of MAPK pathway activation, has been demonstrated in Langerhans cell histiocytosis by IHC [185].

MDM2 Amplification in Low-Grade Osteosarcomas

Low-grade surface and central osteosarcomas, namely, parosteal osteosarcoma and low-grade central osteosarcoma, are characterized genetically by amplification of chromosome 12q13-15 via supernumerary ring chromosomes, resulting in gain or amplification of *MDM2* and *CDK4* genes [186]. Like ALT/WDL/DDLPS in soft tissue, amplification of 12q13-15 can be detected by FISH for the MDM2 locus and/or by surrogate IHC showing nuclear overexpression of MDM2 protein [41]. Histologically, both low-grade osteosarcomas are characterized by the presence of parallel-arranged trabeculae of woven or lamellar bone, surrounded by moderately cellular fibroblastic-type spindle cells. A cartilaginous component of parosteal osteosarcoma is sometimes present as a cap covering the periphery of the tumor [187]. Because of the bland morphology, low-grade osteosarcomas can be easily mistaken for its benign mimics such as fibrous dysplasia, myositis ossificans, and rarely osteochondroma, especially in small needle biopsies. Detection of *MDM2* amplification by either FISH or IHC for MDM2 and CDK4 can be therefore useful in distinguishing low-grade osteosarcomas from benign fibro-osseous lesions [41].

T (Brachyury) Duplication/Amplification in Chordoma

Chordoma is a malignant neoplasm of notochordal differentiation and characterized by axial skeletal location and typical cytomorphology of physaliferous cells within a myxoid background [164]. Brachyury (gene product of *T*) is an important transcription factor in notochord differentiation [188] and a sensitive and specific marker of notochordal tumors including more recently recognized benign notochordal cell tumor (BNCT), and even in small biopsies [189]. Recent NGS studies not only have confirmed the presence of *T (Brachyury)* duplication/amplification in a small fraction of chordoma cases but also identified molecular alterations involving the elements in the P13K signaling pathway and chromatin modeling [190]. Interestingly, deletions at the *SMARCB1* (INI1) locus, with associated loss of INI1 nuclear expression, commonly seen in malignant rhabdoid tumor and epithelioid sarcoma, have recently been demonstrated in a subset of pediatric chordoma cases with a poorly differentiated histology [191, 192].

Bone Tumors with Recurrent Translocations

Aneurysmal bone cyst (ABC) is a benign but locally destructive multicystic lesion of the bone. Histologically, it is characterized by blood-filled spaces surrounded by septa of bland spindle cells and osteoclastic-like giant cells [167]. Diagnosing ABC on FNA is particularly problematic due to the high insufficient rate and non-specific cytomorphology with a very broad differential diagnosis including many giant cell-rich neoplasms and telangiectatic osteosarcoma [193]. The majority of primary ABCs harbor a t(16;17) translation [194], resulting in a fusion transcript *CDH11-USP6*, which does not result in a fusion protein and instead leads to constitutive activation of *USP6* under the control of the *CDH11* promoter [195]. Many other fusion partners (*OMD, COL1A1, ZNF9, TRAP*) identified so far function in a similar manner [196]. FISH with break-apart probes for *USP6* can detect all fusion transcript variants in ABCs, which may be helpful in distinguishing ABC from telangiectatic osteosarcoma. However, the caveat is that *USP6* rearrangement is only present in neoplastic stromal cells, the fraction of which in ABCs ranges from 8% to 82%; a negative FISH result therefore may not necessarily exclude ABC diagnosis [197].

Mesenchymal chondrosarcoma is characterized genetically by *HEY1-NCOA2* fusion and morphologically by a bimorphic pattern composed of a well-differentiated cartilage component and a primitive round cell component [179]. In small biopsies, both components are not always present; either the primitive round cell component or the cartilaginous element may lead to misinterpretation, making the distinction from Ewing sarcoma or chondroblastic osteosarcoma/chondrosarcoma difficult. Identification of *HEY1-NCOA2* fusion either by FISH using *HEY1* or *NCOA2* probes or by RT-PCR detecting the fusion transcripts can be diagnostically useful [198].

The application of molecular testing in several other primary bone tumors with recurrent translocations, namely, Ewing sarcoma, round cell sarcomas with *CIC-DUX4* or *BCOR-CCNB3*, EHE, and myoepithelioma, is discussed in the soft tissue tumor section in this chapter.

Summary

The numerous advances in understanding the molecular features of tumors of soft tissue and bone have facilitated the development of many useful ancillary tests and have greatly enhanced our abilities to make definitive diagnoses on cytology samples. Diagnosis requires integration of morphologic, clinical, and radiographic features with relevant immunohistochemical and molecular tests. Although IHC, FISH, and sequencing assays can all be performed on all cytologic preparations, ROSE can be helpful to ensure specimen adequacy and to triage material for cell block preparation, which is the preferred substrate for ancillary testing. Most diagnostic work-ups of soft tissue and bone tumors begin with IHC to narrow the differential diagnosis, identify the line of differentiation, and confirm characteristic immunophenotypes to then guide the selection of relevant molecular tests; for many tumor types, there are diagnostic immunomarkers for protein correlates of underlying molecular alterations. For soft tissue tumors that harbor recurrent chromosomal rearrangements of gene amplifications, FISH is often useful although not specific for fusion gene type. RT-PCR and other sequencing-based methods can identify specific fusion genes, which may be helpful given that many tumor types can share common gene rearrangements, such as *EWSR1*. The cytopathologist should be aware that ancillary testing still poses many diagnostic pitfalls, as many tumor types share immunohistochemical and genetic features and no one single marker is perfectly sensitive and specific, which may pose numerous diagnostic pitfalls. Lastly, there have been rapid advances in NGS technologies which have played a large role in tumor discovery and may have potential diagnostic and clinical applications in the future.

References

1. Fletcher CDM, Bridge JA, Hogendoorn PCW, Mertens F, editors. WHO classification of tumours of soft tissue and bone. 4th ed. Lyon: IARC Press; 2013.
2. Dal Cin P, Qian X, Cibas ES. The marriage of cytology and cytogenetics. Cancer Cytopathol. 2013;121(6):279–90.
3. Doyle LA, Wang WL, Dal Cin P, Lopez-Terrada D, Mertens F, Lazar AJ, et al. MUC4 is a sensitive and extremely useful marker for sclerosing epithelioid fibrosarcoma: association with FUS gene rearrangement. Am J Surg Pathol. 2012;36(10):1444–51.

4. Yang EJ, Hornick JL, Qian X. Fine-needle aspiration of soft tissue perineurioma: a comparative analysis of cytomorphology and immunohistochemistry with benign and malignant mimics. Cancer Cytopathol. 2016;124(9):651–8.
5. Hwang DG, Qian X, Hornick JL. DOG1 antibody is a highly sensitive and specific marker for gastrointestinal stromal tumors in cytology cell blocks. Am J Clin Pathol. 2011;135(3):448–53.
6. Foo WC, Cruise MW, Wick MR, Hornick JL. Immunohistochemical staining for TLE1 distinguishes synovial sarcoma from histologic mimics. Am J Clin Pathol. 2011;135(6):839–44.
7. Lazar AJ, Tuvin D, Hajibashi S, Habeeb S, Bolshakov S, Mayordomo-Aranda E, et al. Specific mutations in the beta-catenin gene (CTNNB1) correlate with local recurrence in sporadic desmoid tumors. Am J Pathol. 2008;173(5):1518–27.
8. Miyaki M, Konishi M, Kikuchi-Yanoshita R, Enomoto M, Tanaka K, Takahashi H, et al. Coexistence of somatic and germ-line mutations of APC gene in desmoid tumors from patients with familial adenomatous polyposis. Cancer Res. 1993;53(21):5079–82.
9. Doyle LA, Vivero M, Fletcher CD, Mertens F, Hornick JL. Nuclear expression of STAT6 distinguishes solitary fibrous tumor from histologic mimics. Mod Pathol. 2014;27(3):390–5.
10. Yoshida A, Tsuta K, Ohno M, Yoshida M, Narita Y, Kawai A, et al. STAT6 immunohistochemistry is helpful in the diagnosis of solitary fibrous tumors. Am J Surg Pathol. 2014;38(4):552–9.
11. Chen BJ, Marino-Enriquez A, Fletcher CD, Hornick JL. Loss of retinoblastoma protein expression in spindle cell/pleomorphic lipomas and cytogenetically related tumors: an immunohistochemical study with diagnostic implications. Am J Surg Pathol. 2012;36(8):1119–28.
12. Miettinen M, Wang Z, Sarlomo-Rikala M, Abdullaev Z, Pack SD, Fetsch JF. ERG expression in epithelioid sarcoma: a diagnostic pitfall. Am J Surg Pathol. 2013;37(10):1580–5.
13. Qian X. Soft Tissue. In: Cibas ES, editor. Cytology: diagnostic principles and clinical correlates. 4th ed. Philadelphia: Elsevier; 2014. p. 471–518.
14. Mito JK, Conner JR, Hornick JL, Cibas ES, Qian X. SOX10/keratin dual-color immunohistochemistry: an effective first-line test for the workup of epithelioid malignant neoplasms in FNA and small biopsy specimens. Cancer Cytopathol. 2018;126(3):179–89.

15. Hung YP, Fletcher CD, Hornick JL. FOSB is a useful diagnostic marker for pseudomyogenic hemangioendothelioma. Am J Surg Pathol. 2017;41(5):596–606.
16. Chakrapani A, Warrick A, Nelson D, Beadling C, Corless CL. BRAF and KRAS mutations in sporadic glomus tumors. Am J Dermatopathol. 2012;34(5):533–5.
17. Mosquera JM, Sboner A, Zhang L, Chen CL, Sung YS, Chen HW, et al. Novel MIR143-NOTCH fusions in benign and malignant glomus tumors. Genes Chromosom Cancer. 2013;52(11):1075–87.
18. Brems H, Park C, Maertens O, Pemov A, Messiaen L, Upadhyaya M, et al. Glomus tumors in neurofibromatosis type 1: genetic, functional, and clinical evidence of a novel association. Cancer Res. 2009;69(18):7393–401.
19. Antonescu CR, Yoshida A, Guo T, Chang NE, Zhang L, Agaram NP, et al. KDR activating mutations in human angiosarcomas are sensitive to specific kinase inhibitors. Cancer Res. 2009;69(18):7175–9.
20. Huang SC, Zhang L, Sung YS, Chen CL, Kao YC, Agaram NP, et al. Recurrent CIC gene abnormalities in angiosarcomas: a molecular study of 120 cases with concurrent investigation of PLCG1, KDR, MYC, and FLT4 gene alterations. Am J Surg Pathol. 2016;40(5):645–55.
21. Italiano A, Thomas R, Breen M, Zhang L, Crago AM, Singer S, et al. The miR-17-92 cluster and its target THBS1 are differentially expressed in angiosarcomas dependent on MYC amplification. Genes Chromosom Cancer. 2012;51(6):569–78.
22. Walther C, Tayebwa J, Lilljebjorn H, Magnusson L, Nilsson J, von Steyern FV, et al. A novel SERPINE1-FOSB fusion gene results in transcriptional up-regulation of FOSB in pseudomyogenic haemangioendothelioma. J Pathol. 2014;232(5):534–40.
23. Gebre-Medhin S, Nord KH, Moller E, Mandahl N, Magnusson L, Nilsson J, et al. Recurrent rearrangement of the PHF1 gene in ossifying fibromyxoid tumors. Am J Pathol. 2012;181(3):1069–77.
24. Specht K, Zhang L, Sung YS, Nucci M, Dry S, Vaiyapuri S, et al. Novel BCOR-MAML3 and ZC3H7B-BCOR gene fusions in undifferentiated small blue round cell sarcomas. Am J Surg Pathol. 2016;40(4):433–42.
25. Sandberg AA. Updates on the cytogenetics and molecular genetics of bone and soft tissue tumors: liposarcoma. Cancer Genet Cytogenet. 2004;155(1):1–24.

26. Dei Tos AP, Doglioni C, Piccinin S, Maestro R, Mentzel T, Barbareschi M, et al. Molecular abnormalities of the p53 pathway in dedifferentiated liposarcoma. J Pathol. 1997;181(1):8–13.
27. Mertens F, Fletcher CD, Dal Cin P, De Wever I, Mandahl N, Mitelman F, et al. Cytogenetic analysis of 46 pleomorphic soft tissue sarcomas and correlation with morphologic and clinical features: a report of the CHAMP Study Group. Chromosomes and Morphology. Genes Chromosom Cancer. 1998;22(1): 16–25.
28. Meis-Kindblom JM, Sjogren H, Kindblom LG, Peydro-Mellquist A, Roijer E, Aman P, et al. Cytogenetic and molecular genetic analyses of liposarcoma and its soft tissue simulators: recognition of new variants and differential diagnosis. Virchows Arch. 2001;439(2):141–51.
29. Sirvent N, Coindre JM, Maire G, Hostein I, Keslair F, Guillou L, et al. Detection of MDM2-CDK4 amplification by fluorescence in situ hybridization in 200 paraffin-embedded tumor samples: utility in diagnosing adipocytic lesions and comparison with immunohistochemistry and real-time PCR. Am J Surg Pathol. 2007;31(10):1476–89.
30. Clay MR, Martinez AP, Weiss SW, Edgar MA. MDM2 and CDK4 Immunohistochemistry: should it be used in problematic differentiated lipomatous tumors?: a new perspective. Am J Surg Pathol. 2016;40(12):1647–52.
31. Weaver J, Rao P, Goldblum JR, Joyce MJ, Turner SL, Lazar AJ, et al. Can MDM2 analytical tests performed on core needle biopsy be relied upon to diagnose well-differentiated liposarcoma? Mod Pathol. 2010;23(10):1301–6.
32. Weaver J, Goldblum JR, Turner S, Tubbs RR, Wang WL, Lazar AJ, et al. Detection of MDM2 gene amplification or protein expression distinguishes sclerosing mesenteritis and retroperitoneal fibrosis from inflammatory well-differentiated liposarcoma. Mod Pathol. 2009;22(1):66–70.
33. Marino-Enriquez A, Fletcher CD, Dal Cin P, Hornick JL. Dedifferentiated liposarcoma with "homologous" lipoblastic (pleomorphic liposarcoma-like) differentiation: clinicopathologic and molecular analysis of a series suggesting revised diagnostic criteria. Am J Surg Pathol. 2010;34(8):1122–31.
34. Marino-Enriquez A, Hornick JL, Dal Cin P, Cibas ES, Qian X. Dedifferentiated liposarcoma and pleomorphic liposarcoma: a comparative study of cytomorphology and MDM2/CDK4 expression on fine-needle aspiration. Cancer Cytopathol. 2014;122(2):128–37.

35. Liau JY, Lee JC, Wu CT, Kuo KT, Huang HY, Liang CW. Dedifferentiated liposarcoma with homologous lipoblastic differentiation: expanding the spectrum to include low-grade tumours. Histopathology. 2013;62(5):702–10.
36. Binh MB, Sastre-Garau X, Guillou L, de Pinieux G, Terrier P, Lagace R, et al. MDM2 and CDK4 immunostainings are useful adjuncts in diagnosing well-differentiated and dedifferentiated liposarcoma subtypes: a comparative analysis of 559 soft tissue neoplasms with genetic data. Am J Surg Pathol. 2005;29(10):1340–7.
37. Bode-Lesniewska B, Zhao J, Speel EJ, Biraima AM, Turina M, Komminoth P, et al. Gains of 12q13-14 and overexpression of mdm2 are frequent findings in intimal sarcomas of the pulmonary artery. Virchows Arch. 2001;438(1):57–65.
38. Zhang H, Macdonald WD, Erickson-Johnson M, Wang X, Jenkins RB, Oliveira AM. Cytogenetic and molecular cytogenetic findings of intimal sarcoma. Cancer Genet Cytogenet. 2007;179(2):146–9.
39. Zhao J, Roth J, Bode-Lesniewska B, Pfaltz M, Heitz PU, Komminoth P. Combined comparative genomic hybridization and genomic microarray for detection of gene amplifications in pulmonary artery intimal sarcomas and adrenocortical tumors. Genes Chromosom Cancer. 2002;34(1):48–57.
40. Duhamel LA, Ye H, Halai D, Idowu BD, Presneau N, Tirabosco R, et al. Frequency of Mouse Double Minute 2 (MDM2) and Mouse Double Minute 4 (MDM4) amplification in parosteal and conventional osteosarcoma subtypes. Histopathology. 2012;60(2):357–9.
41. Dujardin F, Binh MB, Bouvier C, Gomez-Brouchet A, Larousserie F, Muret A, et al. MDM2 and CDK4 immunohistochemistry is a valuable tool in the differential diagnosis of low-grade osteosarcomas and other primary fibro-osseous lesions of the bone. Mod Pathol. 2011;24(5):624–37.
42. Mejia-Guerrero S, Quejada M, Gokgoz N, Gill M, Parkes RK, Wunder JS, et al. Characterization of the 12q15 MDM2 and 12q13-14 CDK4 amplicons and clinical correlations in osteosarcoma. Genes Chromosom Cancer. 2010;49(6):518–25.
43. Tarkkanen M, Bohling T, Gamberi G, Ragazzini P, Benassi MS, Kivioja A, et al. Comparative genomic hybridization of low-grade central osteosarcoma. Mod Pathol. 1998;11(5):421–6.
44. Antonescu CR, Dal CP. Promiscuous genes involved in recurrent chromosomal translocations in soft tissue tumours. Pathology. 2014;46(2):105–12.

45. Delattre O, Zucman J, Plougastel B, Desmaze C, Melot T, Peter M, et al. Gene fusion with an ETS DNA-binding domain caused by chromosome translocation in human tumours. Nature. 1992;359(6391):162–5.
46. Delattre O, Zucman J, Melot T, Garau XS, Zucker JM, Lenoir GM, et al. The Ewing family of tumors--a subgroup of small-round-cell tumors defined by specific chimeric transcripts. N Engl J Med. 1994;331(5):294–9.
47. Ginsberg JP, de Alava E, Ladanyi M, Wexler LH, Kovar H, Paulussen M, et al. EWS-FLI1 and EWS-ERG gene fusions are associated with similar clinical phenotypes in Ewing's sarcoma. J Clin Oncol. 1999;17(6):1809–14.
48. Jeon IS, Davis JN, Braun BS, Sublett JE, Roussel MF, Denny CT, et al. A variant Ewing's sarcoma translocation (7;22) fuses the EWS gene to the ETS gene ETV1. Oncogene. 1995;10(6):1229–34.
49. Kaneko Y, Yoshida K, Handa M, Toyoda Y, Nishihira H, Tanaka Y, et al. Fusion of an ETS-family gene, EIAF, to EWS by t(17;22)(q12;q12) chromosome translocation in an undifferentiated sarcoma of infancy. Genes Chromosom Cancer. 1996;15(2):115–21.
50. Peter M, Couturier J, Pacquement H, Michon J, Thomas G, Magdelenat H, et al. A new member of the ETS family fused to EWS in Ewing tumors. Oncogene. 1997;14(10):1159–64.
51. Hung YP, Fletcher CD, Hornick JL. Evaluation of NKX2-2 expression in round cell sarcomas and other tumors with EWSR1 rearrangement: imperfect specificity for Ewing sarcoma. Mod Pathol. 2016;29(4):370–80.
52. Wang WL, Patel NR, Caragea M, Hogendoorn PC, Lopez-Terrada D, Hornick JL, et al. Expression of ERG, an Ets family transcription factor, identifies ERG-rearranged Ewing sarcoma. Mod Pathol. 2012;25(10):1378–83.
53. Shing DC, McMullan DJ, Roberts P, Smith K, Chin SF, Nicholson J, et al. FUS/ERG gene fusions in Ewing's tumors. Cancer Res. 2003;63(15):4568–76.
54. Berg T, Kalsaas AH, Buechner J, Busund LT. Ewing sarcoma-peripheral neuroectodermal tumor of the kidney with a FUS-ERG fusion transcript. Cancer Genet Cytogenet. 2009;194(1):53–7.
55. Argatoff LH, O'Connell JX, Mathers JA, Gilks CB, Sorensen PH. Detection of the EWS/WT1 gene fusion by reverse transcriptase-polymerase chain reaction in the diagnosis of intra-abdominal desmoplastic small round cell tumor. Am J Surg Pathol. 1996;20(4):406–12.

56. Ladanyi M, Gerald W. Fusion of the EWS and WT1 genes in the desmoplastic small round cell tumor. Cancer Res. 1994;54(11):2837–40.
57. Wang WL, Mayordomo E, Zhang W, Hernandez VS, Tuvin D, Garcia L, et al. Detection and characterization of EWSR1/ATF1 and EWSR1/CREB1 chimeric transcripts in clear cell sarcoma (melanoma of soft parts). Mod Pathol. 2009;22(9):1201–9.
58. Kosemehmetoglu K, Folpe AL. Clear cell sarcoma of tendons and aponeuroses, and osteoclast-rich tumour of the gastrointestinal tract with features resembling clear cell sarcoma of soft parts: a review and update. J Clin Pathol. 2010;63(5):416–23.
59. Antonescu CR, Nafa K, Segal NH, Dal Cin P, Ladanyi M. EWS-CREB1: a recurrent variant fusion in clear cell sarcoma--association with gastrointestinal location and absence of melanocytic differentiation. Clin Cancer Res. 2006;12(18):5356–62.
60. Stockman DL, Miettinen M, Suster S, Spagnolo D, Dominguez-Malagon H, Hornick JL, et al. Malignant gastrointestinal neuroectodermal tumor: clinicopathologic, immunohistochemical, ultrastructural, and molecular analysis of 16 cases with a reappraisal of clear cell sarcoma-like tumors of the gastrointestinal tract. Am J Surg Pathol. 2012;36(6):857–68.
61. Antonescu CR, Dal Cin P, Nafa K, Teot LA, Surti U, Fletcher CD, et al. EWSR1-CREB1 is the predominant gene fusion in angiomatoid fibrous histiocytoma. Genes Chromosom Cancer. 2007;46(12):1051–60.
62. Qian X, Hornick JL, Cibas ES, Dal Cin P, Domanski HA. Angiomatoid fibrous histiocytoma a series of five cytologic cases with literature review and emphasis on diagnostic pitfalls. Diagn Cytopathol. 2012;40(Suppl 2):E86–93.
63. Attwooll C, Tariq M, Harris M, Coyne JD, Telford N, Varley JM. Identification of a novel fusion gene involving hTAFII68 and CHN from a t(9;17)(q22;q11.2) translocation in an extraskeletal myxoid chondrosarcoma. Oncogene. 1999;18(52):7599–601.
64. Panagopoulos I, Mertens F, Isaksson M, Domanski HA, Brosjo O, Heim S, et al. Molecular genetic characterization of the EWS/CHN and RBP56/CHN fusion genes in extraskeletal myxoid chondrosarcoma. Genes Chromosom Cancer. 2002;35(4):340–52.
65. Flucke U, Tops BB, Verdijk MA, van Cleef PJ, van Zwam PH, Slootweg PJ, et al. NR4A3 rearrangement reliably distinguishes between the clinicopathologically overlapping entities

myoepithelial carcinoma of soft tissue and cellular extraskeletal myxoid chondrosarcoma. Virchows Arch. 2012;460(6):621–8.
66. Hornick JL, Fletcher CD. Myoepithelial tumors of soft tissue: a clinicopathologic and immunohistochemical study of 101 cases with evaluation of prognostic parameters. Am J Surg Pathol. 2003;27(9):1183–96.
67. Gleason BC, Fletcher CD. Myoepithelial carcinoma of soft tissue in children: an aggressive neoplasm analyzed in a series of 29 cases. Am J Surg Pathol. 2007;31(12):1813–24.
68. Brandal P, Panagopoulos I, Bjerkehagen B, Gorunova L, Skjeldal S, Micci F, et al. Detection of a t(1;22)(q23;q12) translocation leading to an EWSR1-PBX1 fusion gene in a myoepithelioma. Genes Chromosom Cancer. 2008;47(7):558–64.
69. Brandal P, Panagopoulos I, Bjerkehagen B, Heim S. t(19;22)(q13;q12) Translocation leading to the novel fusion gene EWSR1-ZNF444 in soft tissue myoepithelial carcinoma. Genes Chromosom Cancer. 2009;48(12):1051–6.
70. Antonescu CR, Zhang L, Chang NE, Pawel BR, Travis W, Katabi N, et al. EWSR1-POU5F1 fusion in soft tissue myoepithelial tumors. A molecular analysis of sixty-six cases, including soft tissue, bone, and visceral lesions, showing common involvement of the EWSR1 gene. Genes Chromosom Cancer. 2010;49(12):1114–24.
71. Flucke U, Palmedo G, Blankenhorn N, Slootweg PJ, Kutzner H, Mentzel T. EWSR1 gene rearrangement occurs in a subset of cutaneous myoepithelial tumors: a study of 18 cases. Mod Pathol. 2011;24(11):1444–50.
72. Jo VY, Antonescu CR, Zhang L, Dal Cin P, Hornick JL, Fletcher CD. Cutaneous syncytial myoepithelioma: clinicopathologic characterization in a series of 38 cases. Am J Surg Pathol. 2013;37(5):710–8.
73. Puls F, Arbajian E, Magnusson L, Douis H, Kindblom LG, Mertens F. Myoepithelioma of bone with a novel FUS-POU5F1 fusion gene. Histopathology. 2014;65(6):917–22.
74. Agaram NP, Chen HW, Zhang L, Sung YS, Panicek D, Healey JH, et al. EWSR1-PBX3: a novel gene fusion in myoepithelial tumors. Genes Chromosom Cancer. 2015;54(2):63–71.
75. Huang SC, Chen HW, Zhang L, Sung YS, Agaram NP, Davis M, et al. Novel FUS-KLF17 and EWSR1-KLF17 fusions in myoepithelial tumors. Genes Chromosom Cancer. 2015;54(5):267–75.
76. Aman P, Ron D, Mandahl N, Fioretos T, Heim S, Arheden K, et al. Rearrangement of the transcription factor gene

CHOP in myxoid liposarcomas with t(12,16)(q13;p11). Genes Chromosom Cancer. 1992;5(4):278–85.
77. Dal Cin P, Sciot R, Panagopoulos I, Aman P, Samson I, Mandahl N, et al. Additional evidence of a variant translocation t(12;22) with EWS/CHOP fusion in myxoid liposarcoma: clinicopathological features. J Pathol. 1997;182(4):437–41.
78. Panagopoulos I, Hoglund M, Mertens F, Mandahl N, Mitelman F, Aman P. Fusion of the EWS and CHOP genes in myxoid liposarcoma. Oncogene. 1996;12(3):489–94.
79. Panagopoulos I, Storlazzi CT, Fletcher CD, Fletcher JA, Nascimento A, Domanski HA, et al. The chimeric FUS/CREB3l2 gene is specific for low-grade fibromyxoid sarcoma. Genes Chromosom Cancer. 2004;40(3):218–28.
80. Mertens F, Fletcher CD, Antonescu CR, Coindre JM, Colecchia M, Domanski HA, et al. Clinicopathologic and molecular genetic characterization of low-grade fibromyxoid sarcoma, and cloning of a novel FUS/CREB3L1 fusion gene. Lab Investig. 2005;85(3):408–15.
81. Guillou L, Benhattar J, Gengler C, Gallagher G, Ranchere-Vince D, Collin F, et al. Translocation-positive low-grade fibromyxoid sarcoma: clinicopathologic and molecular analysis of a series expanding the morphologic spectrum and suggesting potential relationship to sclerosing epithelioid fibrosarcoma: a study from the French Sarcoma Group. Am J Surg Pathol. 2007;31(9):1387–402.
82. Arbajian E, Puls F, Magnusson L, Thway K, Fisher C, Sumathi VP, et al. Recurrent EWSR1-CREB3L1 gene fusions in sclerosing epithelioid fibrosarcoma. Am J Surg Pathol. 2014;38(6):801–8.
83. Rubin BP, Heinrich MC, Corless CL. Gastrointestinal stromal tumour. Lancet. 2007;369(9574):1731–41.
84. Schaefer IM, Marino-Enriquez A, Fletcher JA. What is new in gastrointestinal stromal tumor? Adv Anat Pathol. 2017;24(5):259–67.
85. Medeiros F, Corless CL, Duensing A, Hornick JL, Oliveira AM, Heinrich MC, et al. KIT-negative gastrointestinal stromal tumors: proof of concept and therapeutic implications. Am J Surg Pathol. 2004;28(7):889–94.
86. West RB, Corless CL, Chen X, Rubin BP, Subramanian S, Montgomery K, et al. The novel marker, DOG1, is expressed ubiquitously in gastrointestinal stromal tumors irrespective of KIT or PDGFRA mutation status. Am J Pathol. 2004;165(1):107–13.

87. Espinosa I, Lee CH, Kim MK, Rouse BT, Subramanian S, Montgomery K, et al. A novel monoclonal antibody against DOG1 is a sensitive and specific marker for gastrointestinal stromal tumors. Am J Surg Pathol. 2008;32(2):210–8.
88. Gill AJ, Chou A, Vilain R, Clarkson A, Lui M, Jin R, et al. Immunohistochemistry for SDHB divides gastrointestinal stromal tumors (GISTs) into 2 distinct types. Am J Surg Pathol. 2010;34(5):636–44.
89. Gill AJ, Chou A, Vilain RE, Clifton-Bligh RJ. "Pediatric-type" gastrointestinal stromal tumors are SDHB negative ("type 2") GISTs. Am J Surg Pathol. 2011;35(8):1245–7. author reply 7–8.
90. Rege TA, Wagner AJ, Corless CL, Heinrich MC, Hornick JL. "Pediatric-type" gastrointestinal stromal tumors in adults: distinctive histology predicts genotype and clinical behavior. Am J Surg Pathol. 2011;35(4):495–504.
91. Doyle LA, Nelson D, Heinrich MC, Corless CL, Hornick JL. Loss of succinate dehydrogenase subunit B (SDHB) expression is limited to a distinctive subset of gastric wild-type gastrointestinal stromal tumours: a comprehensive genotype-phenotype correlation study. Histopathology. 2012;61(5):801–9.
92. Miettinen M, Wang ZF, Sarlomo-Rikala M, Osuch C, Rutkowski P, Lasota J. Succinate dehydrogenase-deficient GISTs: a clinicopathologic, immunohistochemical, and molecular genetic study of 66 gastric GISTs with predilection to young age. Am J Surg Pathol. 2011;35(11):1712–21.
93. Dwight T, Benn DE, Clarkson A, Vilain R, Lipton L, Robinson BG, et al. Loss of SDHA expression identifies SDHA mutations in succinate dehydrogenase-deficient gastrointestinal stromal tumors. Am J Surg Pathol. 2013;37(2):226–33.
94. Wagner AJ, Remillard SP, Zhang YX, Doyle LA, George S, Hornick JL. Loss of expression of SDHA predicts SDHA mutations in gastrointestinal stromal tumors. Mod Pathol. 2013;26(2):289–94.
95. Mason EF, Hornick JL. Conventional risk stratification fails to predict progression of Succinate Dehydrogenase-deficient gastrointestinal stromal tumors: a clinicopathologic study of 76 cases. Am J Surg Pathol. 2016;40(12):1616–21.
96. Pasini B, McWhinney SR, Bei T, Matyakhina L, Stergiopoulos S, Muchow M, et al. Clinical and molecular genetics of patients with the Carney-Stratakis syndrome and germline mutations of the genes coding for the succinate dehydrogenase subunits SDHB, SDHC, and SDHD. Eur J Hum Genet. 2008;16(1):79–88.

97. Haller F, Moskalev EA, Faucz FR, Barthelmess S, Wiemann S, Bieg M, et al. Aberrant DNA hypermethylation of SDHC: a novel mechanism of tumor development in Carney triad. Endocr Relat Cancer. 2014;21(4):567–77.
98. Folpe AL, Schmidt RA, Chapman D, Gown AM. Poorly differentiated synovial sarcoma: immunohistochemical distinction from primitive neuroectodermal tumors and high-grade malignant peripheral nerve sheath tumors. Am J Surg Pathol. 1998;22(6):673–82.
99. Barr FG. Gene fusions involving PAX and FOX family members in alveolar rhabdomyosarcoma. Oncogene. 2001;20(40):5736–46.
100. Sorensen PH, Lynch JC, Qualman SJ, Tirabosco R, Lim JF, Maurer HM, et al. PAX3-FKHR and PAX7-FKHR gene fusions are prognostic indicators in alveolar rhabdomyosarcoma: a report from the children's oncology group. J Clin Oncol. 2002;20(11):2672–9.
101. Agaram NP, Chen CL, Zhang L, LaQuaglia MP, Wexler L, Antonescu CR. Recurrent MYOD1 mutations in pediatric and adult sclerosing and spindle cell rhabdomyosarcomas: evidence for a common pathogenesis. Genes Chromosom Cancer. 2014;53(9):779–87.
102. Szuhai K, de Jong D, Leung WY, Fletcher CD, Hogendoorn PC. Transactivating mutation of the MYOD1 gene is a frequent event in adult spindle cell rhabdomyosarcoma. J Pathol. 2014;232(3):300–7.
103. Rekhi B, Upadhyay P, Ramteke MP, Dutt A. MYOD1 (L122R) mutations are associated with spindle cell and sclerosing rhabdomyosarcomas with aggressive clinical outcomes. Mod Pathol. 2016;29(12):1532–40.
104. Mosquera JM, Sboner A, Zhang L, Kitabayashi N, Chen CL, Sung YS, et al. Recurrent NCOA2 gene rearrangements in congenital/infantile spindle cell rhabdomyosarcoma. Genes Chromosom Cancer. 2013;52(6):538–50.
105. Alaggio R, Zhang L, Sung YS, Huang SC, Chen CL, Bisogno G, et al. A molecular study of pediatric spindle and Sclerosing rhabdomyosarcoma: identification of novel and recurrent VGLL2-related fusions in infantile cases. Am J Surg Pathol. 2016;40(2):224–35.
106. Paulson V, Chandler G, Rakheja D, Galindo RL, Wilson K, Amatruda JF, et al. High-resolution array CGH identifies common mechanisms that drive embryonal rhabdomyosarcoma pathogenesis. Genes Chromosom Cancer. 2011;50(6):397–408.

107. Shukla N, Ameur N, Yilmaz I, Nafa K, Lau CY, Marchetti A, et al. Oncogene mutation profiling of pediatric solid tumors reveals significant subsets of embryonal rhabdomyosarcoma and neuroblastoma with mutated genes in growth signaling pathways. Clin Cancer Res. 2012;18(3):748–57.
108. Robinson DR, Wu YM, Kalyana-Sundaram S, Cao X, Lonigro RJ, Sung YS, et al. Identification of recurrent NAB2-STAT6 gene fusions in solitary fibrous tumor by integrative sequencing. Nat Genet. 2013;45(2):180–5.
109. Chmielecki J, Crago AM, Rosenberg M, O'Connor R, Walker SR, Ambrogio L, et al. Whole-exome sequencing identifies a recurrent NAB2-STAT6 fusion in solitary fibrous tumors. Nat Genet. 2013;45(2):131–2.
110. Tani E, Wejde J, Astrom K, Wingmo IL, Larsson O, Haglund F. FNA cytology of solitary fibrous tumors and the diagnostic value of STAT6 immunocytochemistry. Cancer. 2018;126(1):36–43.
111. O'Brien KP, Seroussi E, Dal Cin P, Sciot R, Mandahl N, Fletcher JA, et al. Various regions within the alpha-helical domain of the COL1A1 gene are fused to the second exon of the PDGFB gene in dermatofibrosarcomas and giant-cell fibroblastomas. Genes Chromosom Cancer. 1998;23(2):187–93.
112. Patel KU, Szabo SS, Hernandez VS, Prieto VG, Abruzzo LV, Lazar AJ, et al. Dermatofibrosarcoma protuberans COL1A1-PDGFB fusion is identified in virtually all dermatofibrosarcoma protuberans cases when investigated by newly developed multiplex reverse transcription polymerase chain reaction and fluorescence in situ hybridization assays. Hum Pathol. 2008;39(2):184–93.
113. Pedeutour F, Simon MP, Minoletti F, Barcelo G, Terrier-Lacombe MJ, Combemale P, et al. Translocation, t(17;22)(q22;q13), in dermatofibrosarcoma protuberans: a new tumor-associated chromosome rearrangement. Cytogenet Cell Genet. 1996;72(2–3):171–4.
114. Bridge JA, Kanamori M, Ma Z, Pickering D, Hill DA, Lydiatt W, et al. Fusion of the ALK gene to the clathrin heavy chain gene, CLTC, in inflammatory myofibroblastic tumor. Am J Pathol. 2001;159(2):411–5.
115. Cook JR, Dehner LP, Collins MH, Ma Z, Morris SW, Coffin CM, et al. Anaplastic lymphoma kinase (ALK) expression in the inflammatory myofibroblastic tumor: a comparative immunohistochemical study. Am J Surg Pathol. 2001;25(11):1364–71.

116. Marino-Enriquez A, Wang WL, Roy A, Lopez-Terrada D, Lazar AJ, Fletcher CD, et al. Epithelioid inflammatory myofibroblastic sarcoma: an aggressive intra-abdominal variant of inflammatory myofibroblastic tumor with nuclear membrane or perinuclear ALK. Am J Surg Pathol. 2011;35(1):135–44.
117. Lee JC, Wu JM, Liau JY, Huang HY, Lo CY, Jan IS, et al. Cytopathologic features of epithelioid inflammatory myofibroblastic sarcoma with correlation of histopathology, immunohistochemistry, and molecular cytogenetic analysis. Cancer Cytopathol. 2015;123(8):495–504.
118. Hornick JL, Dal Cin P, Fletcher CD. Loss of INI1 expression is characteristic of both conventional and proximal-type epithelioid sarcoma. Am J Surg Pathol. 2009;33(4):542–50.
119. Flucke U, Slootweg PJ, Mentzel T, Pauwels P, Hulsebos TJ. Re: infrequent SMARCB1/INI1 gene alteration in epithelioid sarcoma: a useful tool in distinguishing epithelioid sarcoma from malignant rhabdoid tumor: Direct evidence of mutational inactivation of SMARCB1/INI1 in epithelioid sarcoma. Hum Pathol. 2009;40(9):1361–2. author reply 2-4.
120. Sullivan LM, Folpe AL, Pawel BR, Judkins AR, Biegel JA. Epithelioid sarcoma is associated with a high percentage of SMARCB1 deletions. Mod Pathol. 2013;26(3):385–92.
121. Le Loarer F, Zhang L, Fletcher CD, Ribeiro A, Singer S, Italiano A, et al. Consistent SMARCB1 homozygous deletions in epithelioid sarcoma and in a subset of myoepithelial carcinomas can be reliably detected by FISH in archival material. Genes Chromosom Cancer. 2014;53(6):475–86.
122. Hollmann TJ, Hornick JL. INI1-deficient tumors: diagnostic features and molecular genetics. Am J Surg Pathol. 2011;35(10):e47–63.
123. Errani C, Zhang L, Sung YS, Hajdu M, Singer S, Maki RG, et al. A novel WWTR1-CAMTA1 gene fusion is a consistent abnormality in epithelioid hemangioendothelioma of different anatomic sites. Genes Chromosom Cancer. 2011;50(8):644–53.
124. Doyle LA, Fletcher CD, Hornick JL. Nuclear expression of CAMTA1 distinguishes epithelioid Hemangioendothelioma from histologic mimics. Am J Surg Pathol. 2016;40(1):94–102.
125. Antonescu CR, Le Loarer F, Mosquera JM, Sboner A, Zhang L, Chen CL, et al. Novel YAP1-TFE3 fusion defines a distinct subset of epithelioid hemangioendothelioma. Genes Chromosom Cancer. 2013;52(8):775–84.

126. Chamberlain BK, McClain CM, Gonzalez RS, Coffin CM, Cates JM. Alveolar soft part sarcoma and granular cell tumor: an immunohistochemical comparison study. Hum Pathol. 2014;45(5):1039–44.
127. Schoolmeester JK, Lastra RR. Granular cell tumors overexpress TFE3 without corollary gene rearrangement. Hum Pathol. 2015;46(8):1242–3.
128. Folpe AL, Mentzel T, Lehr HA, Fisher C, Balzer BL, Weiss SW. Perivascular epithelioid cell neoplasms of soft tissue and gynecologic origin: a clinicopathologic study of 26 cases and review of the literature. Am J Surg Pathol. 2005;29(12):1558–75.
129. Argani P, Aulmann S, Illei PB, Netto GJ, Ro J, Cho HY, et al. A distinctive subset of PEComas harbors TFE3 gene fusions. Am J Surg Pathol. 2010;34(10):1395–406.
130. Yoshimoto M, Graham C, Chilton-MacNeill S, Lee E, Shago M, Squire J, et al. Detailed cytogenetic and array analysis of pediatric primitive sarcomas reveals a recurrent CIC-DUX4 fusion gene event. Cancer Genet Cytogenet. 2009;195(1):1–11.
131. Graham C, Chilton-MacNeill S, Zielenska M, Somers GR. The CIC-DUX4 fusion transcript is present in a subgroup of pediatric primitive round cell sarcomas. Hum Pathol. 2012;43(2):180–9.
132. Italiano A, Sung YS, Zhang L, Singer S, Maki RG, Coindre JM, et al. High prevalence of CIC fusion with double-homeobox (DUX4) transcription factors in EWSR1-negative undifferentiated small blue round cell sarcomas. Genes Chromosom Cancer. 2012;51(3):207–18.
133. Choi EY, Thomas DG, McHugh JB, Patel RM, Roulston D, Schuetze SM, et al. Undifferentiated small round cell sarcoma with t(4;19)(q35;q13.1) CIC-DUX4 fusion: a novel highly aggressive soft tissue tumor with distinctive histopathology. Am J Surg Pathol. 2013;37(9):1379–86.
134. Pierron G, Tirode F, Lucchesi C, Reynaud S, Ballet S, Cohen-Gogo S, et al. A new subtype of bone sarcoma defined by BCOR-CCNB3 gene fusion. Nat Genet. 2012;44(4):461–6.
135. Cohen-Gogo S, Cellier C, Coindre JM, Mosseri V, Pierron G, Guillemet C, et al. Ewing-like sarcomas with BCOR-CCNB3 fusion transcript: a clinical, radiological and pathological retrospective study from the Societe Francaise des Cancers de L'Enfant. Pediatr Blood Cancer. 2014;61(12):2191–8.
136. Puls F, Niblett A, Marland G, Gaston CL, Douis H, Mangham DC, et al. BCOR-CCNB3 (Ewing-like) sarcoma: a clinicopathologic

analysis of 10 cases, in comparison with conventional Ewing sarcoma. Am J Surg Pathol. 2014;38(10):1307–18.
137. Peters TL, Kumar V, Polikepahad S, Lin FY, Sarabia SF, Liang Y, et al. BCOR-CCNB3 fusions are frequent in undifferentiated sarcomas of male children. Mod Pathol. 2015;28(4):575–86.
138. Chebib I, Jo VY. Round cell sarcoma with CIC-DUX4 gene fusion: discussion of the distinctive cytomorphologic, immunohistochemical, and molecular features in the differential diagnosis of round cell tumors. Cancer Cytopathol. 2016;124(5):350–61.
139. Specht K, Sung YS, Zhang L, Richter GH, Fletcher CD, Antonescu CR. Distinct transcriptional signature and immunoprofile of CIC-DUX4 fusion-positive round cell tumors compared to EWSR1-rearranged Ewing sarcomas: further evidence toward distinct pathologic entities. Genes Chromosom Cancer. 2014;53(7):622–33.
140. Hung YP, Fletcher CD, Hornick JL. Evaluation of ETV4 and WT1 expression in CIC-rearranged sarcomas and histologic mimics. Mod Pathol. 2016;29(11):1324–34.
141. Le Guellec S, Velasco V, Perot G, Watson S, Tirode F, Coindre JM. ETV4 is a useful marker for the diagnosis of CIC-rearranged undifferentiated round-cell sarcomas: a study of 127 cases including mimicking lesions. Mod Pathol. 2016;29(12):1523–31.
142. Shibayama T, Okamoto T, Nakashima Y, Kato T, Sakurai T, Minamiguchi S, et al. Screening of BCOR-CCNB3 sarcoma using immunohistochemistry for CCNB3: a clinicopathological report of three pediatric cases. Pathol Int. 2015;65(8):410–4.
143. Kao YC, Owosho AA, Sung YS, Zhang L, Fujisawa Y, Lee JC, et al. BCOR-CCNB3 fusion positive sarcomas: a clinicopathologic and molecular analysis of 36 cases with comparison to morphologic spectrum and clinical behavior of other round cell sarcomas. Am J Surg Pathol. 2018;42(5):604–15.
144. Bhattacharya B, Dilworth HP, Iacobuzio-Donahue C, Ricci F, Weber K, Furlong MA, et al. Nuclear beta-catenin expression distinguishes deep fibromatosis from other benign and malignant fibroblastic and myofibroblastic lesions. Am J Surg Pathol. 2005;29(5):653–9.
145. Carlson JW, Fletcher CD. Immunohistochemistry for beta-catenin in the differential diagnosis of spindle cell lesions: analysis of a series and review of the literature. Histopathology. 2007;51(4):509–14.
146. Lee W, Teckie S, Wiesner T, Ran L, Prieto Granada CN, Lin M, et al. PRC2 is recurrently inactivated through EED or SUZ12

loss in malignant peripheral nerve sheath tumors. Nat Genet. 2014;46(11):1227–32.
147. Zhang M, Wang Y, Jones S, Sausen M, McMahon K, Sharma R, et al. Somatic mutations of SUZ12 in malignant peripheral nerve sheath tumors. Nat Genet. 2014;46(11):1170–2.
148. Cleven AH, Sannaa GA, Briaire-de Bruijn I, Ingram DR, van de Rijn M, Rubin BP, et al. Loss of H3K27 tri-methylation is a diagnostic marker for malignant peripheral nerve sheath tumors and an indicator for an inferior survival. Mod Pathol. 2016;29(6):582–90.
149. Prieto-Granada CN, Wiesner T, Messina JL, Jungbluth AA, Chi P, Antonescu CR. Loss of H3K27me3 expression is a highly sensitive marker for sporadic and radiation-induced MPNST. Am J Surg Pathol. 2016;40(4):479–89.
150. Schaefer IM, Fletcher CD, Hornick JL. Loss of H3K27 trimethylation distinguishes malignant peripheral nerve sheath tumors from histologic mimics. Mod Pathol. 2016;29(1):4–13.
151. Le Guellec S, Macagno N, Velasco V, Lamant L, Lae M, Filleron T, et al. Loss of H3K27 trimethylation is not suitable for distinguishing malignant peripheral nerve sheath tumor from melanoma: a study of 387 cases including mimicking lesions. Mod Pathol. 2017;30(12):1677–87.
152. Mito JK, Qian X, Doyle LA, Hornick JL, Jo VY. Role of histone H3K27 Trimethylation loss as a marker for malignant peripheral nerve sheath tumor in fine-needle aspiration and small biopsy specimens. Am J Clin Pathol. 2017;148(2):179–89.
153. Erickson-Johnson MR, Chou MM, Evers BR, Roth CW, Seys AR, Jin L, et al. Nodular fasciitis: a novel model of transient neoplasia induced by MYH9-USP6 gene fusion. Lab Investig. 2011;91(10):1427–33.
154. Delaney D, Diss TC, Presneau N, Hing S, Berisha F, Idowu BD, et al. GNAS1 mutations occur more commonly than previously thought in intramuscular myxoma. Mod Pathol. 2009;22(5):718–24.
155. Willems SM, Mohseny AB, Balog C, Sewrajsing R, Briaire-de Bruijn IH, Knijnenburg J, et al. Cellular/intramuscular myxoma and grade I myxofibrosarcoma are characterized by distinct genetic alterations and specific composition of their extracellular matrix. J Cell Mol Med. 2009;13(7):1291–301.
156. Kirschner LS, Carney JA, Pack SD, Taymans SE, Giatzakis C, Cho YS, et al. Mutations of the gene encoding the protein

kinase A type I-alpha regulatory subunit in patients with the Carney complex. Nat Genet. 2000;26(1):89–92.
157. Park KU, Kim HS, Lee SK, Jung WW, Park YK. Novel mutation in PRKAR1A in carney complex. Korean J Pathol. 2012;46(6):595–600.
158. West RB, Rubin BP, Miller MA, Subramanian S, Kaygusuz G, Montgomery K, et al. A landscape effect in tenosynovial giant-cell tumor from activation of CSF1 expression by a translocation in a minority of tumor cells. Proc Nat Acad Sci U S A. 2006;103(3):690–5.
159. Cupp JS, Miller MA, Montgomery KD, Nielsen TO, O'Connell JX, Huntsman D, et al. Translocation and expression of CSF1 in pigmented villonodular synovitis, tenosynovial giant cell tumor, rheumatoid arthritis and other reactive synovitides. Am J Surg Pathol. 2007;31(6):970–6.
160. Szuhai K, Cleton-Jansen AM, Hogendoorn PC, Bovee JV. Molecular pathology and its diagnostic use in bone tumors. Cancer Gene Ther. 2012;205(5):193–204.
161. Hameed M. Clinical applications of molecular markers in bone tumors. Adv Anat Pathol. 2015;22(6):337–44.
162. van de Rijn M, Guo X, Sweeney RT, Beck AH, West RB. Molecular pathological analysis of sarcomas using paraffin-embedded tissue: current limitations and future possibilities. Histopathology. 2014;64(1):163–70.
163. Marino-Enriquez A, Bovee JV. Molecular pathogenesis and diagnostic, prognostic and predictive molecular markers in sarcoma. Surg Pathol Clin. 2016;9(3):457–73.
164. Cardona DM, Dodd LG. Bone cytology: a realistic approach for clinical use. Surg Pathol Clin. 2012;5(1):79–100.
165. Domanski HA, Qian X, Stanley DE. Chapter 16: Bone. In: Atlas of fine needle aspiration cytology. 2nd ed. London: Springer; 2018.
166. Kilpatrick SE, Pike EJ, Geisinger KR, Ward WG. Chondroblastoma of bone: use of fine-needle aspiration biopsy and potential diagnostic pitfalls. Diagn Cytopathol. 1997;16(1):65–71.
167. Orosz Z, Athanasou NA. Giant cell-containing tumors of bone. Surg Pathol Clin. 2017;10(3):553–73.
168. Al-Ibraheemi A, Inwards CY, Zreik RT, Wenger DE, Jenkins SM, Carter JM, et al. Histologic spectrum of Giant Cell Tumor (GCT) of bone in patients 18 years of age and below: a study of 63 patients. Am J Surg Pathol. 2016;40(12):1702–12.

169. Behjati S, Tarpey PS, Presneau N, Scheipl S, Pillay N, Van Loo P, et al. Distinct H3F3A and H3F3B driver mutations define chondroblastoma and giant cell tumor of bone. Nat Genet. 2013;45(12):1479–82.
170. Cleven AH, Hocker S, Briaire-de Bruijn I, Szuhai K, Cleton-Jansen AM, Bovee JV. Mutation analysis of H3F3A and H3F3B as a diagnostic tool for Giant cell tumor of bone and Chondroblastoma. Am J Surg Pathol. 2015;39(11):1576–83.
171. Kervarrec T, Collin C, Larousserie F, Bouvier C, Aubert S, Gomez-Brouchet A, et al. H3F3 mutation status of giant cell tumors of the bone, chondroblastomas and their mimics: a combined high resolution melting and pyrosequencing approach. Mod Pathol. 2017;30(3):393–406.
172. Nohr E, Lee LH, Cates JM, Perizzolo M, Itani D. Diagnostic value of histone 3 mutations in osteoclast-rich bone tumors. Hum Pathol. 2017;68:119–27.
173. Yamamoto H, Iwasaki T, Yamada Y, Matsumoto Y, Otsuka H, Yoshimoto M, et al. Diagnostic utility of histone H3.3 G34W, G34R, and G34V mutant-specific antibodies for giant cell tumors of bone. Hum Pathol. 2018;73:41–50.
174. Schaefer IM, Fletcher JA, Nielsen GP, Shih AR, Ferrone ML, Hornick JL, Qian X. Immunohistochemistry for histone H3G34W and H3K36M is highly specific for giant cell tumor of bone and chondroblastoma, respectively, in Fine Needle Aspiration and core needle biopsy. Cancer Cytopathol. 2018; https://doi.org/10.1002/cncy.22000. [Epub ahead of print].
175. Amary F, Berisha F, Ye H, Gupta M, Gutteridge A, Baumhoer D, et al. H3F3A (Histone 3.3) G34W immunohistochemistry: a reliable marker defining benign and malignant Giant Cell Tumor of bone. Am J Surg Pathol. 2017;41(8):1059–68.
176. Amary MF, Berisha F, Mozela R, Gibbons R, Guttridge A, O'Donnell P, et al. The H3F3 K36M mutant antibody is a sensitive and specific marker for the diagnosis of chondroblastoma. Histopathology. 2016;69(1):121–7.
177. Presneau N, Baumhoer D, Behjati S, Pillay N, Tarpey P, Campbell PJ, et al. Diagnostic value of H3F3A mutations in giant cell tumour of bone compared to osteoclast-rich mimics. J Pathol Clin Res. 2015;1(2):113–23.
178. Tsiatis AC, Norris-Kirby A, Rich RG, Hafez MJ, Gocke CD, Eshleman JR, et al. Comparison of Sanger sequencing, pyrosequencing, and melting curve analysis for the detection of KRAS

mutations: diagnostic and clinical implications. J Mol Diagn. 2010;12(4):425–32.
179. de Andrea CE, San-Julian M, Bovee J. Integrating morphology and genetics in the diagnosis of cartilage tumors. Surg Pathol Clin. 2017;10(3):537–52.
180. Amary MF, Bacsi K, Maggiani F, Damato S, Halai D, Berisha F, et al. IDH1 and IDH2 mutations are frequent events in central chondrosarcoma and central and periosteal chondromas but not in other mesenchymal tumours. J Pathol. 2011;224(3):334–43.
181. Tarpey PS, Behjati S, Cooke SL, Van Loo P, Wedge DC, Pillay N, et al. Frequent mutation of the major cartilage collagen gene COL2A1 in chondrosarcoma. Nat Genet. 2013;45(8):923–6.
182. Kerr DA, Lopez HU, Deshpande V, Hornicek FJ, Duan Z, Zhang Y, et al. Molecular distinction of chondrosarcoma from chondroblastic osteosarcoma through IDH1/2 mutations. Am J Surg Pathol. 2013;37(6):787–95.
183. Chen S, Fritchie K, Wei S, Ali N, Curless K, Shen T, et al. Diagnostic utility of IDH1/2 mutations to distinguish dedifferentiated chondrosarcoma from undifferentiated pleomorphic sarcoma of bone. Hum Pathol. 2017;65:239–46.
184. Badalian-Very G, Vergilio JA, Degar BA, MacConaill LE, Brandner B, Calicchio ML, et al. Recurrent BRAF mutations in Langerhans cell histiocytosis. Blood. 2010;116(11):1919–23.
185. Shanmugam V, Craig JW, Hornick JL, Morgan EA, Pinkus GS, Pozdnyakova O. Cyclin D1 is expressed in neoplastic cells of Langerhans cell Histiocytosis but not reactive Langerhans cell proliferations. Am J Surg Pathol. 2017;41(10):1390–6.
186. Gisselsson D, Palsson E, Hoglund M, Domanski H, Mertens F, Pandis N, et al. Differentially amplified chromosome 12 sequences in low- and high-grade osteosarcoma. Genes Chromosom Cancer. 2002;33(2):133–40.
187. Zhang Y, Rosenberg AE. Bone-forming tumors. Surg Pathol Clin. 2017;10(3):513–35.
188. Vujovic S, Henderson S, Presneau N, Odell E, Jacques TS, Tirabosco R, et al. Brachyury, a crucial regulator of notochordal development, is a novel biomarker for chordomas. J Pathol. 2006;209(2):157–65.
189. Jo VY, Hornick JL, Qian X. Utility of brachyury in distinction of chordoma from cytomorphologic mimics in fine-needle aspiration and core needle biopsy. Diagn Cytopathol. 2014;42(8):647–52.

190. Tarpey PS, Behjati S, Young MD, Martincorena I, Alexandrov LB, Farndon SJ, et al. The driver landscape of sporadic chordoma. Nat Commun. 2017;8(1):890.
191. Mobley BC, McKenney JK, Bangs CD, Callahan K, Yeom KW, Schneppenheim R, et al. Loss of SMARCB1/INI1 expression in poorly differentiated chordomas. Acta Neuropathol. 2010;120(6):745–53.
192. Antonelli M, Raso A, Mascelli S, Gessi M, Nozza P, Coli A, et al. SMARCB1/INI1 involvement in pediatric Chordoma: a mutational and immunohistochemical analysis. Am J Surg Pathol. 2017;41(1):56–61.
193. Creager AJ, Madden CR, Bergman S, Geisinger KR. Aneurysmal bone cyst: fine-needle aspiration findings in 23 patients with clinical and radiologic correlation. Am J Clin Pathol. 2007;128(5):740–5.
194. Panoutsakopoulos G, Pandis N, Kyriazoglou I, Gustafson P, Mertens F, Mandahl N. Recurrent t(16;17)(q22;p13) in aneurysmal bone cysts. Genes Chromosom Cancer. 1999;26(3):265–6.
195. Oliveira AM, Perez-Atayde AR, Inwards CY, Medeiros F, Derr V, Hsi BL, et al. USP6 and CDH11 oncogenes identify the neoplastic cell in primary aneurysmal bone cysts and are absent in so-called secondary aneurysmal bone cysts. Am J Pathol. 2004;165(5):1773–80.
196. Oliveira AM, Perez-Atayde AR, Dal Cin P, Gebhardt MC, Chen CJ, Neff JR, et al. Aneurysmal bone cyst variant translocations upregulate USP6 transcription by promoter swapping with the ZNF9, COL1A1, TRAP150, and OMD genes. Oncogene. 2005;24(21):3419–26.
197. Oliveira AM, Chou MM. USP6-induced neoplasms: the biologic spectrum of aneurysmal bone cyst and nodular fasciitis. Hum Pathol. 2014;45(1):1–11.
198. Wang L, Motoi T, Khanin R, Olshen A, Mertens F, Bridge J, et al. Identification of a novel, recurrent HEY1-NCOA2 fusion in mesenchymal chondrosarcoma based on a genome-wide screen of exon-level expression data. Genes Chromosom Cancer. 2012;51(2):127–39.

Chapter 19 Molecular Diagnostics in Pediatric Cytopathology

Maren Y. Fuller and Sara E. Monaco

Abbreviations

BRAF	v-Raf murine sarcoma viral oncogene homolog B
CNS	Central nervous system
CSF	Cerebrospinal fluid
ECD	Erdheim-Chester disease
FFPE	Formalin-fixed paraffin-embedded
FISH	Fluorescence *in situ* hybridization
FNA	Fine-needle aspiration
IGH	Immunoglobulin heavy chain
IHC	Immunohistochemistry
LCH	Langerhans cell histiocytosis

M. Y. Fuller
Department of Pathology, Children's Hospital of Pittsburgh of University of Pittsburgh Medical Center (UPMC), Pittsburgh, PA, USA

S. E. Monaco (✉)
Department of Pathology, University of Pittsburgh Medical Center, Children's Hospital of Pittsburgh of UPMC, Pittsburgh, PA, USA
e-mail: monacose@upmc.edu

S. Roy-Chowdhuri et al. (eds.), *Molecular Diagnostics in Cytopathology*, https://doi.org/10.1007/978-3-319-97397-5_19

NGS	Next-generation sequencing
PCR	Polymerase chain reaction
PTC	Papillary thyroid carcinoma
RPMI	Roswell Park Memorial Institute

Key Points

- The clinical context such as patient age, gender, biopsy location, family history, and presentation can greatly help guide your diagnostic workup, particularly in pediatric pathology
- Although collecting material for ancillary testing (FISH, cytogenetics, NGS) is suggested for nearly all pediatric tumors, it is essential to first obtain adequate material to establish the diagnosis (FNA smears and cell block) and then to reserve sufficient material for triage for the appropriate ancillary testing
- Consideration of the three main histologic patterns (small round blue cell, large epithelioid, and spindle cell) can help guide your diagnostic workup and determine the need for specific ancillary testing
- A few clinical scenarios encountered in pediatric pathology and of special significance are also discussed in this chapter, as the approach to testing in children can differ from that in adults, and many cytopathologists may not see a large volume of these pediatric specimens

Introduction

Childhood cancer is rare, with an estimated 10,000 cases diagnosed each year in the United States [1]. An estimated 1190 children will die from their disease each year, and death rates of childhood cancer have declined by nearly 70% in the past

40 years. However, cancer remains the leading cause of death for children in the United States [1–3]. The most common childhood cancers are leukemia/lymphoma and solid tumors of the brain/central nervous system (CNS), bone/soft tissue, kidney, and eye. However, most cytopathologists are unlikely to encounter specimens from the two most common malignancies, leukemia and CNS tumors, apart from screening for cerebrospinal fluid (CSF) involvement. This chapter will focus on lymphomas and solid tumors, as these are more likely to be encountered by the practicing cytopathologist. As in the adult setting, molecular techniques are often important for diagnosis, specific subtyping, prognosis, and therapeutic decisions.

Approach to Pediatric Fine-Needle Aspirations and Triage

As malignancy is quite rare in children, the majority of pediatric fine-needle aspiration (FNA) biopsies will be benign and serve as a minimally invasive way to provide reassurance to the ordering provider, patient, and family that a lesion with a low clinical suspicion for malignancy is indeed benign [4]. However, it is important to be prepared for a potentially malignant pediatric FNA in order to promptly triage the specimen for the appropriate ancillary studies and to obtain a specific diagnosis [5, 6]. In order to triage appropriately, rapid on-site evaluation (ROSE) is important, particularly in children, given that the spectrum of entities is quite vast. Some of the triage considerations at the time of ROSE include potentially collecting material in RPMI (Roswell Park Memorial Institute) media for flow cytometry and/or cytogenetics, additional unstained aspirate smears for FISH studies or special stains, procuring fresh material for additional testing, collecting in a sterile container for microbiology studies, as well as collecting material for a formalin-fixed paraffin-embedded (FFPE) cell block. When uncertain of the diagnosis, but potentially considering a hematolymphoid malignancy, fresh material can be collected in RPMI media and held in the refrigerator until the initial immunohistochemistry (IHC) stains help to define the type of cells. Then, after evaluating additional material (cell block slides, Papanicolaou-stained slides, IHC), the stored RPMI material can be sent for additional testing or simply used to create another FFPE cell block. In addition, many ancillary tests such as FISH and most molecular tests, including next-generation sequencing (NGS), can be performed on FFPE material, including cell blocks. Thus, it is not always necessary to order all potential ancillary tests at the time of ROSE, as material could be exhausted on unnecessary testing. Thus, a stepwise approach using an initial IHC panel to guide your testing can be beneficial, particularly in small biopsies from pediatric patients.

Cytomorphologic Patterns in Pediatric Fine-Needle Aspirations

When encountering a potentially neoplastic pediatric FNA, there are three major morphologic patterns that, when recognized, will help guide triage for potential molecular and other ancillary testing (Fig. 19.1). These three patterns are small round blue cell morphology, large epithelioid morphology, and spindle cell morphology (Table 19.1). Of the small round blue cell lesions, it is important to look for lymphoglandular bodies and other features that would help to favor a hematolymphoid process and impact triage of the specimen. In pediatric malignancies in particular, there are a variety of scenarios where it is important to consider procuring fresh material, in RPMI media, nucleic acid preservative, or fresh frozen for specialized additional testing (Table 19.2). Of course, having sufficient material for diagnosis always takes precedent.

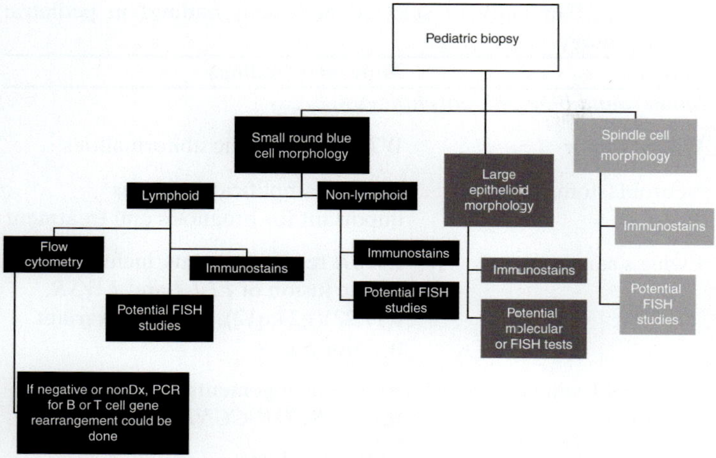

FIGURE 19.1 Algorithm for ancillary studies in pediatric pathology

Small Round Blue Cell Morphology

The small round blue cell morphology is one of the most commonly encountered in pediatric cytopathology. As previously mentioned, the first distinction to make is to determine if the predominant cellular population is lymphoid, in order to triage for flow cytometry, in addition to material for cell block. At the time of ROSE, acute inflammatory processes with neutrophils can mimic lymphoid aspirates if overstained and poorly prepared; thus, excluding a neutrophil-rich aspirate is important as material should be allocated for microbial cultures at ROSE if an acute inflammatory process is present. IHC stains on cell block material can help provide an immunophenotype to confirm and subtype a lymphoproliferative process. Flow cytometry is also helpful for determining an immunophenotype and clonality; however, some important testing, such as Epstein-Barr virus (EBV) status

Table 19.1 Summary of selected molecular findings in pediatric cytopathology

Tumor	Molecular findings
Small round blue cell morphology	
Wilms' tumor	*WT1* or *WT2* gene abnormalities
Neuroblastoma	*MYC-N* amplification status important for prognosis and treatment
Ewing's sarcoma	*EWSR* rearrangements, including classic fusion of *FLI-1* and *EWSR*, t(11;22)(q24;q12), as well as variant translocations
"Atypical Ewing's sarcoma"	*FUS* rearrangements, *CIC-DUX4* fusion, *BCOR-CCNB3* fusion
Alveolar rhabdomyosarcoma	*FOXO1 (FKHR)* rearrangements
Desmoplastic small round cell tumors	t(11;22)(p13;q12)
Clear cell sarcoma	t(12;22)(q13,q12)
Extraskeletal myxoid chondrosarcoma	t(9;22)(q22–23, q11–12)
Burkitt lymphoma	*MYC* alterations, classic rearrangement of translocation of *MYC* to *IGH,* t(8;14)(q24;q32)
Myoepithelial tumors	Varied may include *EWSR* rearrangements
Large epithelioid morphology	
Malignant melanoma	*BRAF*, *NF1* mutations
Large B-cell lymphoma	*IgH* gene rearrangement to prove clonality; assessment of *MYC*, *BCL2*, and *BCL6* to look for double−/triple-hit lymphomas
Pleomorphic adenoma	*PLAG1* rearrangement

TABLE 19.1 (continued)

Tumor	Molecular findings
Langerhans cell histiocytosis	*BRAF* V600E mutation
Translocation renal cell carcinoma	t(X;17) or t(X;1)
Rhabdoid tumor	*INI1* mutations/deletions
Carcinomas	Various molecular testing guidelines
Spindle cell morphology	
Nodular fasciitis	t(17;22) with increased USP6 expression
Synovial sarcoma	*SS18 (SYT)* translocation, t(X;18)(p11;q11)
Congenital infantile fibrosarcoma	t(12;15)(p13,q25)
Inflammatory myofibroblastic tumors	*ALK* rearrangements; t(1,2)(q25;p23) and others
Giant cell fibroblastoma (juvenile form of DFSP)	t(17;22)(q22;q13)
Desmoid fibromatosis	*Wnt*/beta-catenin pathway alterations
Mesoblastic nephroma	t(12;15)(p13;q25)

and proliferation index, cannot be determined via flow cytometry. In scant samples or in samples with nondiagnostic flow cytometry results, molecular techniques, such as polymerase chain reaction (PCR)-based B-cell or T-cell gene rearrangement studies or FISH studies for IgH gene rearrangements, can be useful to establish clonality and can be performed on FFPE cell block material or unstained aspirate smears (Fig. 19.2). This is particularly important when trying to establish clonality in a first-time diagnosis of lym-

Table 19.2 Common/uncommon scenarios for the pediatric pathologist/cytopathologist with ancillary testing correlations

Pediatric FNA scenario and/or ancillary testing result	Molecular correlation and additional testing
Next-generation sequencing or other molecular testing detected a variant of uncertain significance in a tumor specimen	Could collect peripheral blood for testing, in order to determine if mutation is germ line (e.g., present in blood and in tumor) or sporadic (e.g., present in tumor only)
Flow cytometry shows a small, possibly clonal B-cell population with excess lambda/kappa light chain	Review morphology to see if there is an immature-appearing lymphoid population with poor preservation or necrosis that could account for only small viable population by flow cytometry Check flow cytometry report to look at viability, to see if sample was a poorly viable sample If concerned for B-cell lymphoproliferative process and sample contains sufficient abnormal cells in FFPE block, can try B-cell IgH rearrangement PCR studies
Flow cytometry shows a T-cell population with TdT staining of uncertain significance	Review morphology to see if "blastoid" or immature appearing, to exclude a T-lymphoblastic leukemia/lymphoma Perform immunostains to exclude thymic sampling, such as CD1a, CD3, and TdT, cytokeratin, PAX8, p63 Review flow cytometry scattergrams to see if the TdT-positive T-cell population shows a maturational spectrum typical of thymic T-cells

TABLE 19.2 (continued)

Pediatric FNA scenario and/or ancillary testing result	Molecular correlation and additional testing
Limited material from a biopsy in a young patient shows a small round blue cell tumor of uncertain etiology: how to triage for ancillary studies?	Consider splitting material into two containers (one with RPMI and one with formalin). Hold the container with RPMI in the refrigerator overnight, while ordering a very limited immunopanel on the FFPE material (LCA/CD45, CD99, synaptophysin, cytokeratin). If it is lymphoid (LCA positive), send the specimen in RPMI to flow cytometry. If it is not lymphoid (LCA negative), spin down the RPMI specimen into a second cell block for potential immunostains or molecular testing if the other FFPE cell block gets exhausted or is less representative
	Order blank slides to be cut upfront and saved for additional immunostains to avoid trimming the block each time immunostains are ordered
	Save any slides with scant material from smearing during the procedure or rapid on-site evaluation, as these could be used for FISH studies, like IgH gene rearrangement studies to confirm a clonal lymphoid population. Aspirate smears could also be utilized for molecular studies, if necessary

(continued)

Table 19.2 (continued)

Pediatric FNA scenario and/or ancillary testing result	**Molecular correlation and additional testing**
Pediatric thyroid FNA shows high cellularity or features suspicious for a follicular or oncocytic neoplasm, medullary carcinoma, or papillary thyroid carcinoma	Consider obtaining aspirates for cell block (opposed to ThinPrep) to do a limited panel of immunostains (synaptophysin, calcitonin, TTF1) for excluding a medullary thyroid carcinoma or for beta-catenin staining if considering a cribriform-morular variant of papillary thyroid carcinoma (particularly in patients with known Familial Adenomatous Polyposis (FAP) Syndrome)
	Obtain fresh aspirate material in a nucleic acid preservative for potential molecular studies or other appropriate media for sendout molecular testing, which may be helpful in certain scenarios, such as indeterminate categories in *The Bethesda System for Reporting Thyroid Cytology* (TBSRTC)
	Consider genetic testing if familial syndromes are in the differential diagnosis, particularly for medullary thyroid carcinoma (associated with multiple endocrine neoplasia (MEN) syndrome) and cribriform-morular variant of papillary thyroid carcinoma (associated with familial adenomatous polyposis (FAP) syndrome)

phoma or in locations where larger biopsies are challenging or unsafe (e.g., lymph nodes near large blood vessels).

Lymphoid proliferations with a high-grade B-cell morphology include Burkitt lymphoma, diffuse large B-cell lymphoma, and other high-grade B-cell lymphomas, which includes double-hit and triple-hit lymphomas. Burkitt lym-

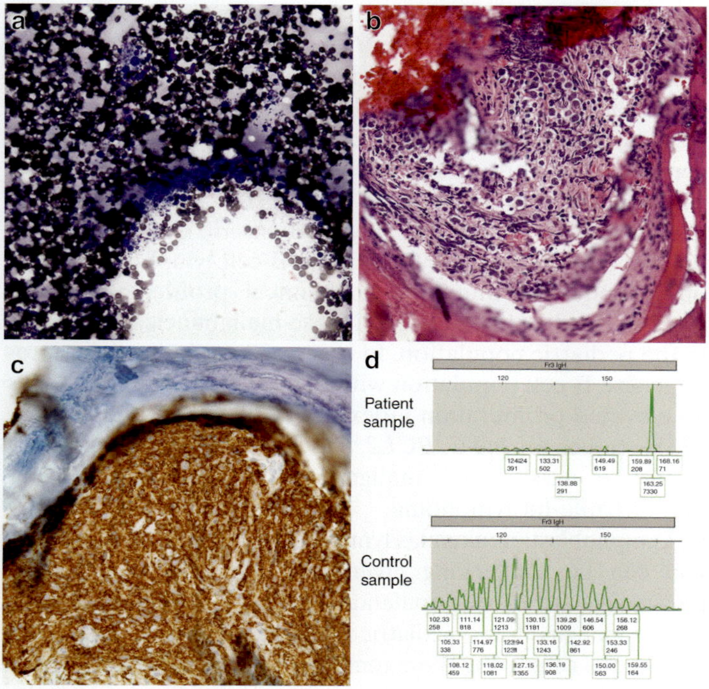

FIGURE 19.2 Large B-cell lymphoma. A 15-year-old girl with left lower leg pain, presented with imaging showing a discrete bone lesion. CT-guided fine-needle aspiration and core biopsy showed a population of CD20-positive lymphoid cells with large nuclei and immature features (**a**–**c**). Given the focal nature of the lymphoid cells, flow cytometry was nondiagnostic. However, PCR studies for the B-cell gene rearrangement were positive (**d**), supporting a clonal B-cell population, compatible with a primary large B-cell lymphoma of bone. (Image 19.2D courtesy of Dr. Somak Roy)

phoma has aberrations in *MYC*, and the classic rearrangement is the translocation of *MYC* to the *IGH* region, t(8;14)(q24;q32). Due to variant translocations, the more specific test is the *MYC* break-apart FISH probe, which is more commonly done if considering other rearrangements of the *MYC* gene or when considering a double- or triple-hit lymphoma. The revised 4th edition of the *WHO Classification of Tumours of Haematopoietic and Lymphoid Tissues* includes a diagnostic algorithm for high-grade B-cell lymphomas based on morphology, immunohistochemical profile, and FISH results [7]. Although very rare, these malignancies may occur in the pediatric population. In cases with an intermediate-to-large size B-cell population with high-grade features (such as an elevated proliferation index or IHC positivity for c-myc), FISH studies for *MYC*, *BCL2*, and *BCL6* are often necessary to further classify these malignancies and to exclude a double- or triple-hit lymphoma.

Lymphoblastic leukemias/lymphomas are also a consideration and can be challenging given that they have a small-to-intermediate sized cell population that may not be readily identified as malignant in a pediatric FNA, particularly in those with suboptimal cellularity. These tumors can occur almost anywhere, but T-cell lymphoblastic leukemia/lymphoma has a particular predilection for occurring in the mediastinum of young adolescent patients. One caveat is that immature T-cells of the thymus will also be TdT positive and thus need to be distinguished from a lymphoblastic leukemia/lymphoma. For this distinction, a combination of cytomorphology and flow cytometry, in addition to the clinical and radiological findings, can be helpful in reaching a definitive diagnosis.

If one encounters a nonlymphoid small round blue cell pattern, the differential diagnosis is wide and includes the Ewing's sarcoma family of tumors, synovial sarcoma, rhabdomyosarcoma, neuroblastoma, blastemal-predominant Wilms' tumor, osteosarcoma, desmoplastic small round cell tumor, and others. Although many of the tumors in this differential can be resolved with a combination of patient presentation, tumor location, and IHC results, there are occasions when ancillary molecular studies are necessary to establish the diagnosis or to provide specific subtyping. In cases of neuroblastoma, *MYC-N* amplification is important for both treatment and risk stratification, and can be determined via FISH testing. Ewing's sarcoma has a characteristic translocation that creates a fusion of *FLI-1* and *EWSR*, t(11;22)(q24;q12) [8, 9]. However, there are also variant translocations of the *EWSR* gene with different partner genes [10], which is why the *EWSR* break-apart FISH probe is commonly performed since it has greater sensitivity for detecting any *EWSR* rearrangement (Fig. 19.3).

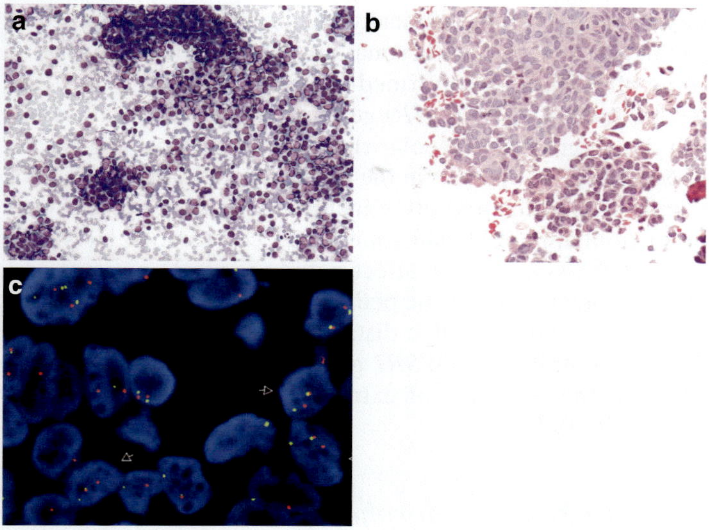

FIGURE 19.3 Primitive neuroectodermal tumor (PNET)/Ewing's sarcoma. A 1-year-old girl presented with a left neck mass that showed a small round blue cell tumor that was positive for CD99 (**a, b**). FISH studies confirmed the presence of an *EWSR1* gene rearrangement (**c**) (LSI *EWSR1* Dual-color break-apart probe 22q12; Abbott Molecular, Des Plaines, IL)

In the past, some tumors that histologically resembled Ewing's sarcoma, but lacked *EWSR* gene rearrangements via the standard FISH panels, had been referred to as atypical Ewing's sarcoma. Increasingly, alternative fusions have been identified, such as *FUS* rearrangements (Fig. 19.4) [11, 12]. Other recently described small round blue cell sarcomas include *CIC-DUX4* fusion sarcoma and *BCOR-CCNB3* Ewing-like sarcoma [13–16]. In some cases, the differential diagnosis may also include monophasic synovial sarcoma. In such scenarios, it may be prudent to order the *EWSR* and *SS18* FISH studies simultaneously and then to consider other tests or IHC stains if both of those results are negative.

A suspected diagnosis of rhabdomyosarcoma can often be confirmed by positive immunostaining for myogenin or myoD1. However, the clinically and prognostically important distinction between embryonal and alveolar rhabdomyosarcoma often must be confirmed by ancillary studies [17]. FISH testing for *FOXO1* (*FKHR)* gene rearrangements can establish the diagnosis of alveolar rhabdomyosarcoma (Fig. 19.5).

Soft tissue neoplasms in the pediatric population also have a wide differential and often include significant overlap with other nonlymphoid small round blue cell tumors. However, many soft tissue tumors affect a wide range of patients and may be encountered in the pediatric population. For example, in a 16-year-old girl with a distal leg soft tissue tumor, a positive FISH study for *EWSR1* gene rearrangement helped to establish the diagnosis of extraskeletal myxoid chondrosarcoma (Fig. 19.6).

Large Epithelioid Morphology

As opposed to adult malignancies, only a minority of pediatric tumors have a large epithelioid morphology. These include some salivary gland, thyroid, hepatic, and head and neck neoplasms, as well as the rare instances of adult-type malignancies such as melanoma and carcinoma occurring in children and adolescents. As has been discussed in previous chapters, there are many recently described translocations

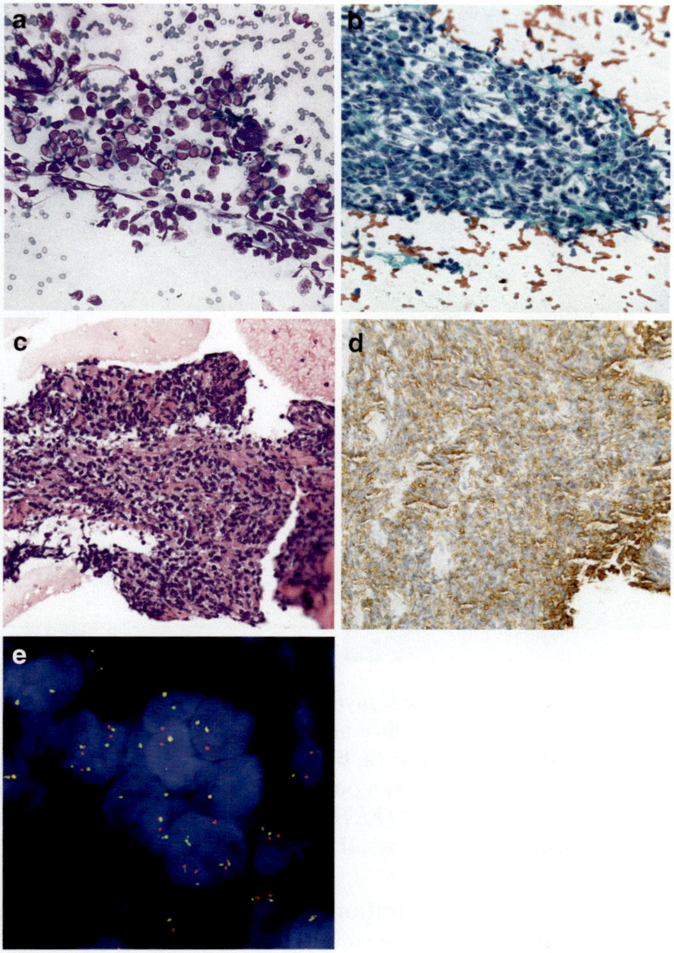

FIGURE 19.4 Small round blue cell tumor with *FUS* gene rearrangement. A 25-year-old girl with a large pelvic mass measuring about 13 cm had an FNA showing a small round blue cell tumor (**a–c**) with positivity for CD99 (**d**). FISH studies confirmed that the tumor was positive for a *FUS* gene rearrangement in 100% of cells (**e**). The *EWSR1* and *SS18 (SYT)* FISH studies were negative (LSI *SS18 (SYT)* dual-color break-apart Probe and LSI *EWSR1* dual-color break-apart probe 22q12; Abbott Molecular, Des Plaines, IL)

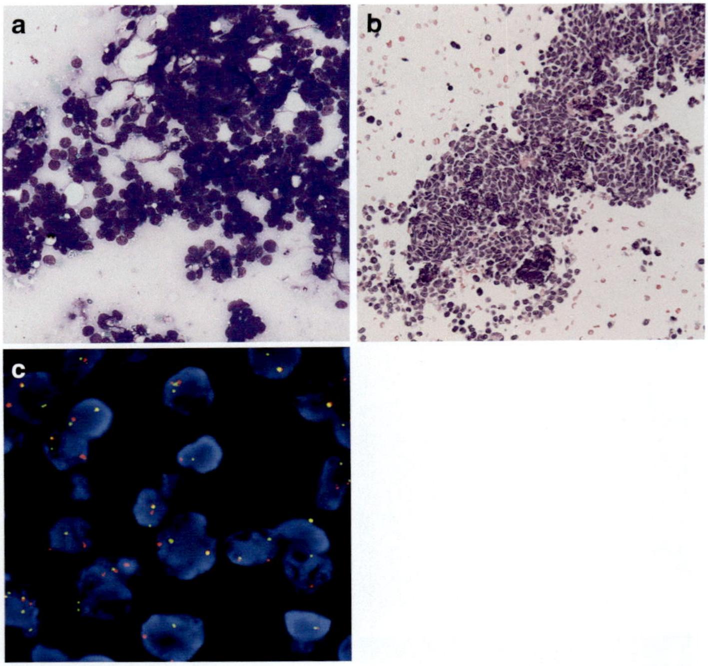

FIGURE 19.5 Alveolar rhabdomyosarcoma. 22-year-old girl with a posterior abdominal wall tumor and ascites. The aspirates showed a small round blue cell tumor (**a**, **b**) with strong staining for desmin and myogenin, in addition to a positive *FOX01* (*FKHR*) gene rearrangement (**c**) (LSI *FOX01* (*FKHR*) dual-color break-apart probe; Abbott Molecular, Des Plaines, IL)

and other molecular alterations in salivary gland neoplasms [18]. Many of these tumors can also be found in the pediatric population with similar morphologic and molecular findings. For example, FISH for *PLAG1* rearrangement can be used to confirm a benign diagnosis of a pleomorphic adenoma in a parotid FNA (Fig. 19.7). Furthermore, routine testing for *BRAF* and other genes should be performed in young patients with malignant melanoma [19]. In patients with thyroid nodules undergoing FNA, material should also be triaged for the appropriate collection media if there is atypia or findings potentially concerning for a neoplasm that may warrant molecular testing or sendout testing.

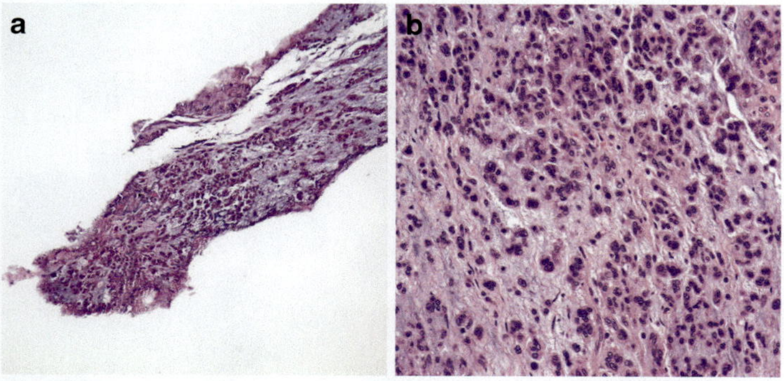

FIGURE 19.6 Extraskeletal myxoid chondrosarcoma. A 16-year-old girl with a left distal leg soft tissue tumor found to be extraskeletal myxoid chondrosarcoma (**a, b**) with positive FISH studies for an *EWSR1* gene rearrangement (LSI *EWSR1* dual-color break-apart probe 22q12; Abbott Molecular, Des Plaines, IL)

In rare cases of adult-type tumors occurring in the young patient, a similar diagnostic workup as in an adult patient is typically utilized. For example, a 21-year-old woman was found to have a lung mass and the CT-guided FNA showed a papillary neoplasm with uniform round nuclei, intranuclear inclusions, and small nucleoli. The tumor cells were positive for TTF1 and negative for thyroglobulin and PAX8, confirming the diagnosis of well-differentiated papillary adenocarcinoma of the lung and excluding a metastasis from the thyroid. The standard lung adenocarcinoma molecular testing was ordered and found a *ROS1* gene rearrangement (Fig. 19.8).

Although molecular testing for thyroid FNAs has been well described and clinically validated, there is still limited data in the pediatric population. Pediatric papillary thyroid carcinoma (PTC) has a different molecular landscape than that of adults, and recent studies have described an increasing number of molecular alterations [20–25]. A positive molecular result in an FNA of a pediatric thyroid lesion can be clinically useful to guide surgical planning [21]. There are also ways to resolve unusual molecular findings in the pediatric thyroid FNA. For example, a 4-year-old girl with a history of neuroblastoma, status post treatment with radiation and chemotherapy over 1.5 years prior, presented with a thyroid

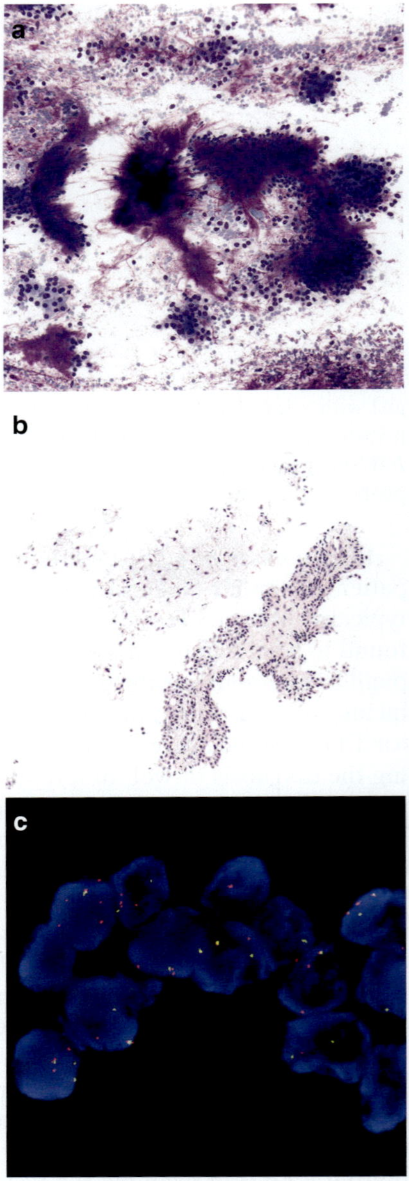

Figure 19.7 Pleomorphic adenoma of the salivary gland. 18-year-old boy with a round, discrete parotid gland lesion that underwent FNA and revealed a mixed population of epithelioid cells and metachromatic stromal material (**a**, **b**). FISH studies were positive for the *PLAG1* gene rearrangement (**c**) (LSI *PLAG1* dual-color break-apart probe 8q12.1; Empire Genomics, Buffalo, NY), confirming the impression of a pleomorphic adenoma or benign mixed tumor

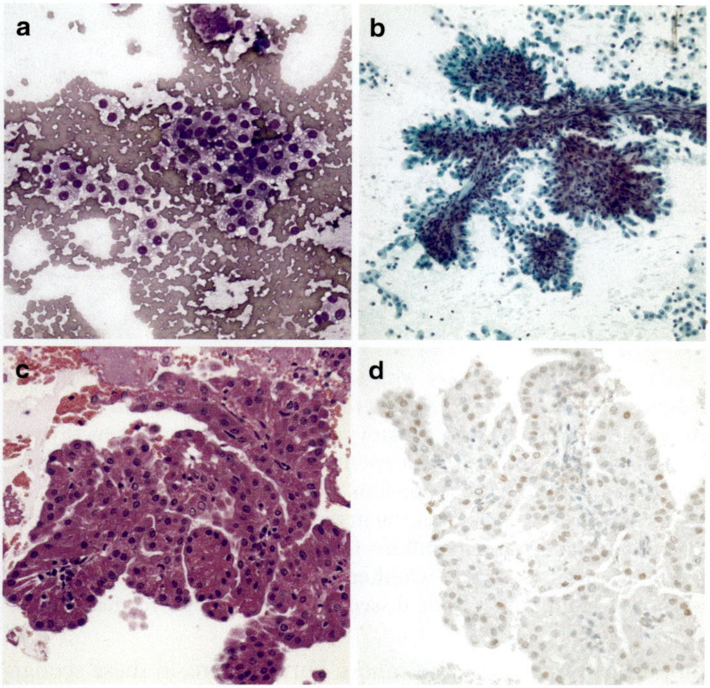

FIGURE 19.8 Adenocarcinoma of the lung with *ROS1* rearrangement. 21-year-old female with a lung mass with papillary features on FNA (**a–c**) and positive TTF1 IHC (**d**), confirmed to be primary lung adenocarcinoma. Thus, molecular testing was ordered, and a *ROS1* gene rearrangement was identified

nodule that showed cytologic features suspicious for a follicular neoplasm by *The Bethesda System for Reporting Thyroid Cytology*. Molecular testing on the thyroid FNA material revealed an *STK11* and *MET* gene variant of uncertain clinical significance. Follow-up testing on a peripheral blood sample showed that the variants were also present in the peripheral blood, supporting the interpretation that these variants were a germ line event (Fig. 19.9).

Other pediatric large cell tumors that may not have a truly "epithelioid" morphology include high-grade large B-cell lymphomas as discussed previously, histiocytoses, alveolar rhabdomyosarcoma, melanoma, alveolar soft part sarcoma, germ cell

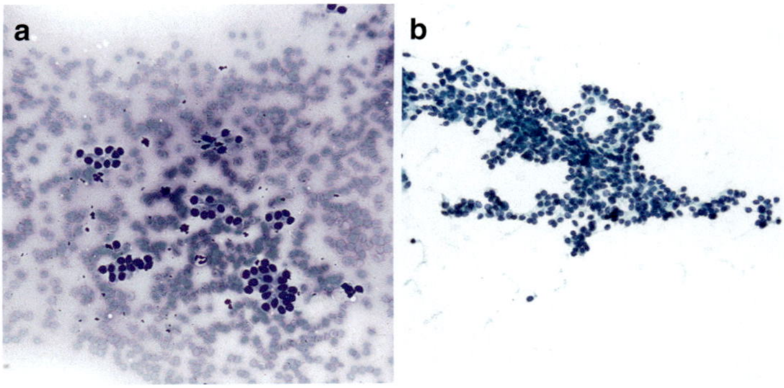

FIGURE 19.9 Thyroid FNA with suspicious for follicular neoplasm diagnosis by the *Bethesda System for Reporting of Thyroid Cytology*. In this 4-year-old girl with a history of neuroblastoma, a new thyroid lesion was detected and underwent aspiration showing a predominance of microfollicles, suspicious for a follicular neoplasm (**a**, **b**). Molecular testing can be helpful in these cases to look for molecular alterations favoring a papillary thyroid carcinoma or other neoplasm, in order to decide whether a partial or total thyroidectomy with or without lymph node dissection should be performed

tumors, osteosarcoma, and others. Furthermore, in these scenarios, performing an INI1 immunohistochemical stain should be considered, as many of the tumors with INI1-loss, including rhabdoid tumor, epithelioid sarcoma, and renal medullary carcinoma, are seen in the pediatric population. Histiocytic neoplasms such as Langerhans cell histiocytosis (LCH) and Erdheim-Chester disease (ECD) have a high prevalence of *BRAF* V600E mutations and should also be considered when there is an abnormal histiocytic population [26] (Fig. 19.10). One consideration to bear in mind is that histiocytic neoplasms such as LCH frequently have a very low allelic frequency due to the relatively low burden of neoplastic cells that carry the mutation. This may lead to a false-negative molecular testing result. Traditional molecular testing such as Sanger sequencing is especially susceptible to a false-negative result, but the allelic burden is often so low in histiocytic neoplasms that even the more sensitive next-generation sequencing (NGS) techniques may also give a false-negative result. In these cases, a well-validated *BRAF* V600E immunohistochemical stain can be a very useful adjunct test.

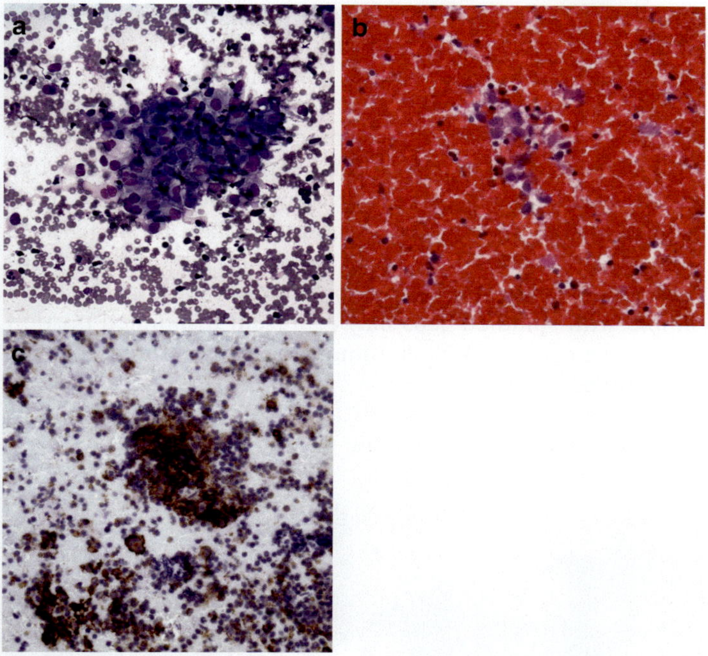

FIGURE 19.10 Langerhans cell histiocytosis. 19-year-old girl with fatigue presented with an enlarged neck mass. Aspirates revealed abnormal histiocytic cells with deep nuclear clefts, imparting a lobulated or cleaved look to the nuclei, intermixed with numerous eosinophils (**a**, **b**). The histiocytic cells were positive for C1a (**c**) and Langerin, compatible with Langerhans cell histiocytosis. Molecular testing confirmed a *BRAF* V600E mutation

Spindle Cell Morphology

The differential diagnosis of a pediatric FNA with spindle cell morphology is broad and includes benign lesions such as fibroma, schwannoma, and nodular fasciitis, as well as malignancies such as synovial sarcoma, malignant peripheral nerve sheath tumor, and spindle cell rhabdomyosarcoma. In many cases, using a combination of clinical history, morphology, and IHC profile is sufficient to arrive at an accurate diagnosis. However, in non-straightforward cases, additional ancillary testing can help confirm the diagnosis. Although previously considered a reactive lesion, studies of nodular fasciitis have identified a recurrent translocation t(17;22) with increased USP6 expression, which can be confirmed by FISH or PCR [27, 28]. Synovial sarcoma can have either monophasic or biphasic morphology and can be confirmed with FISH for *SS18 (SYT)* gene translocation (Fig. 19.11). Other rarer translocation-associated pediatric spindle cell malignancies include the *NTRK*-associated mesenchymal tumors [29]. As with FNA biopsy of any tumor, there may be tumor heterogeneity. One must also take into consideration that the FNA sample with spindled cells may represent a spindled portion of a heterogeneous Wilms' tumor, hepatoblastoma, or other pediatric neoplasm.

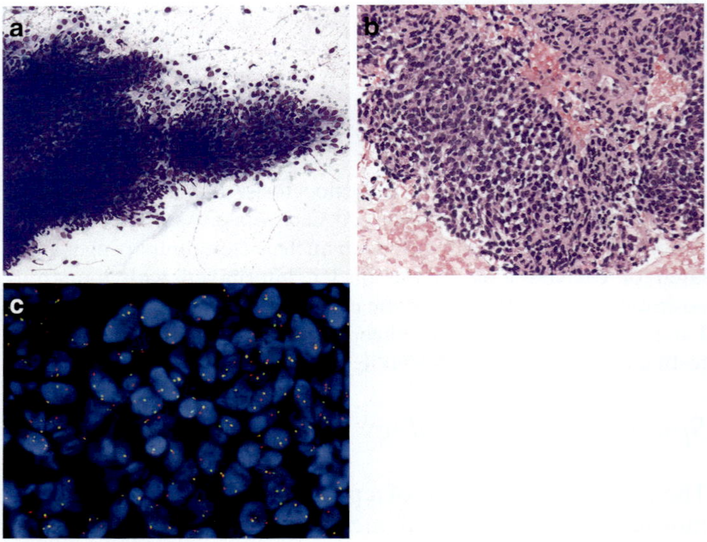

FIGURE 19.11 Synovial sarcoma. 16-year-old girl with a thoracic mass showing a mixed spindle and epithelioid neoplasm (**a**, **b**) that was positive for CD99, bcl2, and cytokeratin. FISH studies confirmed an *SS18 (SYT)* gene translocation (**c**), compatible with a synovial sarcoma (LSI *SS18 (SYT)* dual-color break-apart probe; Abbott Molecular, Des Plaines, IL)

Similar to many FNA biopsies in adults, ancillary testing such as FISH, NGS, conventional molecular testing, and others, is becoming increasingly important for prognosis, theranostics, and diagnosis. Although the variety of pediatric malignancies is broad, many diagnoses require ancillary testing; thus, it is prudent to consider collecting material for cell block, in RPMI, and frozen in many cases.

Acknowledgments Special thanks to all of the staff in the UPMC molecular pathology and ISH/FISH laboratories for their assistance with the preparation of the images in this chapter.

References

1. National Cancer Institute. Childhood cancers [Internet]. [cited 2018 Jan 6]. Available from: https://www.cancer.gov/types/childhood-cancers.
2. Howlander N, Noone A, Krapcho M, Miller D, Bishop K, Kosary C, et al., editors. SEER cancer statistics review, 1975–2014. Bethesda: National Cancer Institute; 2017.
3. Ward E, DeSantis C, Robbins A, Kohler B, Jemal A. Childhood and adolescent cancer statistics, 2014. CA Cancer J Clin. 2014;64(2):83–103.
4. Monaco SE, Teot LA. Cytopathology of pediatric malignancies. Cancer Cytopathol. 2014;122(5):322–36.
5. Barroca H, Bom-Sucesso M. Fine needle biopsy with cytology in paediatrics: the importance of a multidisciplinary approach and the role of ancillary techniques. Cytopathology. 2014;25(1):6–20.
6. Barroca H. Fine needle biopsy and genetics, two allied weapons in the diagnosis, prognosis, and target therapeutics of solid pediatric tumors. Diagn Cytopathol. 2008;36(9):678–84.
7. Kluin P, Harris N, Stein H, Leoncini L, Campo E, Jaffe E, et al. High-grade B-cell lymphoma. In: Swerdlow S, Campo E, Harris N, Jaffe E, Pileri S, Stein H, et al., editors. WHO classification of tumours of haematopoietic and lymphoid tissues. Revised 4th ed. Lyon: International Agency for Research on Cancer; 2017. p. 335–41.
8. Delattre O, Zucman J, Plougastel B, Desmaze C, Melot T, Peter M, et al. Gene fusion with an ETS DNA-binding domain caused by chromosome translocation in human tumours. Nature. 1992;359(6391):162–5.

9. May WA, Gishizky ML, Lessnick SL, Lunsford LB, Lewis BC, Delattre O, et al. Ewing sarcoma 11;22 translocation produces a chimeric transcription factor that requires the DNA-binding domain encoded by FLI1 for transformation. Proc Natl Acad Sci U S A. 1993;90(12):5752–6.
10. Sorensen PH, Lessnick SL, Lopez-Terrada D, Liu XF, Triche TJ, Denny CT. A second Ewing's sarcoma translocation, t(21;22), fuses the EWS gene to another ETS-family transcription factor. ERG Nat Genet. 1994;6(2):146–51.
11. Ng TL, O'Sullivan MJ, Pallen CJ, Hayes M, Clarkson PW, Winstanley M, et al. Ewing sarcoma with novel translocation t(2;16) producing an in-flame fusion of FUS and FEV. J Mol Diagnostics. 2007;9(4):459–63.
12. Tsokos M, Alaggio RD, Dehner LP, Dickman PS. Ewing sarcoma/peripheral primitive neuroectodermal tumor and related tumors. Pediatr Dev Pathol. 2012;15(1 Suppl):108–26.
13. Kawamura-Saito M, Yamazaki Y, Kaneko K, Kawaguchi N, Kanda H, Mukai H, et al. Fusion between CIC and DUX4 up-regulates PEA3 family genes in Ewing-like sarcomas with t(4;19)(q35;q13) translocation. Hum Mol Genet. 2006;15(13):2125–37.
14. Italiano A, Sung YS, Zhang L, Singer S, Maki RG, Coindre J-M, et al. High prevalence of CIC fusion with double-homeobox (DUX4) transcription factors in EWSR1-negative undifferentiated small blue round cell sarcomas. Genes Chromosomes Cancer. 2012;51(3):207–18.
15. Pierron G, Tirode F, Lucchesi C, Reynaud S, Ballet S, Cohen-Gogo S, et al. A new subtype of bone sarcoma defined by BCOR-CCNB3 gene fusion. Nat Genet. 2012;44(4):461–6.
16. Puls F, Niblett A, Marland G, Gaston CLL, Douis H, Mangham DC, et al. BCOR-CCNB3 (Ewing-like) sarcoma: a clinicopathologic analysis of 10 cases, in comparison with conventional Ewing sarcoma. Am J Surg Pathol. 2014;38(10):1307–18.
17. Williamson D, Missiaglia E, de Reyniès A, Pierron G, Thuille B, Palenzuela G, et al. Fusion gene–negative alveolar rhabdomyosarcoma is clinically and molecularly indistinguishable from embryonal rhabdomyosarcoma. J Clin Oncol. 2010 May 1;28(13):2151–8.
18. Pusztaszeri MP, Faquin WC. Update in salivary gland cytopathology: recent molecular advances and diagnostic applications. Semin Diagn Pathol. 2015;32(4):264–74.
19. Lu C, Zhang J, Nagahawatte P, Easton J, Lee S, Liu Z, et al. The genomic landscape of childhood and adolescent melanoma. J Invest Dermatol. 2015;135(3):816–23.

20. Monaco SE, Pantanowitz L, Khalbuss WE, Benkovich VA, Ozolek J, Nikiforova MN, et al. Cytomorphological and molecular genetic findings in pediatric thyroid fine-needle aspiration. Cancer Cytopathol. 2012;120(5):342–50.
21. Buryk MA, Monaco SE, Witchel SF, Mehta DK, Gurtunca N, Nikiforov YE, et al. Preoperative cytology with molecular analysis to help guide surgery for pediatric thyroid nodules. Int J Pediatr Otorhinolaryngol. 2013;77(10):1697–700.
22. Picarsic JL, Buryk MA, Ozolek J, Ranganathan S, Monaco SE, Simons JP, et al. Molecular characterization of sporadic pediatric thyroid carcinoma with the DNA/RNA ThyroSeq v2 next-generation sequencing assay. Pediatr Dev Pathol. 2016;19(2):115–22.
23. Ballester LY, Sarabia SF, Sayeed H, Patel N, Baalwa J, Athanassaki I, et al. Integrating molecular testing in the diagnosis and management of children with thyroid lesions. Pediatr Dev Pathol. 2016;19(2):94–100.
24. Agrawal N, Akbani R, Aksoy BA, Ally A, Arachchi H, Asa SL, et al. Integrated genomic characterization of papillary thyroid carcinoma. Cell. 2014;159(3):676–90.
25. Mostoufi-Moab S, Labourier E, Sullivan L, LiVolsi VA, Li Y, Xiao R, et al. Molecular testing for oncogenic gene alterations in pediatric thyroid lesions. Thyroid. 2018;28(1):60–7.
26. Haroche J, Charlotte F, Arnaud L, von Deimling A, Hélias-Rodzewicz Z, Hervier B, et al. High prevalence of BRAF V600E mutations in Erdheim-Chester disease but not in other non-Langerhans cell histiocytoses. Blood. 2012;120(13):2700–3.
27. Erickson-Johnson MR, Chou MM, Evers BR, Roth CW, Seys AR, Jin L, et al. Nodular fasciitis: a novel model of transient neoplasia induced by MYH9-USP6 gene fusion. Lab Investig. 2011;91(10):1427–33.
28. Patel NR, Chrisinger JSA, Demicco EG, Sarabia SF, Reuther J, Kumar E, et al. USP6 activation in nodular fasciitis by promoter-swapping gene fusions. Mod Pathol. 2017;30(11):1577–88.
29. Davis JL, Lockwood CM, Albert CM, Tsuchiya K, Hawkins DS, Rudzinski ER. Infantile NTRK -associated Mesenchymal tumors. Pediatr Dev Pathol. 2018;21(1):68–78.

Chapter 20
Molecular Cytopathology: Final Thoughts and Future Directions

Sinchita Roy-Chowdhuri

Abbreviations

BRAF	v-Raf murine sarcoma viral oncogene homolog B
cfDNA	Cell-free DNA
CSF	Cerebrospinal fluid
ctDNA	Circulating tumor DNA
DNA	Deoxyribonucleic acid
ddPCR	Droplet digital PCR
EBUS-TBNA	Endobronchial ultrasound-guided transbronchial needle aspiration
EGFR	Epidermal growth factor receptor
EUS	Endoscopic ultrasound
FDA	United States Food and Drug Administration
FNA	Fine-needle aspiration
FISH	Fluorescence *in situ* hybridization
HPV	Human papillomavirus

S. Roy-Chowdhuri
MD Anderson Cancer Center, The University of Texas, Houston, TX, USA
e-mail: sroy2@mdanderson.org

S. Roy-Chowdhuri et al. (eds.), *Molecular Diagnostics in Cytopathology*, https://doi.org/10.1007/978-3-319-97397-5_20

KRAS	Kirsten rat sarcoma viral oncogene homolog
LBC	Liquid-based cytology
LOH	Loss of heterozygosity
NGS	Next-generation sequencing
NRAS	Neuroblastoma RAS viral oncogene
PCR	Polymerase chain reaction
PPAR-γ	Peroxisome proliferator-activated receptor γ
PTC	Papillary thyroid carcinoma
RET	Proto-oncogene tyrosine-protein kinase receptor Ret
RNA	Ribonucleic acid

Key Terminology

Cell-free DNA (cfDNA)	DNA freely circulating in the system and usually refers to free circulating DNA in the blood. Circulating tumor DNA (ctDNA) is a fraction of the cfDNA in neoplastic conditions, where tumor-derived fragmented DNA is released from tumor cells into the circulation and can be extracted from the serum/plasma fraction of blood. cfDNA or ctDNA can be quantified and used for sequencing/mutation analysis, commonly referred to as a "liquid biopsy" assay
Cell pellet	Aggregate of cellular elements at the bottom of a tube after centrifugation of cytology specimen
Droplet digital PCR	PCR-based technology to directly quantify and clonally amplify nucleic acids by dividing the PCR reaction into smaller reactions through a water oil emulsion technique and amplified individually

Liquid-based cytology	Cytopathology preparation method using a proprietary collection media and fixative followed by automated processing to obtain a monolayered slide for morphologic evaluation
Liquid biopsy	A fluid phase biopsy and usually refers to the sampling and analysis of circulating tumor cells or cell-free DNA in blood or other fluids such as amniotic fluid, cerebrospinal fluid, and urine. Liquid biopsies provide a noninvasive, easily accessible alternative to tissue biopsy analysis when the latter is unavailable
Molecular cytopathology	Discipline of cytopathology based on the integration of morphologic changes with the genomic alterations/molecular features underlying the development, progression, and prognosis of neoplastic diseases
Next-generation sequencing	High-throughput molecular platform that allows sequencing multiple gene sequences in parallel and interrogating various genetic alterations for multiple patients in a single run
Residual LBC	Specimen collected in LBC proprietary collection media (such as CytoLyt or CytoRich Red) that remains after processing of monolayered LBC slide for morphologic evaluation
Supernatant	Fluid that separates above the pelleted cellular elements after centrifugation of a cytology specimen

Key Points

- The integration of molecular diagnostic assays in cytopathology has added a genomic dimension to the world of diagnostic cytopathology
- The variety and versatility of cytology specimen preparations provide multiple options for performing molecular assays, as long as the pre-analytic aspects of specimen processing and handling are optimized and the tests are appropriately validated
- Novel applications of cytology specimens for molecular diagnostic assays have redefined and expanded the role of cytopathology in patient care
- Cytopathologists must evolve with the changing landscapes of molecular medicine, embrace new technological advancements, and optimize these methods into routine cytopathology practice

Molecular cytopathology is defined as the application of molecular studies to any type of cytology specimen, whether gynecological, exfoliative, or fine-needle aspiration cytology [1]. Molecular test results are only meaningful when appropriately interpreted in context of the cytomorphology. The importance of standardizing pre-analytical and analytical aspects of molecular testing to obtain relevant and reliable results that can be translated into clinical care cannot be overemphasized. The various chapters of this book have outlined the basic principles of molecular diagnostics currently used in the practice of cytopathology, focusing on the applications of these techniques for diagnosis, prognosis, as well as for assessing therapeutic targets.

Cytopathology as a specialty has been at the forefront of adapting new technology and incorporating new techniques into clinical practice. As discussed in earlier chapters, the advantages of using cytology material over histologic tissue for molecular studies are many, including better-preserved and higher-quality nucleic acids, ease of obtaining fresh whole cells, and the ability to perform on-site evaluation for adequacy. With the advent of high-throughput technologies such as next-generation sequencing (NGS), the clinical applications of molecular cytopathology has expanded from the more conventional tests, such as human papillomavirus (HPV) testing of cervicovaginal specimens and fluorescence *in situ* hybridization (FISH) in urine samples, to a multitude of DNA/RNA and protein-based assays that are routinely used in clinical decision-making. The rapid development of molecular diagnostic assays in surgical pathology has revolutionized the practice of cytopathology with the adoption of these same tests in cytology samples, thereby adding a genomic dimension to the world of diagnostic cytopathology.

This has specific implications when cytology is the primary mode of diagnosis (such as thyroid fine-needle aspiration (FNA) and endoscopic ultrasound (EUS)-guided FNA of pancreaticobiliary tumors and/or pancreatic cysts) as well as in advanced stage patients when cytology is the only specimen available for testing (for instance, malignant effusions, endobronchial ultrasound-guided transbronchial needle aspiration [EBUS-TBNA], and FNA of metastatic sites not amenable to more invasive procedures). A concise summary of relevant molecular testing in cytology specimens is provided in Chap. 1 with more organ-specific molecular diagnostics detailed elsewhere in this book (Chaps. 9, 10, 11, 12, 13, 14, 15, 16, 17, 18, and 19).

As discussed in previous chapters, the versatility of cytology specimen preparations provide a variety of options for performing these molecular tests, as long as the pre-analytic aspects of specimen processing and handling are optimized and the tests are appropriately validated [2–9]. In recent years, liquid biopsy assays interrogating tumor-derived cell-free DNA (cfDNA) from patient plasma samples have gained popularity, especially when tumor tissue is not available or insufficient for molecular testing [10]. NGS and ultrasensitive assays such as droplet digital PCR (ddPCR) have been successfully applied as liquid biopsy assays for personalized cancer therapy leading to the recent approval of these tests by the United States Food and Drug Administration (FDA) for specific situations [11, 12]. With the increasing use of liquid biopsy assays, several groups have explored the use of mutational assays using tumor-derived cfDNA in cytology samples such as cerebrospinal fluid (CSF) and urine [13–19]. The ability to detect clinically relevant genetic alterations in these cytology samples provides a less invasive and easily accessible alternative to obtaining tumor genomic information via a tissue biopsy. This novel application not only aids with diagnosis (e.g., CSF samples in patients with suspected leptomeningeal disease) but also can be used for serial monitoring of patients for therapeutic response and/or disease relapse and development of resistance mutations [15, 16].

More recently, cytopathologists are discovering novel ways to better utilize their specimens by repurposing previously discarded samples to provide additional genomic information in cases that would otherwise warrant an additional biopsy. For years the residual liquid-based cytology (LBC) preparation from cervicovaginal gynecological samples has been utilized for detection of high-risk HPV. Recent studies have explored the utility of molecular testing of residual LBC from non-gynecological FNA samples with promising results [20–25]. The LBC media not only provides optimal preservation of cellular morphology for diagnosis but also preserves nucleic acids for downstream DNA-/RNA-based assays as well as FISH assays. Furthermore, post-centrifuged FNA needle rinse supernatants have been evaluated by some investigators and noted to yield substantial amounts of DNA, sufficient for molecular assays such as microsatellite fragment analysis for loss of heterozygosity (LOH), mutational analysis for multi-gene panels by NGS, and/or hotspot-based testing using PCR/capillary electrophoresis, pyrosequencing, and ddPCR [26–31]. Table 20.1 lists some of the relevant studies reporting molecular testing using residual/supernatant FNA needle rinse substrates. Given that these residual needle rinses and supernatant fluids are routinely discarded, the implications of providing critical genomic-based testing from these samples are far-reaching.

TABLE 20.1 Recent studies reporting molecular testing using unfixed cytology material (residual FNA needle rinses and supernatant fluids)

	Specimen source	Methodology	Genetic alteration evaluated
Finkelstein et al. [28]	Pancreaticobiliary brushing cytology supernatant	LOH of microsatellites Sanger sequencing	1p, 3p, 5q, 9p, 10q, 17p, 17q, 21q, 22q *KRAS*
Finkelstein et al. [27] Deftereos et al. [26]	Pancreas: Supernatant from FNA needle rinse	LOH of microsatellites Sanger sequencing	1p, 3p, 5q, 9p, 10q, 17p, 17q, 21q, 22q *KRAS*
Krane et al. [24]	Thyroid: Residual LBC FNA needle rinse	PCR/pyrosequencing Quantitative PCR	*BRAF, RAS, PAX8/ PPARγ, RET/PTC1, RET/PTC3*
Wei et al. [20]	Residual LBC FNA needle rinse and effusion cytology	NGS	47 gene NGS panel
Kwon et al. [25]	Thyroid: Residual LBC FNA needle rinse	Real-time PCR Pyrosequencing	*BRAF, RAS, PAX8/ PPARγ, RET/PTC1, RET/PTC3*

(continued)

Table 20.1 (continued)

	Specimen source	Methodology	Genetic alteration evaluated
Brown et al. [29]	Thyroid: Supernatant from FNA needle rinse	Pyrosequencing	*BRAF*
Fuller et al. [21]	Thyroid: Residual LBC FNA needle rinse	NGS	50 gene NGS panel
Tian et al. [23]	Residual LBC and supernatant from FNA needle rinse (various sites)	NGS	410 gene NGS panel
Roy-Chowdhuri et al. [30]	Supernatant from FNA needle rinse (various sites)	NGS ddPCR	50 gene NGS panels *EGFR, KRAS, BRAF, PIK3CA, NRAS*
Doxtader et al. [22]	EBUS-TBNA residual cell pellet from LBC	NGS	50 gene NGS panel

Abbreviations: *LOH* loss of heterozygosity, *LBC* liquid-based cytology, *NGS* next-generation sequencing, *ddPCR* droplet digital PCR, *EBUS-TBNA* endobronchial ultrasound-guided transbronchial needle aspiration

As the world of molecular medicine continues to evolve, cytopathologists need to be increasingly involved in the preanalytical and analytical aspects of specimen collection, processing, adequacy evaluation, and molecular testing [2, 3, 32]. Continuing to embrace new advancements in technology together with optimizing and validating these methodologies in cytology samples will be essential to adopting a molecular diagnostic armamentarium into routine cytopathology practice.

References

1. Schmitt FC. Demystifying molecular cytopathology. Int J Surgical Pathol. 2010;18:213S–5S.
2. Bellevicine C, Malapelle U, Vigliar E, Pisapia P, Vita G, Troncone G. How to prepare cytological samples for molecular testing. J Clin Pathol. 2017;70:819–26.
3. da Cunha Santos G. Standardizing preanalytical variables for molecular cytopathology. Cancer Cytopathol. 2013;121:341–3.
4. Maxwell P, Salto-Tellez M. Validation of immunocytochemistry as a morphomolecular technique. Cancer Cytopathol. 2016;124:540–5.
5. Roy-Chowdhuri S, Stewart J. Preanalytic variables in cytology: lessons learned from next-generation sequencing-the MD Anderson experience. Arch Pathol Lab Med. 2016;140:1191–9.
6. Fischer AH, Schwartz MR, Moriarty AT, Wilbur DC, Souers R, Fatheree L, et al. Immunohistochemistry practices of cytopathology laboratories: a survey of participants in the College of American Pathologists Nongynecologic Cytopathology Education Program. Arch Pathol Lab Med. 2014;138(9):1167–72.
7. Berry AB. Analytic inquiry: validation and practical considerations. Cancer. 2017;125:465–9.
8. Fitzgibbons PL, Bradley LA, Fatheree LA, Alsabeh R, Fulton RS, Goldsmith JD, et al.; College of American Pathologists Pathology and Laboratory Quality Center. Principles of analytic validation of immunohistochemical assays: guideline from the College of American Pathologists Pathology and Laboratory Quality Center. Arch Pathol Lab Med. 2014;138(11):1432–43.
9. Jennings LJ, Arcila ME, Corless C, Kamel-Reid S, Lubin IM, Pfeifer J, et al. Guidelines for validation of next-generation

sequencing-based oncology panels: a joint consensus recommendation of the Association for Molecular Pathology and College of American Pathologists. J Mol Diagn. 2017;19(3): 341–65.
10. Stewart CM, Kothari PD, Mouliere F, Mair R, Somnay S, Benayed R, et al. The value of cell-free DNA for molecular pathology. J Pathol. 2018;244(5):616–27.
11. Krishnamurthy N, Spencer E, Torkamani A, Nicholson L. Liquid biopsies for cancer: coming to a patient near you. J Clin Med. 2017;6(1):pii: E3.
12. Kwapisz D. The first liquid biopsy test approved. Is it a new era of mutation testing for non-small cell lung cancer? Ann Transl Med. 2017;5(3):46.
13. Janku F, Vibat CR, Kosco K, Holley VR, Cabrilo G, Meric-Bernstam F, et al. BRAF V600E mutations in urine and plasma cell-free DNA from patients with Erdheim-Chester disease. Oncotarget. 2014;5(11):3607–10.
14. Li Y, Pan W, Connolly ID, Reddy S, Nagpal S, Quake S, Gephart MH. Tumor DNA in cerebral spinal fluid reflects clinical course in a patient with melanoma leptomeningeal brain metastases. J Neuro-Oncol. 2016;128(1):93–100.
15. Li YS, Jiang BY, Yang J, Zhang XC, Zhang Z, Ye JY, et al. Unique genetic profiles from cerebrospinal fluid cell-free DNA in leptomeningeal metastases of EGFR-mutant non-small-cell lung cancer: a new medium of liquid biopsy. Annals Oncol. 2018;29(4):945–52.
16. Momtaz P, Pentsova E, Abdel-Wahab O, Diamond E, Hyman D, Merghoub T, et al. Quantification of tumor-derived cell free DNA(cfDNA) by digital PCR (DigPCR) in cerebrospinal fluid of patients with BRAFV600 mutated malignancies. Oncotarget. 2016;7(51):85430–6.
17. Russo IJ, Ju Y, Gordon NS, Zeegers MP, Cheng KK, James ND, et al. Toward personalised liquid biopsies for urothelial carcinoma: characterisation of ddPCR and urinary cfDNA for the detection of the TERT 228 G>A/T mutation. Bladder Cancer. 2018;4(1):41–8.
18. Togneri FS, Ward DG, Foster JM, Devall AJ, Wojtowicz P, Alyas S, et al. Genomic complexity of urothelial bladder cancer revealed in urinary cfDNA. Eur J Hum Genet. 2016;24(8):1167–74.
19. Xia Y, Huang CC, Dittmar R, Du M, Wang Y, Liu H, et al. Copy number variations in urine cell free DNA as biomarkers in advanced prostate cancer. Oncotarget. 2016;7(24): 35818–31.

20. Wei S, Lieberman D, Morrissette JJ, Baloch ZW, Roth DB, McGrath C. Using "residual" FNA rinse and body fluid specimens for next-generation sequencing: an institutional experience. Cancer Cytopathol. 2016;124(5):324–9.
21. Fuller MY, Mody D, Hull A, Pepper K, Hendrickson H, Olsen R. Next-generation sequencing identifies gene mutations that are predictive of malignancy in residual needle rinses collected from fine-needle aspirations of thyroid nodules. Arch Pathol Lab Med. 2018;142(2):178–83.
22. Doxtader EE, Cheng YW, Zhang Y. Molecular testing of non-small cell lung carcinoma diagnosed by endobronchial ultrasound-guided transbronchial fine-needle aspiration. Arch Pathol Lab Med. 2018. https://doi.org/10.5858/arpa.2017-0184-RA.
23. Tian SK, Killian JK, Rekhtman N, Benayed R, Middha S, Ladanyi M, et al. Optimizing workflows and processing of cytologic samples for comprehensive analysis by next-generation sequencing: Memorial Sloan Kettering Cancer Center experience. Arch Pathol Lab Med. 2016;140(11):1200–5.
24. Krane JF, Cibas ES, Alexander EK, Paschke R, Eszlinger M. Molecular analysis of residual ThinPrep material from thyroid FNAs increases diagnostic sensitivity. Cancer Cytopathol. 2015;123(6):356–61.
25. Kwon H, Kim WG, Eszlinger M, Paschke R, Song DE, Kim M, et al. Molecular diagnosis using residual liquid-based cytology materials for patients with nondiagnostic or indeterminate thyroid nodules. Endocrinol Metab (Seoul). 2016;31(4):586–91.
26. Deftereos G, Finkelstein SD, Jackson SA, Ellsworth EM, Krishnamurti U, Liu Y, et al. The value of mutational profiling of the cytocentrifugation supernatant fluid from fine-needle aspiration of pancreatic solid mass lesions. Mod Pathol. 2014;27(4):594–601.
27. Finkelstein SD, Bibbo M, Kowalski TE, Loren DE, Siddiqui AA, Solomides C, Ellsworth E. Mutational analysis of cytocentrifugation supernatant fluid from pancreatic solid mass lesions. Diagn Cytopathol. 2014;42(8):719–25.
28. Finkelstein SD, Bibbo M, Loren DE, Siddiqui AA, Solomides C, Kowalski TE, Ellsworth E. Molecular analysis of centrifugation supernatant fluid from pancreaticobiliary duct samples can improve cancer detection. Acta Cytol. 2012;56(4):439–47.
29. Brown AE, Lim KS, Corpus G, Hustek MT, Tran TA, Chang CC. Detection of BRAF mutation in the cytocentrifugation supernatant fluid from fine-needle aspiration of thyroid lesions may enhance the diagnostic yield. Cytojournal. 2017;14:4.

30. Roy-Chowdhuri S, Mehrotra M, Bolivar AM, Kanagal-Shamanna R, Barkoh BA, Hannigan B, et al. Salvaging the supernatant: next generation cytopathology for solid tumor mutation profiling. Mod Pathol. 2018;31:1036–45.
31. Malhotra N, Jackson SA, Freed LL, Styn MA, Sidawy MK, Haddad NG, Finkelstein SD. The added value of using mutational profiling in addition to cytology in diagnosing aggressive pancreaticobiliary disease: review of clinical cases at a single center. BMC Gastroenterol. 2014;14(1):135.
32. da Cunha Santos G, Saieg MA. Preanalytic specimen triage: smears, cell blocks, cytospin preparations, transport media, and cytobanking. Cancer Cytopathol. 2017;125:455–64.

Index

S. Roy-Chowdhuri et al. (eds.), *Molecular Diagnostics in Cytopathology*, https://doi.org/10.1007/978-3-319-97397-5